Praise for

BEYOND THE CHECKLIST

"The deeper I progressed into this terrific book, the more embarrassed I became for my profession of medicine. Behind our casual assumption as airline customers that we will arrive safely lies an enormously complex process that addresses all human and system issues that could possibly affect safety in air travel. With a few notable exceptions, we in medicine do not come anywhere remotely close to where we need to be to assure our patients of this same kind of safety commitment. There can be no excuse for medicine not pursuing this same all-engaging, relentless process. Our patients deserve nothing less. This is a must-read book for anyone with any connection at all to the delivery of health care services."
—TERRY R. ROGERS, MD, The Foundation for Health Care Quality

"*Beyond the Checklist* takes us behind an apparently simple tool to lay out the complex social and organizational transformation that makes the checklist effective in aviation and to argue for a similar top-to-bottom transformation of health care. By shifting our attention to the detailed, sustained, and careful work that will be required to make health care safer, the book moves us forward on a long, difficult, but ultimately rewarding journey."
—ROBERT L. WEARS, MD, University of Florida and Imperial College London

"*Beyond the Checklist* provides a timely and insightful assessment of crew resource management (CRM), a key tool for averting disaster in the airline industry. The authors make a compelling case for its application to health care delivery. This book should become an essential text for health care professionals, educators, and policymakers seeking to improve interprofessional training and practice."
—SCOTT REEVES, University of California, San Francisco

"The ideas presented in this book are so clearly developed and the writing so engaging that its audience will not be limited to patient safety experts. Patients, their families, and health care providers of all kinds will also benefit from the authors' insight into hospital safety improvement. The case studies are rich in detail and full of critical reflections on the connection between quality care and optimally functioning teams. The tone of *Beyond the Checklist* is hopeful but, for good reason, very urgent as well."
—SEAN P. CLARKE, RN, PhD, FAAN, McGill University School of Nursing

"Some experts downplay the parallels between health care and aviation, but there is much we can learn from the system-wide change that greatly improved passenger safety on commercial airlines. This excellent book highlights the innovative programs of pioneering hospitals where better teamwork and effective communication guide every interaction—from the bedside to the boardroom."
—JULIA HALLISY, DDS, The Empowered Patient Coalition

"This important book brings both a sense of urgency and the hope of clarity in addressing a fundamental and widespread problem in health care. It is a must-read for clinicians and students who deliver care and a call for leadership from every member of the interprofessional team. Leadership is required to change the culture and systems of care delivery. *Beyond the Checklist* provides the inspiration and a path for that change."
—HEATHER M. YOUNG, RN, FAAN, Betty Irene Moore School of Nursing, University of California, Davis

"*Beyond the Checklist* shows us that Crew Resource Management principles help us deal with our human inability to always perform 'perfectly' while operating in a complex work environment. Little mistakes in aviation compound into huge problems. In commercial airlines, virtual strangers routinely solve complex problems without making critical mistakes. The culture of CRM provides for this as a normal way of operation. If embraced by the field of medicine, it will totally transform the way the industry operates."
—CAPTAIN GREGORY S. NOVOTNY

Beyond the Checklist

A VOLUME IN THE SERIES

The Culture and Politics of Health Care Work

edited by Suzanne Gordon and Sioban Nelson

A list of titles in this series is available at www.cornellpress.cornell.edu.

Beyond the Checklist

What Else Health Care Can Learn from Aviation Teamwork and Safety

Suzanne Gordon,

Patrick Mendenhall, and

Bonnie Blair O'Connor

Foreword by Captain Chesley "Sully" Sullenberger

ILR Press
an imprint of Cornell University Press
Ithaca and London

First published 2013 by Cornell University Press
First printing, Cornell Paperbacks, 2013

Printed in the United States of America

Library of Congress Cataloging-in-Publication Data

Gordon, Suzanne, 1945–
    Beyond the checklist : what else health care can learn from aviation teamwork and safety / Suzanne Gordon, Patrick Mendenhall, and Bonnie Blair O'Connor.
        p. cm.
    Includes bibliographical references and index.
    ISBN 978-0-8014-5160-7 (cloth : alk. paper) —
    ISBN 978-0-8014-7829-1 (pbk. : alk. paper)
1. Health care teams.   2. Patients—Safety measures.   3. Medical errors—Prevention.   4. Aeronautics—Safety measures.   5. Aircraft accidents—Prevention.   I. Mendenhall, Patrick.   II. O'Connor, Bonnie Blair.   III. Title.
    R729.5.H4G67   2013
    363.12'492—dc23   2012034342

Cornell University Press strives to use environmentally responsible suppliers and materials to the fullest extent possible in the publishing of its books. Such materials include vegetable-based, low-VOC inks and acid-free papers that are recycled, totally chlorine-free, or partly composed of nonwood fibers. For further information, visit our website at www.cornellpress.cornell.edu.

Cloth printing   10 9 8 7 6 5 4 3 2 1

Paperback printing   10 9 8 7 6 5 4 3 2 1

Contents

Foreword

The moment a flock of Canada geese hit the aircraft and we were forced to land US Airways Flight 1549 in the Hudson River, on January 15, 2009, I knew that my life would change forever and I would gain public attention that I had never sought or imagined.

What I could not know, but only hope, is that this challenge, successfully handled, would serve as a catalyst for my becoming a consultant on the problems of patient safety.

Aviation safety is a field I know well. But what connection could it have to patient safety? Why would workplace protocols and training practices designed to save lives in the airline industry have any relevance to health care?

As this book makes clear, the teamwork required to deliver hundreds of passengers to their destination safely is the same kind of teamwork needed to avoid life-threatening mistakes in hospitals. In the aviation industry, I was part of the effort to implement the safety methodology known as crew resource management (CRM) at US Airways. It was our CRM training that enabled my crew—which included my first officer, Jeff Skiles, and three flight attendants—to land on the Hudson River that frigid January day and then safely evacuate 150 passengers without a life-threatening injury or fatality. As the authors of *Beyond the Checklist* point out, there was a method behind this "miracle." Our unscheduled landing was greatly assisted by the much-changed practices in our industry related to communication and cooperation among all members of the crew, regardless of their rank or job responsibility.

As I have spoken with and observed those who work in the health care field, I have been struck by the many similarities between the early days of CRM formation and developments happening today in the patient safety movement.

Not long ago, there were captains in our cockpits who acted like gods with a little "g" and cowboys with a capital "C." You questioned the captain's authority at your own peril, even if you were a fellow pilot. When I was a young first officer, I witnessed many of my colleagues carrying around little notebooks so they could keep track of the quirks and preferences of particular captains they flew with, just as some nurses today record and share such information about the surgeons they assist in the operating room.

When CRM first emerged—in the wake of aircraft crashes that were due to failures in crew communication, teamwork, and workload management—some captains worried they would be deprived of their decision-making authority. Others, like some doctors today, felt they didn't need to learn the "soft skills" of better communication and respectful interaction with coworkers. Over time, we have learned that our cockpit management decisions are far better when we have regular input and information from all members of our aviation team, in the air and on the ground.

Because of CRM's sea change in our workplace culture, flying—which is inherently dangerous—has become remarkably safe. Travel through the world of high-tech medicine, which can be hazardous for individual patients, is now being made safer wherever hospitals truly embrace similar methods of interprofessional teamwork and training.

Beyond the Checklist correctly argues that aviation safety was improved through more than just checklists, as important as those are. Checklists alone cannot cure the current fragmentation of patient care or avert tragedies like the loss of twelve-year-old Rory Staunton, who died from undetected septic shock after being discharged by New York University Medical Center in summer 2012. As I noted in the *New York Times* after Rory's death, some in the medical field regard such fatalities as an unavoidable consequence of delivering care in any complex, high-stress, high patient volume environment. In aviation, such rationalizations for avoidable human error were rejected long ago and replaced with the creation of a robust safety system that has now become the culture of the field. I hope that readers of this book can learn from our experiences in aviation and join our common effort to apply its best practices to the challenge of providing quality patient care in the safest possible manner.

CAPTAIN CHESLEY "SULLY" SULLENBERGER

Acknowledgments

This is a book about teamwork, and it took a team to write it. As coauthors newly relating to each other, we had to employ the methods of any successful safety-related endeavor: communication, team building, workload balancing, and threat and error management. None of that was easy. In book writing and editing, egos are always involved—in our case, the usual authorial ego quotient was multiplied by three. Marshaling the "team intelligence" necessary to produce what we hope is a useful and credible book became our overriding, collective goal.

We were assisted by many far-flung helpers who advanced our thinking, connected us to the right resources, guided and advised us, and grabbed us by the collar when we sometimes strayed down the wrong path. We all benefited from the different personal and professional support networks that each of us brought to this work. The respective individual and joint acknowledgments of Suzanne, Bonnie, and Patrick are as follows:

Along with Patrick and Bonnie—who were a joy to work with—Suzanne thanks several special people. Susan Bianchi Sands was her initial link to Robert Francis, whose explanation of the changes wrought by Crew Resource Management (CRM) led to the enlistment of Bonnie and Patrick as coauthors. Robert Francis, in turn, put us in touch with airline industry experts long involved with CRM. Jim Pitisci was an invaluable guide to the Airbus Training Center and provided much insight into understanding how pilots think. Jan Von Flatern also facilitated Suzanne's very educational visit to Airbus in Miami. Steve Predmore provided important explanations of how CRM is implemented in a major airline like JetBlue. Suzanne's contribution to the book owes much to three University of Maryland friends and colleagues: Jeff Johnson, Kate McPhaul, and Jane Lipscomb.

Suzanne also thanks Sioban Nelson, Brian Hodges, Maria Tassone, and others at the Centre for Interprofessional Education and the Wilson Centre at the University of Toronto. Particular thanks also go to Helen Caroulanis and Mariana Arteaga for their help in arranging schedules and meetings. Scott Reeves's research and writing on teamwork in health care was also a significant influence on this book.

At Maimonides Medical Center, Pamela Brier, a truly unusual hospital CEO, provided unflagging assistance and invaluable institutional access. Also many thanks go to her always-helpful colleagues Barry Ensminger, Sondra Olendorf, David Feldman, and Kathryn Kaplan for enabling us to understand and report on the process of change in their model hospital. Suzanne particularly thanks Tom Smith at Maimonides. In her view, he is the best Chief Nursing Officer not just in New York City but in the entire universe as well.

Suzanne's many conversations with Emily Cole, Margo Woods, Gordy Schiff and Mardge Cohen, Mike McGillion, and many others have enriched her writing about health care, in this book and others. Sioban Nelson, as Suzanne's coeditor for Cornell University Press's series on the Culture and Politics of Health Care Work, consistently acts as an amazing copilot. On this particular flight deck there is no assignment of captain and copilot but a constant exchange of roles (co-captains, if you will) that has helped produce books that they are very proud of.

Finally, Suzanne thanks her husband, Steve Early, who has cheerfully endured more impromptu lectures about health care and the airline industry than he ever expected to hear when he married Suzanne thirty-three years ago. Their daughters, Alexandra Early and Jessica Early, have been equally good listeners. Jessica has even opted to become a nurse notwithstanding her youthful overexposure to many kitchen-table discussions about the problems facing RNs and health care today.

Bonnie would like to express her heartfelt thanks to her coauthors for their insights, wisdom, energy, and teamwork; to all of the clinicians and staff members of the Osher Clinical Center at Brigham and Women's Hospital for the best days of every workweek for the past nine years and for the compassion, warmth, and clinical skill from which she benefited. She also expresses her thanks to Mal O'Connor for unending love, support, and encouragement.

Patrick wishes to express his deepest gratitude to his wife, Martha, for her unwavering support and encouragement for this project. Throughout twenty-five years of marriage and the raising of three wonderful children, she epitomizes the ideologies of teamwork in action that are addressed in this book.

To his partners in this effort, Suzanne and Bonnie, without whom this would never have happened: This project is living proof of what can be achieved when very different individuals come together to form an authentic team with a well-defined, shared, and common vision. Suzanne has been a true inspiration to us all: Through remarkable drive, energy, and leadership, she has led (not pushed) us across the finish line. Thank you for your patience and especially for your friendship.

To Captains Gary Allen, Don Keating, and Tom Perillo, Patrick's partners in Crew Resource Management LLC (CriticalCRM.com), thank you for your CRM wisdom and the opportunity to contribute to this effort. You have each blazed a trail in this industry and leave an enduring mark through your contributions to CRM training.

And to the thousands of pilots and flight attendants with whom Patrick has had the pleasure of working for over forty years of flying airplanes, "my education continues" each and every time we meet: thank you not only for the flying lessons but for the life lessons as well.

We all thank Sean Clarke and Bob Wears for their careful and thorough reviews of this book and for all the comments that have helped to strengthen it. Finally, we thank the team at Cornell University Press that has brought this book safely to publication. Fran Benson maintained the situational awareness that brought the project through years of development. Ange Romeo-Hall did her usual exquisite cross-monitoring and course correction. Nathan Gemignani, Mahinder Kingra, and Jonathan Hall have been on the ground—and sometimes in the air traffic control center—managing our flight plan. And Kitty Liu patiently put up with too many delays, altitude deviations, and almost-end-of-the-runway landings.

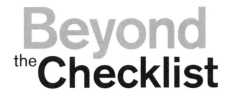

Introduction

PROOF OF LIFE

There is practically no member of the flying public who does not recall the amazing news of a flight that made a safe emergency landing in the middle of the Hudson River without harm to passengers or crew. At 3:25 p.m. on January 15, 2009, US Airways Flight 1549 took off on what was supposed to be a routine flight from New York's LaGuardia Airport en route to Charlotte, North Carolina, with five crew members and 150 passengers on board. One hundred seconds later, the aircraft, commanded by Captain Chesley "Sully" Sullenberger, crossed paths with a flock of migrating Canada geese. And then—BOOM!—the aircraft collided with several of the large birds, which pelted both engines. As the giant turbines, spinning at over ten thousand revolutions per minute, began to disintegrate, the engines were irreparably damaged and shut down. Captain Sullenberger and his first officer, Jeffrey B. Skiles, experienced a feeling, Sullenberger wrote later, that was "unlike anything I'd ever experienced in a cockpit before. . . . Without the normal engine noises it became eerily quiet," a quiet that turned the aircraft's cabin, as the flight attendants would later describe, "as silent as a library," only one that weighed 150,000 pounds and was 2,900 feet above New York City.[1]

In the next three minutes and twenty-eight seconds, Sullenberger and Skiles, neither of whom had ever experienced the simultaneous loss of both jet engines, had to function in the most catastrophic conditions to save their passengers, flight attendants, and themselves. With only seconds to react, they landed the jetliner in the middle of the frigid river, and then they and the crew proceeded to get every person safely out of the aircraft and onto rafts or the wings of the crippled plane. From there, NY Waterway ferries, Coast Guard and New York fire and police department vessels, well-trained in emergency rescues, along with passing sightseeing cruise boats, quickly retrieved them all.

In the initial reporting of what could have been a major disaster, the emphasis was on the miraculous. Later, the reality of what happened on that cold January day began to emerge, and it had nothing to do with miracles or solo heroic action. The successful landing, evacuation, and rescue of Flight 1549 was the direct result of a concerted effort to make flying safer by refining communication and teamwork, as well as workload and threat and error management—a program commonly known in the aviation industry as Crew Resource Management (CRM).

The story of US Airways Flight 1549 is perhaps the ultimate proof of life of the success of decades' worth of safety efforts in the aviation industry. The Airbus 320 landed safely and its passengers managed to get to shore without a single serious injury not simply because of Sullenberger's and Skiles's knowledge, judgment, and skill but because, in the commercial aviation industry, thirty years of research, training, and commitment has taught groups of individuals how to function as teams. As Sullenberger recently said, "creating a team out of a collection of individuals was incredibly important that day." As an industry, aviation is now indisputably safer than it was thirty years ago, in large part because the industry has systematically moved beyond individual intelligence to embrace and foster what we call "team intelligence" (TI). CRM has resocialized and reeducated everyone who works in aviation (not only flight deck, cabin, and ground crew but also management and many others) to stop thinking, deciding, acting, and learning *alone* and to think, decide, act, and learn *together*.

During the airline industry transition to the jet age in the 1960s and 1970s, a series of disastrous crashes took place: among them, two planes colliding in Tenerife, Canary Islands; a "controlled flight into terrain," or CFIT—straight into the Florida Everglades; and a perfectly airworthy craft simply running out of fuel and crashing near Portland, Oregon. In response, CRM began in the early 1980s. Its goal was to transform a culture in which error was defined as "weakness"—which, in turn, led to shame, blame, and punishment—into a culture of learning and teamwork. Now human errors are immediately dealt with and then evaluated for what they can teach about preventing, managing, or containing their effects. Critical to this endeavor was redefining the roles of the team leader and team members. In aviation, the captain is still the captain of the ship, but his or her focus as the team leader is on the efficient and effective management and functioning of the entire team and not simply on accomplishing the tasks of the captain and copilot. Similarly, the job of the team members is not to blindly obey orders but to inquire, contribute, advocate, and assert; in the most extreme conditions, it is also to intervene if necessary to assure the safety of the aircraft and its passengers.

Rather than exhorting people to work in teams or simply declaring that the cockpit, cabin, ground, and other personnel are a team by virtue of their presence together at the same time and in the same place, the airline industry recognized early on that true teams are deliberately created and that an institutional infrastructure that supports teamwork must also be created and continually maintained. The industry has devoted extensive resources to team socialization and education, followed up by frequent retraining to keep teamwork skills current. As we shall describe, in the aviation industry, protocols are established so that team leaders create functional teams rapidly, sometimes expanding them in crisis situations. Like the crew on flight 1549, more often than not, these teams are made up of people who have never worked together as a group but nonetheless routinely find themselves responsible for the safety of hundreds of passengers, as well as one another, on any given flight. Like Captain Sullenberger did when he started the journey that ended in the Hudson, the job of the team leader may be to turn a group of strangers into a high-functioning team in just minutes or hours.

As is suggested by the program's name—Crew Resource Management—the team's job is to utilize all resources and information available. Decisions and information are shared and consistently updated. Crews are taught how to constructively frame, negotiate, and resolve disagreements so that conflicts or problems fuel further collective and individual learning experiences. Team members are redefined not as obstacles to the captain's authority but as crucial human resources who make flight safer and the captain's job easier.

Under this new paradigm people are still given orders to carry out, but every team member is empowered to monitor all others, and all are given a voice in decision making. All members of the team, regardless of rank, status, or position, are authorized and even encouraged to point out to any other team member—with sufficient clarity and urgency—if he or she is making a mistake. The team works to ensure that errors are resolved and do not develop into catastrophes. Captain Sullenberger was the first to state that it was this kind of training—training that he frequently conducted as one of the people who designed and implemented CRM at his own airline and later as founder of his own consulting company—that was responsible for the successful landing and passenger evacuation in January 2009.

As Robert Francis, who worked in the Federal Aviation Administration (FAA) for years before becoming vice chairman of the National Transportation Safety Board (NTSB), has explained,

> The transformation that has made aviation safer is the result of a fundamental shift in perceptions and definitions of authority and deference that has taken place in aviation over the past three decades. Thirty years ago the captain would come in to the cockpit and either directly or indirectly convey the following to the first officer and flight engineer, "I'm the captain. I'm king. Don't do anything, don't say anything. Don't touch anything. Shut up!" Now, it's "I'm the captain, I'm king. Please tell me if you see me making a mistake."

The result: There are fewer airplane crashes and far less tension in workplace relationships.

THE STATE OF PLAY IN HEALTH CARE

Let's contrast commercial aviation with another industry in which millions of people depend on the skill, judgment, and action of a group of highly trained professionals whose historical socialization and education has taught them to think, act, and learn as individuals. In this industry, the long-standing norms regarding socialization and education have yet to be reversed or—in most settings—even minimally challenged. That industry is health care.

Since 1999, when the prestigious Institute of Medicine (IOM) issued its report on patient safety in the United States, *To Err Is Human*, the startling facts of a deeply dysfunctional health care system have become the subject of intense debate. Sadly, there has been little substantive change. According to the IOM, as many as ninety-eight thousand Americans die of medical errors and injuries every year in the United States.[2] Preventable complications are the order of the day in U.S. hospitals, with each patient experiencing on average at least one medication error every single day.[3] Hospital-acquired infections like methicillin-resistant *Staphylococcus aureus* (MRSA) and *Clostriduim difficile* (C-diff) are increasingly common, as are patient falls, bedsores, urinary tract and central venous catheter line infections, and a host of other ills.

Since the IOM report in 1999, billions of dollars have been spent trying to make health care safer. In some instances, these efforts have resulted in improvements for both patients and staff—and we will discuss some of these examples at length. In general, however, too many of the problems highlighted in the IOM report remain. We know, for example, that simple hand washing is the most effective infection-prevention mechanism known to humankind. Yet in health care institutions in industrialized countries, 50 percent of health care workers still do not wash their hands.[4] We now recognize that failures of teamwork and communication are responsible for more than 75 percent of medical errors and injuries, yet heath care professionals and workers still do not communicate with one another routinely and effectively. In one major eastern teaching hospital, an unpublished survey revealed that 40 percent of hospital employees said they were too afraid of reprisals to speak up about a safety issue even if a patient was in imminent danger.[5] Numerous studies show that although health care institutions have spent literally billons of dollars on safety initiatives, our institutions are still not safe. In 2010, several reports from the Agency for Healthcare Research and Quality (AHRQ) showed that rates of bloodstream infections could be reduced dramatically by a series of simple steps, known as the Checklist. At the same time, AHRQ reported, such infections *increased* by 8 percent in one year for most of the nation.[6]

In the same year two professors from Case Western Reserve published an article in the *Berkeley Technology Law Journal* warning doctors about the false promises of health care information technology.[7] Software bugs, inadequate training in complex technology, incessant warnings of drug interactions when no real threats exist, and data-entry errors that generate incorrect outputs can, even in the electronic environment, create significant patient safety hazards for which physicians may be held liable.[8]

Finally, just as we finished writing this book, the U.S. Department of Health and Human Services released results of a study on hospital-error reporting practices. When the investigators looked at hospital records for Medicare patients, they discovered that in spite of requirements, most hospital errors were not reported. When errors were reported, hospitals did not initiate efforts to solve the problems that caused them. What was most disturbing about the study was its discussion of why such reports were not made. Unlike in years past, the failure to report was not because employees were afraid to admit mistakes but because they did not recognize what kinds of events actually harmed patients or were confused about what actually constituted harm. In some cases employees thought common events were isolated ones or that someone else would report the problem. In other words, hospital staff members do not share a common mental model, assumptions, or information about what is and is not harmful to patients. Serious events that either were not reported or were "not captured by incident reporting systems" in hospitals "included hospital-acquired infections, such as a case of septic shock leading to death; and medication-related events, such as four cases of excessive bleeding because of the administration of blood-thinning medication that also led to death."[9]

The injuries and harm that an individual hospital patient experiences may seem far less dramatic than an airplane with 155 people landing in the Hudson River or a crash in the Everglades that killed 101. Still, it is worth contrasting the failures in communication and teamwork that threaten patients with the communication successes that now save passengers and crews every day. Here is an example with which we are quite familiar, but which has not been published in the medical literature:

In March 2010, a sixty-four-year-old woman who had survived several cancers, whom we will call Mrs. Smith, was admitted to a major northeastern teaching hospital with a life-threatening bowel obstruction. She had low blood pressure, was in shock, and had a systemic infection and kidney failure. The hospital was world-renowned for its patient safety; Mrs. Smith's family was confident she would get high-quality care. An emergency colostomy was performed to bypass the affected area of her colon. When the surgeon sewed her up, however, he made an error and left behind some necrotic bowel. Over the next two weeks, the woman ate almost nothing, even after her kidneys started to rebound and she seemed better. Although Mrs. Smith's colostomy output was high—a sign of bowel dysfunction—the many specialists working on her case (internal medicine physicians, kidney doctors, and surgeons) seemed unable to agree about her nutritional status or the significance of the high output. As is common in teaching hospitals, the rotating specialists and hospitalists communicated through notes in the patient's chart but rarely face-to-face.

After three weeks, Mrs. Smith left the hospital for home (her insurance did not cover admission to a rehabilitation facility). There she developed a fungal infection in her mouth and throat, to which doctors quickly attributed her eating problems. After the infection was treated, however, Mrs. Smith still could not eat. One of her closest friends—who happened to be an internist (let's call her Dr. A)—stayed with her when her home care nurse had to be away. Dr. A, who measured her friend's caloric intake, observed that she consumed fewer than three hundred calories over twenty-four hours. She became convinced that Mrs. Smith had a significant bowel problem and was slowly starving to death. When Dr. A discussed the issue with the home care nurse, the nurse said she was frantic because she could not convince the patient's doctors to recognize how serious the eating problem was.

Not surprisingly, several days later Mrs. Smith was readmitted to the hospital. Her care was now transferred to a new group of providers who did not know her at all. After reading her chart, they assumed she was chronically sick and was "on her last legs." Dr. A and Mrs. Smith's daughter tried to convince the new team that Mrs. Smith was actually not "like this," and that there was something seriously wrong. A nutritionist who consulted on the case wrote a strongly worded note recommending that if she did not improve, the patient should receive total parenteral nutrition (TPN)—which delivers complete nutrition intravenously. The physicians' belief that this was "just the way the patient was" contradicted yet another strongly worded note: the patient's oncologist had visited from another hospital and clearly informed the treating physicians that Mrs. Smith had survived her previous cancers and should make a full recovery.

Mrs. Smith did not improve. She was discharged to a long-term acute care facility (LTAC), where her condition deteriorated even further. She was readmitted to the original hospital, where the treating physicians finally met with Dr. A and Mrs. Smith's family. The medical team attributed Mrs. Smith's difficulties to psychological problems, insisting she was simply "not trying hard enough" to eat. Only when Dr. A and her daughter became her health care proxies a week later were they able to arrange for another meeting, where finally a hospitalist (was it the third, fourth, or fifth involved in her care?) listened to the distraught daughter and physician friend, examined the condition of her colon more carefully, discovered the dead bowel, and finally prescribed TPN. Within a day of getting the nutrition, Mrs. Smith was better. Within a week, she could stand. It took two months of TPN before the surgeon could operate to remove her necrotic bowel. She lost considerable bone density and deteriorated from a vigorous woman who could easily walk two miles without effort to one who found it difficult to walk a mile without getting winded.

Dr. A summed it up:

> This took place at one of the best hospitals in the world. Her primary care doctor is a noted patient safety advocate. Yet she was dying of malnutrition in front of everyone's eyes. No one ever talked to anyone else. The teams never met with one another. Things were communicated in the electronic medical record, but there was never a [face-to-face discussion about the patient]. No one would listen to the family, or friends, or even me—and although it shouldn't matter, I am, after all, a physician. My friend went into the hospital on March 11. . . . [I]t wasn't until May 22nd that she was put on TPN. For over two months, she ate no more than 400 calories a day. It's a miracle—and not a medical miracle—that she is alive.

This is not good enough. Health care needs to become a high-reliability industry in more than name. It needs a radical cultural transformation, like the one that has taken place in aviation over the past thirty years.

To help promote that transformation, we decided to write this book: a description and analysis of a major cultural shift that has made one complex and safety-critical industry—never previously known for concern for interpersonal or interprofessional relations—into an exemplary teamwork culture that is arguably now one of the safest in the world.

If aviation could do it, health care can too.

The superficial evidence appears to suggest that more health care administrators and professionals concerned with safety now recognize the parallels between health care and aviation. Yes, there are many differences between these professions, yet people who work in health care seem increasingly to recognize that the similarities with aviation are significant and cannot be ignored. Both are hierarchical settings: one group dominates all other groups; the ones that are dominated have been tutored in deference and their contributions have been traditionally downplayed. In both settings, people's lives depend on the knowledge, skill, and judgment of a host of players who ostensibly work well together. A heroic medical narrative that has obscured the roles of the lower-status professionals whose participation is essential to service provision permeates health care. In both fields this narrative has contributed to a lack of oversight and effective communication that have put its end users at risk.

Finally, there is a huge reliance on advanced technology in both sectors and a deep reluctance to engage in the teamwork and communication that have been demonstrated to save lives. Ironically, failure to embrace and master communication and team-building skills can actually cause enhanced technologies to work *against* success and safety.

As if recognizing all of this, best-selling books and scientific journal articles now promote aviation-inspired checklists and time-outs in ORs and ICUs. We hear about the use of huddles—a series of daily briefings—in labor and delivery.

Simulation centers are popping up in hospitals and medical and nursing schools as effective teaching tools for adult learners, as are efforts to introduce interprofessional education in health care. In hospitals, CNOs, CEOs, and medical leaders are finally recognizing the need to create more respectful relationships in their workplaces and are launching so-called civility initiatives. Pilots are often invited to consult or lecture in hospitals to share the aviation perspective on the safety that comes with teamwork and to describe their successful experiences.

Throughout North America, to one degree or another, the education of health professionals now includes efforts to encourage interprofessional education (IPE) in the service of creating interprofessional practice or care (IPE/IPC) in the clinical setting. These have been under way in Canada for several years. In the United States, IPE/IPC efforts began to gain momentum in 2009 with the founding of the American Interprofessional Health Collaborative (AIHC) and the Interprofessional Education Collaborative (IPEC), the latter comprising representatives from the American Association of Colleges of Nursing, the American Association of Colleges of Osteopathic Medicine, the American Association of Colleges of Pharmacy, the American Dental Education Association, the Association of Schools of Public Health, and the Association of American Medical Colleges. In 2011, IPEC issued two concurrent reports: *Competencies for Interprofessional Practice*, identifying four key competency areas to be mastered in addition to the existing Competencies presently guiding curricula for each individual profession, and its action-strategy companion piece, *Team-Based Competencies: Building a Shared Foundation for Education and Clinical Practice*.[10]

In medicine it seems now to be universally acknowledged that failures of teamwork and communication—not simply failures in technical proficiency—cause the majority of medical errors and injuries in hospitals and other health care facilities. Studies too numerous to cite have now documented that it is not the incompetent surgeon or a small group of bad apples in other disciplines that cause the most harm to patients. It is human factors—the failure of human beings to relate effectively and productively with one another in highly technological settings, to recognize human limitations in performance ability owing to "life factors" such as extreme fatigue and emotional distress, and to actively resist the culture of blame—that are the major cause of patient harm.

In many of the studies published in the most reputable scientific journals, CRM is repeatedly mentioned as a model for how to create safer hospitals and health care institutions. In the mid-1990s, the MedTeams Project was utilized in the emergency room setting.[11] The AHRQ has developed an aviation-inspired TeamSTEPPS curriculum that is used in many facilities, and The Joint Commission (TJC), formerly known as the Joint Commission on Accreditation of Healthcare Organizations (JCAHO), now recommends that teamwork and communication training be incorporated into professional education. The Affordable Care Act also allocates funding to create more interprofessional education in health care professional training programs and to encourage interprofessional practice in healthcare facilities.

Many of these initiatives have created their own small revolutions and promise to create even more. The lessons of aviation and other safety-critical, high-reliability industries are receiving more attention in health care than ever before.[12] In spite of great resistance, some of these initiatives are producing positive models that offer great promise, as described in subsequent chapters. Nevertheless, we write this book out of concern that that there is much more lip service than real systemic change when it comes to making health care a truly high-reliability industry—one in which genuine interprofessional and occupational practice is the norm. This is why it is so important for health care to recognize how much it can learn and adapt from the aviation model of safety and teamwork. Moving beyond the checklist will help advance the efforts of all of those who are working so hard to make health care safer for both patients and those who work in health care settings. For those already familiar with CRM, this book provides a detailed look at the content of CRM training programs that many safety advocates may find of interest.

We've called this book *Beyond the Checklist* because we are convinced that those working for safety in healthcare can benefit from a greater awareness of the enormous breadth and depth of the transformation that has occurred over the past three decades in commercial aviation and of what it actually took to make that happen. As our title suggests, safety in aviation is not just about the creation of checklists or briefing protocols. It is about a major cultural and behavioral shift— one that needs to occur in health care as well.

We explore not only what the CRM model offers—the nuts and bolts of CRM training—but also how aviation has managed, in a relatively short time, to create this massive cultural shift so that those in health care can review its most critical lessons for system-wide change and adapt and apply those lessons to their own settings. We will address the following questions:

- How did the airline safety movement develop?
- How were CRM trainings initially designed and implemented?
- How were they studied, refined, and changed on the basis of research findings?
- How did safety advocates overcome the resistance of pilots who felt their authority was directly challenged by this movement?
- How did they overcome resistance or skepticism from other airline workers?
- How did reformers demonstrate positive impact on work processes and organization?
- How did they demonstrate enhanced safety outcomes?

As we explore how a change of this magnitude took place in aviation, we will also be careful to describe the context in which the transformation occurred. In order to design and implement this new model and help refine and improve it, aviation reformers gathered together *all* involved stakeholders (including unions, researchers, company officials, government officials, and academics). The reformers understood that cultures and practices do not change after a single workshop or presentation; thus the central concepts, safety trainings, oversight, and supervision were designed to be continuous and self-reinforcing. In these trainings the emphasis is not on abstract concepts but on practical application of specific sets of teachable skills. The aviation safety curriculum is undergirded by a strong conceptual framework and supported by decades of human-factors and sociotechnical research; it is evidence-based. CRM training focuses on the kinds of skills and standard operating procedures (SOPs) that produce and reinforce new behaviors, which in turn engender new attitudes. For reinforcement, the new paradigm was also integrated into the work processes—technical, mechanical, and social—and the work organization of the airlines. Over time, CRM has been expanded beyond the crew inside the aircraft (i.e., pilots and flight attendants) to include other specialties—handlers, dispatchers, and mechanics, as well as resources outside the bounds of the company. All of this has produced a keen sense of team intelligence and recognition of "distributed cognition," which has produced greater safety across the industry.

TEAM INTELLIGENCE AND DISTRIBUTED COGNITION

Any discussion of safety in high reliability industries will include the concept of "emotional intelligence" (EI). First articulated by psychologist Howard Gardner in his groundbreaking *Frames of Mind* and later popularized by author Daniel Goleman, EI has become such a popular concept that it now comes with its own set of constructs, promises, management tomes, scoring systems, and inventories (and, of course, critiques).

While EI is certainly an important concept, creating genuine teamwork requires moving beyond the individualized concept of emotional intelligence to that of team intelligence (TI). Emotional intelligence emphasizes self-regulation and monitoring as necessary for one-on-one relationships and what are known as "social skills." It is perhaps a prerequisite of team intelligence, but on its own it is not enough.

As we have defined it, TI is the active capacity of individual members of a team to learn, teach, communicate, reason, and think together, irrespective of position in any hierarchy, in the service of realizing shared goals and a shared mission. TI has the following requisites:

- Team members must develop a shared team identity that allows them to articulate the shared mental model, shared language, and shared assumptions needed to realize their clear and common goals.
- Team members must be willing and able to share information, cross-monitor, and coach all members of the team, as well as to solicit and take into account their input, no matter their position in the occupational hierarchy.
- Team members must understand one another's roles and work imperatives and how these mesh so that common goals can best be accomplished.
- Team members must help and support one another so that each individual member can perform his or her job efficiently and effectively.[13]

Team intelligence produces not only action but also effective interaction.

In high-reliability, safety-critical industries, creation of team intelligence is grounded in the recognition that safe and effective job performance requires individuals to engage in a specific kind of group cognition—what cognitive anthropologist Edwin Hutchins calls "distributed cognition." In his work on aircraft carriers and aviation (in *Cognition in the Wild*), Hutchins lays out a theory of distributed cognition that is crucial to our understanding of CRM—and by extension what it will take to create true teams in health care:

> All divisions of labor, whether the labor is physical or cognitive in nature, require distributed cognition in order to coordinate the activities of the participants. Even a simple system of two men driving a spike with hammers requires some cognition on the part of each to coordinate his own activities with those of the other. When the labor that is distributed is cognitive labor, the system involves the distribution of two kinds of cognitive labor: the cognition that is the task and the cognition that governs the coordination of the elements of the task.[14]

Put in everyday language, what Hutchins is saying is that all the participants in a real team need to know how to do—and how to think about—their individual tasks. But they also need to think about how their tasks, knowledge of their tasks, and knowledge of the changing context in which those tasks are performed affect the activities of those with whom they are working—even if those people are not working right by their side at the moment.

Distributed cognition is much too complex a phenomenon to elaborate on in this short discussion, but one of its fundamental elements is the recognition that the people on your team are in fact *thinking* about their work and not just doing mindless work. On the aircraft carrier that Hutchins describes, those involved in the crucial activity of navigation—the constant effort to figure out where one is and where one is going—combine different "sources of data that are reasonably independent." One crew member plots by means of visual bearings, another by means of radar, another by means of ocean depth. Each crew member, however, values the information gathered by the other—a fact that affords the team as a whole "the opportunity for the detection of error through the comparison of independently [calculated] representations." That is, one crew member does not dismiss the other's data and concerns because that crew member is lower in status or acquired his information through direct observation rather than through "objective measures."

A Danish nurse once told Suzanne about a lecture she'd attended given by a military general to a group of health care professionals: The general told the group that when an army is in battle and a private says, " 'Stop! There's a mine,' we don't say, 'No, we won't stop because the person providing this information is just a private.' *We all stop.* You in health care," he told the audience, "are [also] on a battlefield, but when the equivalent of a private—say a nurse—tells a surgeon to stop, you *don't* ignore the directive because that person giving it is 'just a nurse.' " The point? In the army everyone implicitly if not explicitly recognizes the concept of distributed cognition and acts accordingly. Meanwhile, in health care, concerns about status often lead people to devalue the important information those of lower status actually have. Although team intelligence and distributed cognition were not popular currency in the early aviation safety movement, we believe that the creation of a culture of safety in aviation is a perfect example of both concepts at work.

FLIGHT MAP

The first chapter of *Beyond the Checklist* describes the history of the airline safety movement. Chapters 2 through 9 take you through the content of CRM courses and explain how the key concepts—communication, team building, workload management, and threat and error management—function: how they *shape new behaviors* and *generate new norms*. Interspersed among these four topics are case studies that illustrate how some health care institutions have tried to use teamwork initiatives to transform the problematic aspects of health care training and socialization that put patients at risk. One of these case studies reports on the results of a team-building initiative funded by a National Institute of Health (NIH) grant to Dr. David Eisenberg, who coauthors the case presentation. These chapters describe and analyze positive examples of change in health care that utilize some of the principles of cultural change that have made the aviation model so successful.

The book's penultimate chapter analyzes why the aviation safety model worked. What principles of cultural change does CRM embody, and how might they be adapted and applied to the health care setting? Our conclusion argues that if aviation, with its history of toxic hierarchy and poor communication, can change, so can health care—and suggests how fundamental change can be facilitated.

TO THE SKEPTICS

Many in health care are skeptical that the lessons of the aviation safety movement can be workably applied to their professional settings—particularly to the complex hospital environment. One head of curriculum at a large American medical school once told us, "Health care is so much more complex than aviation. After all, in aviation it's just two guys in a box, and flying a 747 isn't that different than flying a Cessna."

We surely do not agree with the premise that flying hundreds of passengers in a million-pound airplane through turbulence, an engine on fire, and a passenger experiencing a medical emergency is less challenging than performing surgery on one (even very complex) patient in a stable and predictable operating room. Nevertheless, we can all agree that health care and aviation are very, very different in their *particular* demands—and that invidious comparisons lead to fruitless arguments.

To focus only on the differences between the two endeavors, however, is to ignore the very important structural similarities that make the CRM model a useful and readily adaptable foundation for beneficial change in health care. No one can prove who experiences more job stress or complex responsibility, and in the end this is a spurious debate.

It's a pretty safe bet that when Captain Sullenberger was landing his plane in the Hudson, he was not thinking, "Oh this could be so much worse: I could be a neurosurgeon!" Nor would we think that a physician rapidly managing all of the medications, actions, personnel, and supports needed to rally a "crashing" patient is thanking her lucky stars that she's not an airline pilot. The pilot needs to deliver his or her passengers safely to their destination, and the surgeon must deliver his or her patient to wellness. If one industry can benefit from the experience of the other and reduce errors and thus enhance safety, why wouldn't it try?

The real question is, How can the responsible parties in any industry or organization best function to protect those who depend on their skills and professional judgment for survival? We can learn from best practices and relevant models wherever and whenever they are developed and then adapt them to different settings in which they may be useful. What is paramount is how an institution—or, in the case of CRM, an entire global industry—learned to change for the better and for the safer and how it has sustained change over time. What did the airline industry do concretely to transform workplace relationships and create a different model of workplace hierarchy and teamwork? How did it confront power and status differentials and learn to help people speak up about safety without fear of reprisal? What strategies and tactics did it utilize, what obstacles did it confront and overcome, and what values and practices did it change—and how? We also believe that, in spite of the differences between healthcare and aviation, the principles of CRM—learning to communicate more effectively, learning to lead a team and work effectively on a team, as well as learning to manage stressful workloads and anticipate a variety of threats to safety, as well as to prevent, manage or contain error—are crucial in healthcare and can and should be taught to and learned by all who care for the sick and vulnerable.

We ask our readers to suspend the common tendency to react defensively: "If you think your job is bad, look at mine." We invite you to come fly with us and see how an extraordinary experiment in cultural and behavioral change took hold, flourished, and radically increased industry-wide safety in aviation, and how those lessons can be applied to great effect in the health care workplace.

Chapter 1

History of Crew Resource Management

UNITED 173, DECEMBER 28, 1978: A DEFINING MOMENT

18:06:40—First Officer: I think you just lost number four . . . better get some cross-feeds open there or something.

18:06:46—First Officer: We're going to lose an engine. . . .

18:06:49—Captain: Why?

18:06:49—First Officer: We're losing an engine.

Captain: Why?

First Officer: Fuel.

18:07:06—First Officer: It's flamed out.

18:07:12—Captain: to Portland Approach: . . . would like clearance for an approach into two eight left, now.

18:07:27—Flight Engineer: We're going to lose number three in a minute, too.

18:07:31—Flight Engineer: It's showing zero.

Captain: You got a thousand pounds. You got to.

Flight Engineer: Five thousand in there . . . but we lost it.

Captain: All right.

18:07:38—Flight Engineer: Are you getting it back?

18:07:40—First Officer: No number four. You got that cross-feed open?

18:07:41—Flight Engineer: No, I haven't got it open. Which one?

18:07:42—Captain: Open 'em both—get some fuel in there. Got some fuel pressure?

Flight Engineer: Yes sir.

18:07:48—Captain: Rotation. Now she's coming.

18:07:52—Captain: Okay, watch one and two. We're showing down to zero or a thousand.

> Flight Engineer: Yeah.
>
> Captain: On number one?
>
> Flight Engineer: Right.
>
> 18:08:08—First Officer: Still not getting it.
>
> 18:08:11—Captain: Well, open all four cross-feeds.
>
> Flight Engineer: All four?
>
> Captain: Yeah.
>
> 18:08:14—First Officer: All right, now it's coming.
>
> 18:08:19—First Officer: It's going to be—on approach though.
>
> Unknown Voice: Yeah.
>
> 18:08:42—Captain: You gotta keep 'em running. . . .
>
> Flight Engineer: Yes, sir.
>
> 18:08:45—First Officer: Get this [expletive] on the ground.
>
> Flight Engineer: Yeah. It's showing not very much more fuel.
>
> 18:09:16—Flight Engineer: We're down to one on the totalizer. Number two is empty.
>
> 18:13:21—Flight Engineer: We've lost two engines, guys.
>
> 18:13:25—Engineer: We just lost two engines—one and two.
>
> 18:13:38—Captain: They're all going. We can't make Troutdale.
>
> First Officer: We can't make [expletive]![1]

At 6:15 p.m., December 28, 1978, United Airlines Flight 173 crashed into a wooded area near Portland, Oregon, about six miles short of the airport. Incredibly, of 189 souls on board, only 13 were killed (including 2 crew members), and 23 were seriously injured. In addition, two unoccupied homes were destroyed. In part, that was because there was no fire since there was no fuel on board. The aircraft was destroyed, however.

This incident became a defining moment in commercial aviation, a tipping point that captured the attention of aviation safety experts and agencies throughout the industry. Aside from the obvious—the spectacular crash of an aircraft and associated loss of life—UA 173 focused a very bright light on a *culture* that twentieth-century aviators had inherited from the pioneers of the field: a culture that, while purposeful in the past, had become increasingly dysfunctional in the world of modern jet aircraft.

Put very simply, the airline crew culture in 1978 was extremely hierarchical and autocratic. United 173 was flown by a crew that was socialized in what is referred to as the "captain is king" tradition. According to the investigation report written by the National Transportation Safety Board (the federal agency that investigates airline accidents and makes recommendations about how to prevent them), the cause of the crash was the "failure of the captain to monitor properly the aircraft's fuel state and to properly respond to the low fuel state and the crewmembers' advisories regarding the fuel state. . . . Contributing to the accident was the failure of the other two crewmembers to fully comprehend the criticality of the fuel state or to successfully communicate their concern to the captain."[2]

"The captain," the report states, "had a management style that precluded eliciting or accepting feedback." The first officer and the flight engineer (FE) (who paid with his life) failed to "monitor the captain" and give effective feedback and provide sufficient redundancy.[3] It was only when it was too late that the first officer expressed a direct view, 'Get this . . . on the ground!'[4] In this kind of environment, the crisis was neither prevented, managed, nor contained. Why? Because, as the NTSB reported, "the landing gear problem had a seemingly *disorganizing* [our italics] effect on the flight crew's performance. . . . The Safety Board believes that this accident exemplifies a recurring problem—a breakdown in cockpit management and teamwork during a situation involving malfunctions of aircraft systems in flight."[5]

Because of the spectacular nature of aircraft accidents in terms of potential—and actual—loss of life and damage, commercial aircraft accidents get a great deal of attention. In reality, accidents are incredibly rare compared with the high numbers of *positive* outcomes when a flight is challenged by mechanical or other threats. Aviation successes receive scant attention in all but the most stunning cases.

JET BLUE 292, SEPTEMBER 21, 2005: A SUCCESS STORY

One such success occurred on September 21, 2005, when JetBlue Flight 292, an Airbus A-320 with 140 passengers and a crew of 6, took off from Southern California's Bob Hope Airport (Burbank) headed for New York's John F. Kennedy International Airport. After the plane lifted off the runway, when the captain tried to retract the landing gear, a display of two error messages indicated that there was a problem. The first officer (FO) continued to fly the plane while the captain responded to the electronic centralized aircraft monitor (ECAM) prompts.[6] The captain then consulted the flight crew operating manual (COM), which suggested that the nose gear—the wheels directly under the aircraft's cockpit—had somehow rotated ninety degrees from its normal "aligned" position, making it physically impossible to retract it. The captain informed—and later continued to update—the flight attendants (FAs) about the problem. They in turn advised passengers about the development and kept them informed.

In an effort to get a visual confirmation of the situation, the captain decided to do a "fly-by" or "low pass" in front of the air traffic control tower in Long Beach,

California, to see if they could verify the problem with the nose gear. The tower, JetBlue ground personnel, and a local news helicopter verified that the nose gear was indeed cocked ninety degrees to the left. In this situation, the plane could not land safely. There would be no alternative but to execute an emergency landing.

As the FO continued as the "pilot flying," the captain, in consultation with safety personnel in New York, decided to divert the plane to Los Angeles International Airport (LAX), where the airline has a maintenance hub. Because it was making a transcontinental flight, the plane had taken on a large quantity of fuel. All agreed that it would not be safe for it to land with the existing fuel load, and the decision was made to delay the landing until the majority of the fuel on board had been burned off to reduce the possibility of a fire and to make the plane lighter and an emergency landing safer.

The aircraft circled for three hours until the fuel had burned down. During this time, the pilots consulted with JetBlue in New York and with maintenance personnel, as well as with engineers in France at Airbus and Messier-Dowty, the manufacturers of the plane and its landing gear. They also thoroughly briefed the flight attendants on the aircraft status and what they could expect. The captain requested their assistance in trying to shift the center of gravity (CG) of the aircraft as far aft as the structural limits would allow. This would allow the captain to hold the defective nose gear off the ground as long as possible after touchdown. The flight attendants worked with passengers to move them and their luggage toward the rear of the aircraft.

They spoke to all the passengers individually prior to the landing to ensure that they knew the emergency procedures that would take place and how to properly brace themselves. The flight attendants checked and double-checked each other's work to ensure that everything was completed and would go according to plan. This kind of communication is critical in reassuring passengers and preventing panic in the cabin. The captain briefed the FAs that they could not evacuate passengers through the doors in the rear of the aircraft and advised them that they would have to use the forward doors. After three hours, the plane approached LAX for its emergency landing.

With emergency equipment at the ready on the ground, the plane touched down at 120 knots (138.2 miles) an hour.[7] As the aircraft slowed down, the nose gear touched ground. With their nose wheels perpendicular to the direction of motion, the tires quickly shredded until the metal wheels were scraping the ground at such high speed that it created a plume of white smoke, which made it difficult to see the plane. Although no one could see what had happened to the wheels, the flight attendants in the front of the aircraft could smell the strong odor of burning rubber. Air traffic controllers were able to observe that there was no fire and reported this to the captain, who in turn relayed the information to the cabin crew.

While media and airport observers held their collective breaths, the aircraft skittered to a halt a thousand feet short of the end. The nose tires completely shredded during the landing and "about half of the two wheels were ground off." Otherwise the plane was undamaged and none of the 145 people on board were hurt. Because of the clear communication among all parties—air traffic control (ATC), cockpit, FAs, and passengers—regarding the aircraft status once it was on the ground, everyone understood the condition of the aircraft and recognized that it was no longer in danger. There was no panic among the passengers, and it was quickly determined that an emergency evacuation was not necessary.

To understand the significance of this successful outcome, it is necessary to travel back several decades to contrast this incident with a seemingly relentless series of aviation disasters that too often captured the headlines during that time. Let's return to the disaster that was United Flight 173 and compare it with the success of the Jet Blue flight. Like the crew of Jet Blue 292, the United 173 crew had the luxury of time, but the similarities end there. In Portland in 1978, the crew of United Flight 173 failed to monitor the captain; the flight attendants were not alerted to the problem; the captain failed to listen to the flight engineer, who in turn failed to alert the captain to the seriousness of the situation. The crew, as the NTSB report emphasized, became disorganized instead of hyperorganized in a crisis. Why? Why weren't flight attendants made aware of the significance of the problem? Why did no one listen to the first officer, and why did he fail to signal the problem with sufficient urgency? There was a lot of time available to create and utilize crew communication, to enlist the crew as a resource, and to manage the emergency. None of that happened. Again, the question is, Why?

The answer is that, for the most part, the assumption in the cockpit during that era was that the captain was responsible for *everything* and had all the answers. In spite of the fact that there were two other highly qualified and experienced crew members available in the same small space, *one* person made all the decisions.[8] That person apparently did not recognize that others had relevant expertise and could contribute to solving a very pressing problem. The reason that the United 173 scenario did not repeat itself thirty years later is that in the ensuing decades commercial aviation began to reevaluate its modes of operation and to drastically reconsider its dominant hierarchal structure. Reports of flights like United 173—among many others—led to a dramatic reconsideration of the culture of aviation, a culture whose positives had as many negatives and whose heroic aviators had learned a whole lot of "wrong stuff" along with the Right Stuff.

A BIT OF HISTORY

It is almost a cliché to say that flying a plane requires a lot of skill and occasional heroism and is, by its very nature, risky. This statement was certainly true for the early years of powered flight. Statistics from the past fifty years document that today it's considerably safer to fly an airplane at 36,000 feet than to drive a car at sea level. The new cliché is that you have a much greater chance of being struck by lightning (about 1 per million in a given year)[9] or dying in a car crash (1.4 per million miles) than you do of getting harmed in a commercial airliner (0.2 per million miles).[10]

So does that mean that flying is inherently safe? Should we conclude that technology has made it possible for a plane to fly itself or for a smart flight attendant or even passenger—guided, we would assume by a qualified individual on the ground—to land the plane if both pilots are somehow incapacitated? This may be a common Hollywood fantasy, but in actuality it is not likely. As we noted in the introduction, airline safety isn't a result only of better technology but also of hard work with the human beings who train to interface with that technology and with each other. It's the result of a decades-long reassessment of the heroic, "captain-as-king-who-need-not-listen-to-the-commoners" model of aviation. It's also a result of a reevaluation of acceptable risk, of conceptualizations and understandings of human error, and of accepted definitions of who is and who is not a member of the team and how the team is formed. All of this began in the 1970s when crash after crash mobilized the industry for dramatic change.

RISKY BUSINESS

In the early days of aviation, there was a tacitly granted acceptable level of risk associated with the performance of these less-than-perfect air machines. What early aviators experienced were the limitations and challenges of the aircraft, systems, environment, and traffic control of the day. A pilot was expected to show strength and sangfroid in the face of these mechanical uncertainties. Thus emerged the myth of the steely-eyed individual at the controls—sublimely confident, personally in command, and utterly cool under pressure. There was plenty of pressure to be had. By today's standards, the first aircraft were remarkably unreliable, and only the most talented and resourceful aviators made it back to the ground safely. The successful outcome of any flight was believed to be (and may actually have been) due as much to the pilot's stick-and-rudder skills as to any other factor, including the performance of the machine and the presence of some luck.

As aircraft grew and designs evolved requiring two—then three—pilots to operate them, mechanical reliability improved remarkably.[11] In the 1960s jet-powered aircraft allowed human beings to fly higher, faster, and farther with increased reliability—but the cockpit culture did not necessarily evolve to keep pace with these advances.

No matter how many people were in the cockpit or cabin or how well trained they were, in the 1960s and 1970s, the captain was still in charge of every detail. He did not necessarily work closely or collaboratively with his crew to take advantage of the varied resources each crew member brought on board. Hierarchy trumped collaboration in the cockpit, where the captain worked mainly with his copilot and flight engineer, and it certainly trumped any notion of teamwork with flight attendants who worked in the cabin. Mostly female, flight attendants were usually asked to provide coffee and meals but not operational input.

As a series of incidents and accidents in the late 1970s and early 1980s made clear, this model of (what we can now conclude was) a toxic hierarchy was being increasingly revealed as dysfunctional. In the case of United 173, the captain was very much in charge—yet clearly was not really engaged with his crew, who appeared to have been intimidated into "hinting and hoping" their concerns rather than being able to strongly assert their warnings of the impending disaster that they clearly recognized.

A TREND EMERGES

United Flight 173 was the tipping point. To use this term, of course, suggests that a number of other events provided the critical mass that helped tip the scales. And indeed, United 173 was only one of a number of serious commercial airline accidents that occurred over a relatively short period of time. Many of these preceded it and were ultimately found to have been "avoidable" in spite of the presence of mechanical or environmental factors. *Human intervention could have prevented these accidents, and human failures ended up being their ultimate cause.* Let's take a look at a few examples.

Eastern Airlines 401, December 29, 1972

Eastern Airlines Flight 401, a Lockheed L-1011, crashed after an experienced air crew became distracted by a *burned-out landing gear light*. Of 176 passengers and crew on board, 101 lost their lives; the aircraft itself was destroyed. Unbeknownst to the crew, they had inadvertently placed the autopilot in a very slow, shallow descent while troubleshooting the problem. The airplane began a shallow descent and crashed in the Florida Everglades, fatally injuring 94 passengers and 5 crew members. Two others died after the crash. Air traffic controllers had recognized that the aircraft was on a gradual path toward the ground but had only vaguely and nonspecifically inquired, "How's it goin' out there, Eastern?"

So how did a highly trained, professional air crew team in a modern, well-equipped jet end up crashing their airplane over the malfunction of a fifty-nine-cent lightbulb? And why did controllers not inquire more specifically about the airplane's descent or challenge the crew's violation of federal aviation regulations by its departure from assigned altitude without ATC clearance? The aircraft crew had lost "situational awareness," and the air traffic controller addressed their departure from their assigned altitude by failing to express concerns with the requisite urgency. Both of these concepts are addressed as we look at the evolution of Crew Resource Management.

Tenerife, Canary Islands, March 27, 1977

The most deadly aircraft collision in worldwide aviation history occurred in 1977 at Los Rodeos Airport, Tenerife, Canary Islands, when KLM-Royal Dutch Airlines Flight 4805 collided on the runway with Pan American Flight 1736, killing 583 passengers and crew.

Both 747s had diverted to the tiny, mountainous airport because of bomb threats at their destination, Las Palmas, also in the Canary Islands. The weather in Tenerife—heavy fog—was marginal upon their arrival, and it steadily deteriorated as the two large jets loitered around the confines of Tenerife's single runway, waiting for the OK to depart.

One aspect of this crash that was nearly as remarkable as the devastating loss of life was that the KLM captain was literally the poster boy for the airline. As chief training captain for the KLM 747 fleet, Captain Jacob van Zanten was very experienced and was routinely featured in company advertisements. In one KLM magazine (which happened to be on board the very aircraft involved in this crash), van Zanten is seen in the cockpit, his smiling face turned toward the reader. The headline, almost eerily ironic given his actions in Tenerife, trumpets, "KLM: From the people who make punctuality possible."[12] Van Zanten's copilot was also very experienced but was brand new to the 747. In fact, Captain van Zanten had recently given him his 747 checkride (a scripted scenario known only to the simulator instructor that challenges the crew to handle a variety of realistic emergencies in real time during a typical line flight).[13]

The Spanish air traffic controllers on Tenerife had difficulty communicating in English, and the Dutch copilots' nonstandard phraseology exacerbated the numerous misunderstandings. Van Zanten, although a very experienced pilot, was also getting more and more impatient because of various delays that had plagued the flight. After a lengthy delay, Las Palmas reopened, and the two jumbo jets attempted to maneuver for takeoff within the limited confines of the small airport.

KLM taxied down the runway first, turning 180 degrees into position for takeoff. Unbeknownst to the overeager Dutch captain, the Pan Am plane was taxiing in the fog down the runway behind them but now in the opposite direction. As the KLM captain began the takeoff roll, the copilot exclaimed, "Wait a minute, we don't have an ATC clearance." The captain braked, responding, "No . . . I know that. Go ahead and ask." Dutifully the copilot asked for takeoff clearance and was told to "stand by for takeoff."

The KLM captain, his impatience likely overriding his good judgment, apparently misinterpreted the tower's reply, said "Let's go," and initiated his takeoff again.

The copilot, now understandably confused, transmitted meaninglessly over the radio "We are now at takeoff!" further confounding matters between Pan Am and ATC.

The fog was so thick that neither ATC nor the taxiing Pan Am crew could see the end of the runway or KLM accelerating down it. Seconds later the Pan Am crew identified KLM's lights coming out of the fog and frantically attempted to clear the runway as the KLM captain rotated the aircraft for takeoff, forcing the jet into flight. Although KLM's nose gear passed over the other 747, the main landing gear sheered off Pan Am's upper deck and both aircraft were destroyed by fire. Five hundred and eighty-three passengers and crew were killed.

Accident investigators determined that—the dense fog notwithstanding—poor communication and use of nonstandard terminology were the main causes of the collision and the resultant disastrous loss of life. Perhaps even more important, analysts wondered, how could such an experienced KLM crew make such a basic yet catastrophic mistake? Why was the KLM captain so reluctant to accept input and why did the copilot, who clearly knew they had not been issued takeoff clearance, not speak up more assertively to prevent this accident—or to save his own life?

"Safety analysts believed it was possible that the first officer, who had only 95 hours in the 747, and who was flying with the KLM chief 747 instructor, may have been intimidated by the *captain's legendary status.*"[14] In other words, it was an authority issue: the combination of the captain's impressive persona and the copilot's lack of confidence flying a new airplane resulted in an experienced copilot's becoming confused and doubting his own capabilities. Was this example of the powerful influence of authority dynamics over human behavior an anomaly? History proves otherwise.

HOW THE COCKPIT CULTURE DEVELOPED

The cockpit culture on December 28, 1978, was, in a word, dysfunctional. It is certainly understandable how the culture had developed, considering the origins of the human-machine interface that makes a flight crew.[15] Aviation culture has historically concentrated on the pilot and his individual flying skills. At its inception, flying was a risky solo endeavor. Icarus was not the only one who took chances and failed. All the early aircraft pioneers flew alone. There was no radio contact. No crew. Just man and space. These risks were deemed acceptable in part because those who took them were primarily the ones who bore the costs. In what has become known as the Golden Age of Flight, between 1919 and 1939, the aviator was on his—or rarely, as in the case of Amelia Earhart, on *her*—own. Early aviators flew primarily by themselves or were accompanied by only one other person, with whom they were barely in contact because of the exposure to the elements and wind noise in open cockpits. While these well-heeled aviators made the headlines, thousands of lesser-known solo airmen flew the mails. In 1925 Congress passed the Kelly Air Act, which authorized the Post Office Department to make contracts with aviation companies to deliver the mail by air.[16]

Even when early pilots flew with a navigator, contact was difficult and minimal. From aviation's inception as a mode of transport, teamwork was rarely a consideration. A large part of pilot training, whether conducted in military, commercial, or general aviation arenas, is often accomplished one-on-one as flight instructors demonstrate and students unquestioningly mimic technical maneuvers—and especially behaviors. The first major milestone in any pilot's advancement is to fly solo. Until the introduction of CRM in commercial aviation, a pilot's primary demonstration of competency was based almost entirely on technical aptitude: the ability to perform a standard set of maneuvers and handle emergencies (with little or no regard for interaction with the rest of the crew). Although commercial transport pilots flew as crews, competence had little to do with teamwork or error management in the cockpit. The first flight attendants were required to be registered nurses, who would know how to take care of someone who got sick during the flight.

As a reflection of these values, industry leaders developed a training environment that measured "individual proficiency" by requiring "each captain to demonstrate the ability to handle *without assistance*" whatever exigencies might arise. "Copilots, called first officers, had their individual proficiency measured by how well they assisted the captain." In fact, as Robert L. Helmreich and H. Clayton Foushee note, "in 1952 the guidelines for proficiency checks at one major airline *categorically stated* that 'the first officer should not correct errors made by the captain.' "[17] As one pilot who'd trained in this kind of environment in the military told Suzanne, "As a young pilot, you followed the commander and kept your head down. If he flew into the ground, you followed him." Or as Captain Chesley "Sully" Sullenberger recently said, "In the bad old days, when the captain ruled the cockpit by whim and was a god with a small 'g' and a cowboy with a capital 'C,' first officers even carried little notebooks that listed the idiosyncrasies and personal preferences of different captains." This is what operating room nurses do today, as they catalog the varying preferences of myriad surgeons.

As airlines expanded in the Jet Age, the vast majority of airline pilots were trained in the military,[18] and this remained the norm until the mid-1980s. Military pilots were socialized in a strict hierarchy in which error was often attributed to the individual and was considered a sign of weakness or insufficiency. As Tom Wolfe wrote in *The Right Stuff*, "There are no *accidents* and no fatal flaws in the machines, there are only pilots with the wrong stuff."[19] Error was not something people discussed together or learned from. In a sense, it was so shameful that some pilots might have preferred to be buried with their mistakes. Military fighter pilots have been known to jest, "Better to die than to look bad!" The level of acceptable risk that was routinely tolerated by solo aviators moving from the military or mails into commercial passenger flight did not adjust with the technology, cockpit and cabin reconfiguration, or even the times (in the sixties after all, the entire culture was re-reimagining itself, reflecting on traditional views of hierarchy and attitudes toward masculinity).

Here is Wolfe's description of how the fighter pilot was socialized to accept what would normally be considered unacceptable levels of risk:

> One fine day, after he had joined a fighter squadron, it would dawn on the young pilot exactly how the losers in the great fraternal competition were being left behind. Which is to say, not by instructors or other superiors or by failures at prescribed levels of competence, but by death. At this point the essence of the enterprise would begin to dawn on him. Slowly, step by step, the ante had been raised until he was now involved in the grimmest and grandest gamble of manhood. Being a fighter pilot—for that matter, simply taking off in a single-engine jet fighter of the Century series, such as an F-102, or any of the military's other marvelous bricks with fins on them—presented a man, on a perfectly sunny day, with more ways to get himself killed than his wife and children could imagine in their wildest fears.[20]

"THAT'S JUST WHAT WE DO . . ."

When Patrick made the transition from military to commercial aviation in 1989, he observed that the "no limits" attitude that was so much a part of the military pilot persona was still very present with many of his new airline colleagues. Although the pace had slowed considerably, he tells of working and "unwinding " to the point of sheer exhaustion.

> When I first started flying, I was flying to Tokyo up to several times a month. Our flights would usually get in around 4:00 or 5:00 in the afternoon local time. We would usually get checked in at the hotel, wash up, and hit the ground running by 5:00 or 6:00 p.m. Problem is, 5:30 local is already 1:30 a.m. at home!
>
> The routine usually involved dinner at the local flavor of the week: haunts that were given names by the old timers like The Yellow Awning, Ako's, The Spiral Staircase, and The Fishbowl. Of course these names would have absolutely no meaning to the locals in the event that you could even speak the language. But at 1:30 a.m. circadian time (CT—the time according to your body's internal clock), it really helped to keep things simple.
>
> And so it went: dinner at 6:00 (2:00 a.m. CT) (if you were lucky—sometimes these places only held a dozen or so gaijins (foreigners) at a time, so you were left to drink Sapporos (the popular local beer) until the "second seating" at 7:00 or 7:30 (3:00 or 3:30 a.m. CT). Then dinner until 7:00 or 8:00 (3:00 or 4:00 CT), and for the really hard chargers—and there were a lot of them at that time—there might be a couple more hours at the local watering hole drinking beer and swapping flying stories. We would often not make it back to the hotel until 10:00 or 11:00 (6:00 or 7:00 a.m. CT).
>
> I would usually sleep well for at least a few hours, then I'd wake up for what I later learned to be "the 2 o'clock flush." Seriously. I actually heard the term a

number of times before I realized that that is exactly what I was doing, along with about a hundred of my colleagues at around 2:00 am each night. Now considering that 2:00 a.m. in Tokyo is 10:00 a.m. at home, this posed a slight problem: good sleep beyond that point in my circadian day was difficult at best.

When I came home from those trips, I was a mess: exhausted, crabby, impatient, and generally a danger to myself and anyone around me. We used to joke about keeping away from power tools and checkbooks for at least three days after one of these long international trips. I remember remarking about this enervation to one of the "old guys" who had been doing this his entire career. He replied, "That's just what we do." He retired a couple months after that exchange and within a year had passed away from a heart attack!

But by the time that I joined the airline, we were in the midst of a huge cultural shift. In the early 1990s the airline industry in general and my company in particular started into a financial "death spiral." The company had become a takeover victim and was subsequently burdened with massive debt; they came to the employees for some temporary financial relief (which turned out to be only a sneak preview of things to come). That situation, along with completion of the merger with another airline, made for some very unsettling and unhappy times. In addition to these growing pains, there were a number of sexual harassment and age discrimination judgments against the company and certain individuals. And who can forget the famous "Fargo Follies," where a 727 crew flew from Fargo, North Dakota, to Minneapolis quite decidedly under the influence; they were met at the gate in Minneapolis by the FAA, armed with breathalyzers and warrants. The incident was front-page news for weeks and had an unusually long half-life. It impacted the entire transportation industry, making us all subject to random breathalyzer and drug tests, not to mention disparaging remarks from the public for years.

The upshot of all this is that in a relatively short time span that "work hard-play hard" culture that I had experienced as a new hire in 1989 had shifted toward a "work hard—and watch out for yourself (a.k.a. CYA)" culture.

TECHNOLOGICAL ADVANCES

Despite the cavalier attitudes toward human fallibility, it was clear that something was going terribly wrong in the cockpit. The introduction of the "black box" into cockpits greatly enhanced their ability to figure out precisely *what* was wrong. The black box is actually two separate boxes: a flight data recorder (FDR)—which records, at a minimum, time, heading, airspeed and altitude—and the cockpit voice recorder (CVR), which records all cockpit conversation and radio traffic within the cockpit.[21]

This leap in technology allowed investigators a much clearer look into the pathology of accidents like the crash of United 173, as well as several other crashes in the 1960s and 1970s. As jet aircraft became the mainstay of commercial air travel, their vastly improved reliability drastically reduced both maintenance problems and the numbers of aviation accidents. What had not become more reliable, though, was how human beings interacted with one another as they dealt with the technology of the newer, safer aircraft. As more research focused on human error in our increasingly technological society, it became abundantly clear that accidents were related not primarily to failures in technical proficiency but to the interfaces between human beings and technology as well as between human beings and each other. The concept of human factors—a complex concept refined in the 1980s—was increasingly discussed as a key determinant in aviation accidents as well as accidents in other high-risk endeavors.

THE HUMAN FACTOR

The identification of human factors as a significant source of error was truly revolutionary. It reversed the assumption that if a plane went down, it was due primarily to mechanical misfortune and was a quixotic and unfortunate cost of doing business. Until aviation investigated other sources of error—like how the brain works in stressful situations, how human beings interact with one another and with machines, and how systems shape behavior and behavior shapes systems—there was little hope for change.

Fortunately, for both passengers and airline crews, previously cherished notions of how accidents happen were being revised in the 1970s. Although it is difficult to pinpoint the precise beginnings of the CRM movement, one place to start is to consider the work of several aviation researchers. One was John K. Lauber, who is credited with first using the term "cockpit resource management." Lauber was a psychologist who began his research career at the Naval Training Devices Center in Orlando, Florida, in 1969. In that capacity he worked on the Lockheed P-3C Orion, an antisubmarine airplane. In 1973 he began to work with the National Aeronautic and Space Administration's (NASA's) Ames Research Center, where he started to explore how pilots functioned on commercial airplanes. In the early 1970s airlines like Pan Am and United had begun to use high-fidelity flight simulators and direct pilot observation—researchers flying in cockpits on airline flights—to figure out how to improve pilot performance. With the support of Pan American airline's management and NASA, Lauber and several colleagues interviewed line pilots and flight engineers. What they discovered was startling—at least in that era. Pilots didn't complain about lack of technical training. What they were concerned about was, as Lauber recalls, "more difficult to pin down."[22] They were worried about lack of training in leadership, command, communication, decision making, and similar concepts.

Randy Babbitt, former administrator of the Federal Aviation Administration, started his career as a pilot for Eastern Airlines. He eventually became chairman of the Airline Pilots Association during the early days of the aviation safety movement and echoed those complaints: "In the old days, it was like the first officer and captain were going to work for two different airlines. Everyone had his own way of doing things. There was no particular standard. Some pilots read the checklist, some pilots didn't. You had to sit on your hands and watch what was gonna happen, try to anticipate what the captain wanted." Babbit's experiences as a new pilot reflected this:

> I was a new pilot for Eastern on reserve. [Being on reserve is the equivalent of a doctor's being on call. The pilot either carries a cell phone or beeper or must be near a phone so that he or she remains within the company's reach to replace a sick or rescheduled pilot on short notice.] For at least a year, I never flew the same piece of equipment twice; every time I went to work it was different. You just fill in when other people were sick or on vacation. We're going to fly the plane to Tokyo and you and I don't even know each other. We've never worked together and there are no standard operating procedures. . . . As a first officer you had to extract the procedures from some of these grumpy old guys.

In aviation in the late seventies Robert Helmreich confirms, "There was no concept of a team. None whatsoever. Captains looked at first officers and flight engineers not as resources but as kind of like fire extinguishers: 'Break the glass if they're needed.'"

It turned out, however, that not all the captains were "grumpy old guys," and a lot of them, Lauber's study revealed, had serious concerns about the status quo. Often the most vocal complaints, Lauber discovered, were from newly upgraded captains, who were learning the hard way that "being a captain involved something considerably more than adding some gold braid to their uniforms and moving across the cockpit from the right to the left seat."[23]

At this time, other researchers were documenting the same problems. Notable among their studies was the now-classic one by the physician Hugh P. Ruffell Smith.[24] Before these studies it was assumed that pilot training need only concentrate on technical knowledge and skills. The assumption was that pilots' skill and training would result in standardized responses to any situation—including an emergency. The Ruffell Smith study, conducted in 1976 but published by NASA in 1979, put a very large nail into the coffin of that assumption. It presented B-747 pilots in simulators with the following scenario: the pilots were on a Trans-Atlantic flight when early in their journey an engine failed. How should they respond? Far from dealing with the situation in a standard manner and safely maneuvering the aircraft back to land, pilots varied enormously in how they dealt with the emergency, and many of them made errors that it was assumed they would never ever make. "Several seriously overweight landings resulted from errors in fuel-dump calculations made by flight engineers who were given several tasks to complete concurrently," Thomas Chidester writes, describing the study. "It was as if each crewmember knew what he or she was supposed to do but did not know how the duties fit with those of other crewmembers."[25] Sound familiar?

At the same time that Ruffell Smith and Lauber and others were studying aviation errors, another two figures who would prove to be critical to the development of CRM were also observing pilots and airline crews—Robert Helmreich and his graduate student, Clay Foushee. Helmreich got his start as an organizational psychologist at the University of Texas in Austin, where he began to teach in 1966. He was interested in how people functioned on teams. In the 1970s he had contracts and grants with NASA to investigate how people functioned in small groups in stressful situations. As Foushee describes it, "In the post Apollo era, with the space station and [talk of] lunar colonies and trips to Mars, there was an awful lot of concern about isolation and confinement and how you can manage to put together a team of people that can function effectively under very stressful circumstances for long periods of time."

There were a very limited number of environments in which the researchers could observe people in small groups in stressful situations, since, as Foushee points out, "the world was not overflowing with NASA-type long-duration missions." If the researchers were to find out more, they realized they would have to do research in a different setting. Fortuitously, flight simulators were just coming on line, and there was increasing interest in the performance of airline crews. So Helmreich and Foushee began their long careers observing commercial airline pilots and crews. What they discovered was what other researchers were also documenting: put highly trained pilots in the confined space of an airline cockpit (or cockpit simulator), present them with an emergency, and what you got was a "high degree of variance in how people worked together and functioned."

In one of their first publications, Foushee explains, the researchers took transcripts of their flight simulations with multiple crews and "content coded the kinds of communications that had broken down in terms of commands, and inquiries and questions." There were, they reported,

> substantial differences in communications. Overall, crews that communicated more made fewer errors and performed better. As we delved more and more into it, we began to see that there was really a certain type of leadership style that can predict how well a crew functions. Captains who encouraged participation by subordinate crew members tended to notice and catch more mistakes, to function more smoothly as a crew and to be more adherent to procedures and checklists.
>
> The conclusion drawn from these investigations was that "pilot error" in documented accidents and incidents was more likely to reflect failures in team communication and coordination than deficiencies in "stick-and-rudder" proficiency or mechanical failures.[26]

In other words, misunderstandings and miscommunication between crew inside the aircraft, often compounded by others outside the aircraft, were factors in nearly all aircraft accidents.

After the United 173 accident NASA sponsored a workshop in 1979 entitled "Resource Management on the Flightdeck." After close analysis of the accidents discussed above as well as several other accidents, incidents, and events with similar components, members agreed that failures of "interpersonal communications, decision making, and leadership" in particular were underlying factors in the majority of air crashes to that point.[27] This meeting helped provide impetus that led at least some airlines to begin experimenting with pre-CRM initiatives. So, in 1981, United Airlines developed the first comprehensive CRM program, which it called Command/Leadership/Resource Management (C/L/R).

UNITED AIRLINES' CRM PROGRAM

Although Flight 173 became known as the final straw in this unfortunate accident trend, an earlier incident involving a United jet marks one of the first cases where an accident could be definitively traced back to what we now identify as a CRM failure. The dysfunctional crew interaction was captured on recording devices (CVR and FDR) and clearly documented as such in the ensuing accident investigation. On November 11, 1965, United Flight 227, a 727, left New York's LaGuardia Airport headed for San Francisco, making stops in Cleveland, Denver, and Salt Lake City. Salt Lake ended up being its last stop. As Ed Soliday, who was senior staff executive, director of safety, and vice president of safety, quality assurance, and security at United explained, "Probably one of the first real glaring events was the United 727 accident in Salt Lake City in which the copilot [or first officer], who was the pilot flying [PF], multiple times pushed the throttles forward on a 727 and the captain kept closing them [pulling them back]." In other words, recognizing the added performance required for an approach to this high-altitude airport, the FO was "stepping on the gas" and the captain was doing just the opposite, even though the FO was the pilot flying the approach. The captain ultimately took control of the aircraft, which hit the ground 335 feet short of the runway.

After the 1979 NASA meetings and long internal discussions, as well as discussions with the pilots' union, it was clear that some kind of specific training was needed. But the question was what kind would not ruffle the feathers of pilots who, as Soliday recalls, "had a lot of concerns about what would happen to the captain's authority. They didn't want to turn the cockpit into a democracy." United hired a consulting firm and worked with Bob Helmreich's group at the University of Texas and also with NASA to create a program that was, in its initial phases, built around a book called *The New Managerial Grid* by Robert Blake and Jane Mouton.[28] Because, Soliday says, the airline initially thought the problem (and solution) revolved solely around the captain, it began by training captains in a joint effort with the pilots' union, which was involved from the very beginning of the program. In the end, however, the airlines realized that captains were not the only source of error, and so all United pilots were put through a four-day team-building course, designed, Soliday says, "to bring you into the stark reality of what your leadership style and decision-making processes looked like."

In the course's first phase sessions included captains, copilots, and flight engineers who were trained with their peers in rank, not together. Before the pilots met, they were given twenty-five hours of homework that had to be done before they arrived. What happened if pilots didn't do their homework? "They'd just flat take you out of the schedule," Soliday says. "They'd send you home. This was tough-love stuff. We were not putting up with any nonsense; we were gonna do this."

The participants were then divided into teams—not of like-minded people but of opposites. Smokers were put on teams with people who violently objected to smoking. People known not to get along were teamed up with people they couldn't stand. Women—what few there were—were *not* teamed up with all women. The goal was, Soliday says, to break down the walls, to address the kinds of things that he had learned in his twenty years of flying:

> It's the little things that will intimidate other people from speaking up. You've got to break those walls down. You've got to encourage people to tell you everything they know. You've got to show them that you respect them. If you're the smartest guy in the world, you can learn something from the dumbest guy.
>
> The goal was also to teach people that the best team leader was not always the highest-ranking person—particularly not if the designated leader has drifted into a one-one decision mode [i.e., making all decisions himself]. Of the high-risk events we had at United when we almost lost airplanes during my tenure, it was because the copilot failed to recognize that the captain had drifted into a one-one.
>
> To help pilots who'd been taught to revere rank and hierarchy above all else, the teams United assembled were asked a series of twenty nonstructured problem-solving questions that had no black-and-white answers. The instruction was, "make your decisions as a team." To do this, most teams chose a leader—a decider—who was, from their point of view, "the smartest guy in the room." In some teams, the decider would decide with little or no discussion. The competition was to figure out which teams came up with the best answers. As the pilots began to look at which teams scored highest, it became clear that those with the "smartest" team leader and the least discussion were often the losers. This recognition, Soliday says, led to self-critique. Facilitators reinforced this critique with lessons on honesty and openness, willingness to inquire and advocate. Inquiry and advocacy are the keys to problem solving. It's OK to give orders, but one of the things we emphasize is that great decisions are based on the maximum information available in the time available. That means that if you're in a critical situation, you make the decision of what to do based on as much information as you can get at that time.
>
> One of the other things pilots needed to learn was the impact of fatigue and personal problems on performance. In aviation, 'hot sticks' thought they had no problems—or at least not ones that affected performance. All of us carry personal things and we all think we're strong enough to handle it. We don't recognize that we're drifting into self-absorption and we're not paying attention to the task at hand.

Over the course of four years, United put thousands of pilots through the training and quickly added flight attendants. "We thought that it would take us ten years to change that culture at United," Soliday remarks. "We actually began to see the change in six years."

There were two major incidents that validated the CRM culture at United: the first occurred on February 24, 1989, when United Flight 811, a 747, lost its cargo door during climb-out over the Pacific Ocean.

Flight 811 took off from Honolulu International Airport bound for Auckland, New Zealand, with 3 flight crew members, 15 flight attendants, and 337 passengers at approximately 01:52 HST. Sixteen minutes after takeoff, at about 22,000 feet (6,700 meters), a grinding noise was heard, followed by a loud thud that rattled the whole aircraft—one and a half seconds later the forward cargo door blew out abruptly. The pressure differential caved in the main cabin floor above the door, causing ten seats (8G and H through 12G and H) and an individual seated in 9F to be ejected from the cabin, resulting in nine fatalities (seats 8G and 12G were empty) and leaving a gaping hole in the aircraft. The pilots began an emergency descent to get the aircraft rapidly down to breathable air while performing a 180-degree left turn to return to Honolulu.

The decompression had damaged components of the on-board emergency oxygen supply system, which is located primarily in the vicinity of the door, rendering the emergency oxygen system inoperative for the cockpit crew.

The debris ejected from the plane during the explosive decompression caused severe damage to the number three and four engines, causing visible fires in both. The crew declared an emergency and began dumping fuel to get the plane's weight down to an acceptable landing weight.

The flight engineer went to the cabin to inspect the situation and observed severe damage immediately upon leaving the cockpit: the aircraft's skin was peeled off in some areas on the upper deck, revealing the frames and stringers. When he went down to the lower deck, he saw a huge hole in the side of the plane. He reported that a large section of fuselage aft of the number one exit door was open. He thought the damage had been caused by a bomb and, considering the condition of the plane, felt it would be unwise to exceed 250 knots (460 kilometers per hour). The plane's stall speed was around 240 knots (440 km/h), producing a narrow operating envelope.

As the plane neared the airport, the landing gear was extended. The damaged flaps were only partially deployed. This resulted in an unusually high landing speed between 190 and 200 knots (350–370 km/h). Nevertheless, the captain was able to get the plane to a halt without going off the end of the runway. Fourteen minutes had elapsed since the emergency was declared. Evacuation was carried out, and all passengers and flight attendants were off in less than forty-five seconds, though every flight attendant suffered some injury during the evacuation, ranging from scratches to a dislocated shoulder.[29]

According to Soliday:

The written approved FAA procedure, when your airplane is at high altitude and has had a rapid decompression, is to lower the landing gear and descend as rapidly as possible. The captain was doing the procedure by the book, but when that cargo door let go, the debris (from the door and parts around the door, part of the floor of the first class cabin and people who were sucked out of the airplane) went through the two engines on the right side of the aircraft, which severed the hydraulic lines. If they lowered the gear, they couldn't get it back up.[30] The copilot said to the captain, "I know it's procedure but are you sure you want to lower this landing gear? 'Cause we don't know if we can hold altitude."[31] The captain said, "That's a good point. We're going down pretty fast right now. We'll keep the gear up."

   If they had lowered the landing gear, they'd have landed in the water. They didn't lower the landing gear until they had the runway in sight. They could not hold altitude with the landing gear down. When they got on the ground, the first thing that captain said when interviewed by the media, they asked him what it was that he would attribute to the fact that they made it back, he said CRM. I would've followed the procedure if I hadn't been taught to listen to my copilot.[32]

The second big event to validate the impact of CRM training at United occurred July 19, 1989, in Sioux City, when flight 232 had an uncontained turbine failure in the center (tail) engine of a DC-10. In addition to the loss of thrust from the engine, the explosion resulted in a loss of all hydraulic systems on the aircraft—a situation that had never been anticipated or trained for. As Soliday explains,

It was the equivalent to a 4 x 8 sheet of plywood hanging out in the slipstream. No one had ever flown an airplane with all the hydraulics out to a safe landing; no one ever survived that. They had the throttles on two engines so that meant they had to use asymmetrical thrust [to steer the aircraft]. Whenever you move the throttles on an airplane that has engines that are under the wing, the nose pitches up and down. All they had were the throttles; I was talking to them from the ground. Al Haynes, who was the captain, had the sense to ask for—there's a flight instructor on the DC-10s sitting in the back writing. One of the things we teach in CRM is to find and use all of your resources available. So they brought this flight instructor up to the cockpit. He had four crew members, and together they did what no one had ever done before. They flew the airplane to the ground and quite frankly, saved half the people.

   After this landing, Haynes went around the country on his own saying that if he hadn't had CRM training, he'd have lost that airplane. It was a synergistic effort of four guys in the cockpit solving problems that no one had ever trained them on, no one ever anticipated occurring. Once the word got out (there were still a few diehards arguing that CRM was a communistic thing), then CRM became very popular.

United Airlines spent about $4 million and trained all of its pilots. The initial program, which emphasized "providing participants with insights into their personal managerial styles . . . requiring participants to assess their own behaviors and those of peers," eventually shifted to a more systems-based approach.[33] Nonetheless, United's C/L/R program was an overall success, becoming a model for other airlines to emulate. Despite some pilots who denounced the individually focused training as "psycho-babble" and "charm school" or attempts to "manipulate their personalities," CRM was quickly accepted at United.[34]

CRM PROGRAM EVOLUTION

Following United's lead, other airlines began to adopt CRM training programs. They experimented with their own ways of creating trainings. As the CRM model changed at different airlines, safety experts inside the companies were also benefiting from ongoing studies conducted by researchers who closely investigated how crews were functioning. Wiener, Kanki, and Helmreich's excellent source book *Cockpit Resource Management* describes an impressive array of studies that were conducted on how crews work—and don't work—together. Over the course of three decades, organizational, social, and industrial psychologists, as well as sociolinguists and management experts in teamwork, have studied how crews functioned. Their investigations guided how CRM evolved and was taught in the aviation setting. Among the many things they analyzed were how crews communicate, how the different personalities of captains and crews affect performance and error, how crews (not just individuals) make decisions, how teamwork should be defined, the dynamics of authority, and how CRM programs could and should be evaluated. They also studied the impact of fatigue and work intensification on crews' ability to communicate; to prevent, manage, or contain error; and to prevent accidents.

All these studies used the tool of high-fidelity simulation, in which crews go into a virtual airplane and handle virtual problems. Pilot and flight attendant training depends a great deal on simulation, which is not only a remarkably faithful replica of the real thing but allows realistic manipulation of conditions that, because of their danger, could never be attempted in an actual aircraft. In addition, monitoring air crew response, replay, and real-time training optimizes effectiveness. Flight attendants also train in cabin mock-ups, equipped with seats, emergency exits, doors, and equipment. Researchers designed scenarios that would not only test the kinds of emergencies that FAs might normally encounter but also teach FAs how to integrate into the larger team by implementing one of the central tenets of CRM: inquiry, advocacy, and assertion.

Researchers studying decision making in the cockpit designed situations to analyze "crews that differed on their overall performance on simulated flights." What they discovered was that the keys to effective crew decision making included four central elements: (1) good situation awareness, (2) high levels of what is called "metacognition," meaning knowledge of their own thoughts and of factors that influence their thinking, (3) shared mental models based on explicit communication, and (4) efficient resource management.[35] Captains and crews who thought about thinking—that is, thought about problems before they happened (what is called threat and error management, TEM)—were able to deal with a confluence of multiple problems—turbulence, high crosswinds making landing impossible, loss of hydraulics—all of which could be dealt with individually but when combined, made it hard to make decisions. Crews that did better were also more aware of information needed to solve a problem, as well as how to deal with ambiguous problems that could not be solved by the book.

Effective crews, researchers discovered, were those that were able to move beyond understanding and solving problems individually and excelled at developing a shared understanding of the problem. This affected the dynamics of authority. The crews who developed a shared understanding of "ill-defined or non-routine problems" developed "shared problem models" through communication.[36] Captains in these situations did not just bark out orders, which crew members then jumped to obey. Rather, crews became hyperorganized, able to cross-monitor, apportion tasks, and utilize all resources and information, in large part because their captains used low-workload periods to prepare for possible high-workload ones.[37] Other researchers homed in on precisely how communication occurs in cockpits and what makes for more effective communication and teamwork.

As airlines applied this research to their CRM programs, government participation in this effort extended way past the initial NASA meeting in 1979. When CRM training was first developed, the FAA initially only *recommended* that commercial airlines do it. To incentivize the major airlines to develop CRM programs, the FAA agreed to concurrent development of the Advanced Qualification Program, or AQP. AQP reduced overall recurrent training costs for the airlines and incorporated CRM training into the curriculum. AQP has turned out to be a win-win for all parties concerned. On October 2, 1990, the FAA mandated CRM training for commercial airlines.

Although airlines are granted great latitude in CRM program development, a fairly common model has been adapted and promoted by most U.S. commercial airlines. CRM and the closely related derivative concept of TEM have been recognized as being so vital that these programs have been embraced voluntarily by the U.S. military, emergency services (fire, police, EMT), and the energy and medical industries.

THREAT AND ERROR MANAGEMENT

Development of Crew Resource Management has proven to be an extremely effective tool in improving communication, workload management, teamwork—and ultimately, safety. CRM addresses the nuts and bolts of human-to-human and human-to-machine interface. TEM training, by contrast, has been likened to such situations as defensive driving training for motor vehicles. TEM is a tool that enhances safety by anticipating threats as early as possible and dealing with them proactively, either by eliminating each threat or by taking measures to reduce its severity. Should a threat eventually evolve into an actual error, TEM philosophy attempts to mitigate the error in the most effective manner.

SHIFTING THE CULTURAL BIAS IN HIRING PRACTICES

Despite many pilots' resistance, CRM proved durable. In the late 1980s and 1990s, airline hiring practices began to lean very strongly in the direction of recruiting pilots with strong team-building experience rather than the single-seat fighter-pilot types who had often been given preferential hiring in the past.[38] Although basic stick-and-rudder skills are as vital and indispensable as ever, increased cockpit automation in modern airliners requires additional emphasis on interpersonal and team-building skills. When companies began to change hiring policies in favor of team-oriented pilots, a common comment from some of the old-timers was, "If I were being interviewed today, I wouldn't get hired by this company!"

The CRM movement, more appropriately described as a cultural transformation, is referred to as "an evolution, not a revolution." Although its detractors hoped it would merely be a temporary inconvenience, the firm commitment of regulators, managers, and operators ensured that there would be no short-term approach to what had been clearly identified as an entrenched cultural problem. The only way to transform the wrong stuff into the really right stuff would be to create an industry-wide program that would have to evolve, change, and adapt as it developed.

COMMITMENT AND REINFORCEMENT

Today all commercial airline pilots and flight attendants are routinely exposed to the concept of Crew Resource Management at various stages of their respective educational and training programs. At a minimum, CRM training is introduced during initial training and revisited annually during recurrent training.[39] Effective CRM programs emphasize continuous reinforcement of CRM principles by incorporating CRM in all aspects of the operation. CRM philosophy stresses that CRM should encompass the entire flight department. Consequently, flight attendants, airline mechanics, dispatchers, air traffic controllers, and even baggage handlers at some point receive the training.

Recognizing CRM's benefits to commercial airlines, other organizations have enthusiastically adopted the model. To maintain International Standards for

Business Aircraft Operations (IS-BAO) certification, regulators of business aircraft operations have recently made CRM training a requirement for certification as well.[40] The military has similarly adopted versions of the CRM model for flight operations and other departments, as have several other high-reliability organizations (HROs) such as the energy industry and emergency services.

Even the space shuttle program placed a great deal of emphasis on CRM training (called SFRM, spaceflight vernacular for Spaceflight Resource Management). Captain Greg Johnson, STS 125 pilot, stated, "One of the first classes that we had as a new astronaut crew was SFRM." Captain Johnson explained that SFRM was absolutely critical to mission success. He said, "The crews that worked most effectively as teams—that communicated most efficiently—had the fewest 'issues' when under pressure. And there are certain times during launch and reentry where these skills had to be perfected to ensure survival."

But what exactly is CRM? What exactly do pilots, flight attendants, and other personnel learn? There is no one-size-fits-all CRM training. The programs have adapted as they have been developed, and each airline has its own variations. We'll take you through the major components of CRM in a moment, but first we'd like to introduce the broad guidelines with which all these programs have to conform. These guidelines evolved from the initial CRM training plan that came from the 1979 industry summit. To be most effective, CRM training should consist of three parts: initial indoctrination and awareness, recurrent training every one to two years, and continuous reinforcement in day-to-day line operations. In the most recent FAA CRM guidance document,[41] these three parts of CRM training plan are explained.

Indoctrination and Awareness

- Initial indoctrination typically consists of classroom presentations and focuses on communication and decision making, interpersonal relations, crew coordination, leadership, and adherence to SOPs (standard operating procedures), among others.[42] In this component of CRM training, the concepts are developed, defined, and related to the safety of line operations. This component also provides a common conceptual framework and a common vocabulary for identifying crew coordination problems.
- Indoctrination can be accomplished by a combination of training methods. Lectures, audiovisual presentations, discussion groups, role-playing exercises, computer-based instruction, and videotaped examples of good and poor team behavior are commonly used methods.
- Initiating indoctrination/awareness training requires the development of a curriculum that addresses CRM skills that have been demonstrated to influence crew performance. To be most effective, the curriculum should define the concepts involved and relate them directly to operational issues that crews encounter. Many organizations have found it useful to survey crew

members. Survey data have helped identify embedded attitudes regarding crew coordination and cockpit management. The data have also helped to identify operational problems and to prioritize training issues.

- Effective indoctrination/awareness training increases understanding of CRM concepts. That understanding in turn often influences individual attitudes favorably regarding human-factors issues. Often the training also suggests more effective communication practices.

- It is important to recognize that classroom instruction alone does not fundamentally alter crew-member attitudes over the long term. The indoctrination/ awareness training should be regarded as a necessary first step toward effective crew performance training.

Recurrent Training

- The other two parts (as we explain in chapter 2) are *recurrent training* and *continuous reinforcement*. If CRM training is a one-shot event, no matter how thorough, its effectiveness will be limited. The key to its successful implementation in aviation is that once introduced, it was then kept in the forefront through recurrent training, and it has evolved and adapted over time.

Continuous Reinforcement

- CRM concepts not only are continually reinforced and evaluated during training but are key elements of accident and incident investigation and analysis. Part of this process of continuous reinforcement comes in the form of reporting programs. The two primary reporting programs, Aviation Safety Action Program (ASAP) and Flight Operations Quality Assurance (FOQA) (both to be discussed in greater detail later) have been key elements to developing and enhancing CRM and TEM effectiveness.

CREW PERFORMANCE INDICATORS

"CRM training is based on an awareness that a high degree of technical proficiency is essential for safe and efficient operations. Demonstrated mastery of CRM concepts cannot overcome a lack of proficiency. Similarly, high technical proficiency cannot guarantee safe operations in the absence of effective crew coordination."[43] Human-factors analysts have defined several factors, indicators, or measures that represent the core components that must work in concert to have a successful outcome in *any* high-reliability operation. Four such measures, called "crew performance indicators" (CPIs),[44] are described below. First and foremost is *technical proficiency*, which is generally assumed to be high among professionals. The other three CPIs addressed here are *communication, team building,* and *workload management.*

Since the inception of CRM, measurable progress has been made in these subject areas; emphasis is now being placed on threat and error management. Probably the most productive tool in the overall CRM arsenal is the TEM model, which is based upon the early identification of threats and employment of effective mitigation strategies to reduce or eliminate them before they turn into errors.

But before we can manage threats, whether at sea level in health care or at thirty-six thousand feet in aviation, we have to communicate them. So we will start with the communication CPI.

Chapter 2

Communication

"DREAMS"

In 1986 the U.S. Navy's flight demonstration team, the Blue Angels, celebrated its fortieth anniversary. To commemorate the event, the rock group Van Halen produced a dramatic video of "the Blues" featuring six of the navy's finest aviators performing a series of dazzling maneuvers set to the band's hit song "Dreams." When Patrick's company, CRMLLC, presents its CRM course to pilot groups to set the tone, trainers will often introduce the session with this five-minute video of a truly amazing performance. The audience rarely fails to be awestruck by the proficiency of this group of pilots who execute heart-stopping maneuvers, sometimes within inches of one another. Rather than focusing on group proficiency, most participants zero in on the skill of a group of discrete individuals who just happen to be flying in the same airspace. As the video winds down, trainers quickly reframe the experience: "How do you think things would turn out if these guys were not working as a team?" trainers ask. "What would happen if communications between them were ineffective? If they failed to manage their workload properly? If they were proficient as solo aviators but lacked the ability to work as a team, what would this video look like?"

The question is clearly rhetorical. By now pilots all know that unless communication, workload management, teamwork, and technical proficiency—the core precepts of CRM—approached near perfection, there would be no Blue Angels and no inspiring video to view. One of the facilitators for CRMLLC, Scott Anderson, is in fact one of the pilots shown in the video. Anderson emphatically confirms that any breakdown in those four principles would result in disaster—and in fact, it has.

According to Anderson, communication, teamwork, workload management, and technical proficiency were part and parcel of every aspect of the Blue Angels operation.

The team had a thorough briefing before and debriefed after *every* flight—whether for a live show in front of a crowd of half a million or team training over the El Centro, California desert. Each debrief included a "General and Safe" portion that not only involved the six demonstration pilots, but all members of the operation.

The Maintenance Officer was always there, as well as the Fat Albert Crew, Technical Reps (in this case, McDonald Douglas, as the manufacturer of our aircraft), the flight surgeon and any other pertinent ground observers. The boss would go around the room and expect commentary from each person regarding both general observations and *any* safety related issue. These would include general comments, safety "events," voice procedures and so on—anything was fair game. Probably the biggest safety issue that was brought up involved communication. Literally every phrase, checklist, challenge and response was scripted to the point that a "nonresponse" or an inappropriate (or misstated) response was a *major* distraction.

Commenting further on the communications emphasis within the team, Anderson said, "The debriefs could sometimes be brutal. Everything from radio communication errors (known as 'noodles') to a 'low start' or 'low bottom' was covered in the debrief. No error and no person was left untouched; but when we left the room, it was over—done! The learning process was priceless and we took the lessons with us with the understanding that any 'spilled blood'—and there was plenty—was left on the debriefing room floor."[1] As Anderson emphasizes, "Virtually *every* Blue Angel accident that I can recall throughout history was ultimately the result of someone straying from SOP."

CREATING EFFECTIVE COMMUNICATION

Communication noun 1. the act or process of communicating; fact of being communicated; 2. the imparting or interchange of thoughts, opinions, or information by speech, writing, or signs; 3. something imparted, interchanged, or transmitted; 4. a document or message imparting news, views, information, etc.

According to this common definition, a basic send-receive model, the essence of communication is "the activity of conveying information" or "the process of transferring information from a sender to a receiver," as if shooting an arrow into the bull's-eye of a target. Sounds simple: message sent—message received—done. And because so many of us unwittingly accept this simplistic model, we participate in *mis*communication all the time. Successful communication involves a great deal more than senders and receivers. Each party to the attempted communication has his or her own frame of reference, vocabulary (not just of words and specialized terms but of *meanings* that vary by context), sense of proper communication behavior, sense of self in relation to other parties, and scores of other variables that play a role in the success of the communication effort. We may be so intent on what we say, how we say it, our own sense of how difficult it is for us to say it, or of how obvious what we're saying is to us that we can easily forget the many factors that influence the people with whom we are trying to share a message and a meaning. Indeed, we may be so convinced that we've gotten our message across clearly that we are surprised or annoyed that other people have misinterpreted it or failed to take the hint.

This is why aviation accident investigation archives are rife with examples of poor—or nonexistent—communication. No matter where or when such an accident happens, you can almost be certain that a common thread—*and threat*—involved communication. Crew Resource Management addresses the actual, factual, complex nature of successful communication and shows the woeful inadequacy of the simplistic send-receive model. For example, one source of poor communication in aviation can be traced to a social factor: the traditional hierarchies that have for so long been an integral part of aviation culture. In a strict hierarchy, superiors speak (or command) when *they* feel it is important; subordinates remain silent or speak when spoken to. Superiors are presumed to possess all the knowledge and information that counts *about any project or endeavor*, subordinates to possess knowledge or information relevant only to their particular assigned tasks. Given this history of emphasis on the hierarchical command structure, CRM focuses on developing—in *all* air crew members—the attitudes and skill sets that help to ensure that the voices, intelligence, and professional resources of all the members of a flight crew are taken into account and utilized.

To create an effective CRM environment, the focus of the communication CPI is not only on what works but also on what doesn't. Inadequate, inappropriate, or failed communication is analyzed to determine the ways in which, in specific circumstances, individuals' approaches have actually created barriers to the effective transfer of critical information and the ways used to get crew members on the same wavelength. Teaching and learning effective communication has to focus not only on skill building but also on understanding and addressing the barriers we encounter when we try to put these skills into practice. Communication is *the* central element in team building and in effective team*work*. In addition to properly conveying information, effective communication has several other functions. In the CRM framework it serves to

- establish common language, both terminology and meaning;
- establish interpersonal relationships;
- establish predictable behavior patterns;
- maintain attention to overall situation, to task, to self, and to fellow crew members; and
- manage the team—both in the classical supervisory sense and also in terms of self-awareness and intercrew monitoring.[2]

CRM trainings—which may superficially seem to be pragmatic exercises in good collegial manners and common sense—are actually complex constructions that are built on years of study and research. They are founded on what the noted cultural anthropologist Clifford Geertz called "thick descriptions" and detailed analyses' of years of observed crew behavior in which human-factors researchers "have not only analyzed particular behaviors but the context in which those behaviors have been developed or adapted."[3] Grounding the very pragmatic advice and skills taught in CRM trainings is a solid theoretical perspective that has evolved after years of studying how airline crews communicated with each other pre-CRM and how they work in the post-CRM environment. Communication patterns are uncovered by analyzing data from the black boxes installed in all commercial aircraft (but not required on corporate aircraft). These record what happened in the last minutes of flight on fatal journeys like that taken by the crew and passengers on Eastern Flight 401 (December 29, 1972). Researchers present in the cockpit and flight simulators also studied flight crews to discover how people really behaved in commercial aircraft. When United Airlines began its first programs, line-oriented flight training (LOFT) sessions, "one of the major innovations . . . was the use of video cameras in the simulators to record crew interactions in the training environment. By replaying the tape of their LOFT, crews gain[ed] the ability to review their actions and decisions and to obtain insights into their behavior, guided by the LOFT instructor."[4]

Utilizing all the tools at their disposal, researchers analyzed everything from how routine comments could be understood—or misunderstood—depending on whether they were used to verify, repeat, or question information exchanged, to how problem-solving talk functioned in normal or abnormal situations. They also considered how communication could erode or be enhanced as a function of workload and discovered the importance of workload management and regulation to optimal communication and teamwork. Years of such research created an awareness that effective communication was absolutely central to team functioning and leadership. It became clear that rather than following the traditional style of shouting out commands in the service of control, good captains articulated

> plans and strategies, creat[ing] a context in which their commands and information requests take on meaning. This articulation helps to build a shared mental model for the situation. It enables the first officer to make suggestions, coordinate actions, and offer information that contributes to solving the problem and making decisions. Communication analyses help to delineate what information is critical, when it should be solicited, the best way in which it should be integrated, who the possessors of information are, and whether specific patterns can be linked to more effective crew communication and coordination.[5]

Perhaps one of the most important functions of communication in the context of aviation—and one that is also paramount in health care—is understanding how communication can establish predictable behavior in both ordinary and extraordinary situations. These known behavior patterns *in themselves* then communicate information about the nature of a situation, thus helping to support appropriate responses and engagement among team members. Pilots, flight attendants, and others working in aviation share a common challenge with those who work with the sick and vulnerable: the so-called predictable unpredictability of their work. This means that although most of the time things go along according to familiar routines (which already take into account scores of variables at any given time)—any of about a zillion things could also go radically wrong at any moment.

Because plane crashes are extremely rare today, the public perception of commercial aviation is that it is safe and reliable, and not much of consequence generally goes on. It is easy to *imagine* that flying a plane is mostly about two guys in a box executing predictable routines hour after hour, day in and day out. In fact, the process is actually anything but routine. So many unpredictable events occur outside the awareness of the passengers and public (turbulence, thunderstorms, ice, an oil leak, a decompression, a passenger who becomes seriously ill, a terrorist event, or an engine that explodes, etc.) that the illusion of predictability and routine is quite easily maintained. After all, there are almost fifty thousand flights going on in the world every day—about eight thousand in the United States alone. Yet the fact remains that in spite of the multiple layers of safeguards that have been developed throughout the decades—including CRM—flying airplanes is inherently dangerous. Each unpredictable variable has the potential to become a serious incident by itself, and sometimes several of these occur simultaneously.

Sometimes a threat arises from events that are supposed to never happen because technological advances have made them "impossible." (Always remember the maiden voyage of the "unsinkable" Titanic.) Consider Qantas Airways Flight 32 (QF32), an Airbus A-380 that took off from Singapore on November 4, 2010, bound for Sydney with 469 souls on board. During climb-out, the number two (left, inboard) engine encountered an "uncontained turbine failure," which resulted in damage to the adjacent (number one) engine, punctured the left wing and a wing fuel tank, and damaged the wing spar, among other things. This highly automated aircraft has multiple redundant and automated systems designed to ensure the safest and most efficient operation possible. Yet the crew on QF32, much to their surprise and consternation, discovered that even with all this great technology, maneuvering this massive, broken machine successfully back to earth actually came down to the combined efforts of five human beings (who, by the way, made the correct decision to ignore many of the automated messages and directives in favor of their own—human—instincts and judgment).

Why? Because the malfunction resulted in 43 ECAM (engine condition and monitoring) system messages—many contradicting one another—in the first sixty seconds alone; these were followed by even more messages as the situation progressed. Keep in mind that just *one* of these malfunction messages can require twenty or more steps to address the condition that caused it. The messages ranged from "Engine Two Overheat" (which took further—human—investigation to correctly interpret) to engines one and four going to a "degraded" mode, loss of a hydraulic system, and a fuel imbalance resulting from a hole in one of the fuel tanks. Interestingly, the fuel imbalance message typically leads the crew to transfer fuel from one side of the aircraft (the heavy side) to the other. The QF32 crew, obviously understanding that *in this specific context* the imbalance had to have come from a leak, correctly chose *not* to follow that part of the imbalance procedure. Captain David Evans, one of five pilots on the flight deck at the time of the incident, credits the crew's ability to work as a team—and specifically their training in CRM—for the successful outcome of this incident.

In these situations, predictable communication patterns can help people navigate the potentially catastrophic uncertainties that they confront. Health care professionals often claim that predictable communication is impossible because of their constant confrontation with uncertainty. What is not well understood or accepted yet in health care is that predictable communication patterns may be the *best and most effective* way to mitigate the stress that is itself a by-product of the constant ambiguity in their work.

This is precisely what researchers discovered when they studied how pilots and other crew members deal with uncertainty in aviation. One crucial aspect of predictable communication patterns is that sharing of essential information among team members is common practice. Another is use of a shared set of terms, including shorthand names for complex actions or situations. For example, "Increases in crew errors were . . . associated with increases in the amount of communication in which one or more crew members expressed uncertainty about what the others were talking about. In other words, crews appear to perform best in a cockpit environment in which pilots share and acknowledge information about the state of the aircraft and minimize the amount of uncertainty about communication."[6] This kind of performance enhancement obviously extends to anyone on the aviation team, even if they are not inside the aircraft (traffic controllers, ground crews, etc.). What is crucial here is that the standardization of communication patterns allows crews to spend their mental energy on dealing attentively with specific technological problems rather than wasting it trying to figure out what others are saying, thinking, or expecting.

Training people to perform the many functions of communication effectively also allows crew members to sustain the critical function of maintaining their awareness of the individual tasks they have to perform, monitoring the tasks of others, and maintaining situational awareness—an awareness of the bigger picture, such as flying the plane, even while dealing with a smaller-scale, if crucial, demand. Although crew communication in CRM helps establish interpersonal relationships, these exist not to serve the interpersonal needs of crew members but to allow them to coordinate the performance of their workplace tasks safely and effectively. Any glitch in communication is a barrier to people's keeping on task, returning to task, and maintaining situational awareness. This is important not because communication glitches aren't "nice" interpersonally but because they aren't *safe*. "CRM training is not an end in itself, a means of living for consultants, a power structure for management, nor an opportunity to generate research data and statistics. Nor is CRM the last frontier of aviation safety or organizational efficiency—or a frontier of any kind. We provide CRM training to operational personnel so that they are better able to contribute to the aviation system production's goals: the safe and efficient transportation of people and goods."[7]

Loss of situational awareness can be a critical by-product of poor communication. Eastern Flight 401 is an excellent illustration of a loss of situational awareness as a result of poor communication when three highly trained and skilled pilots all forgot to fly their airplane as they focused on dealing with burned-out lightbulb. Like a couple arguing about which exit to take as they travel down a freeway and failing to notice the tractor-trailer truck in their path, these pilots were distracted from noticing the Florida Everglades heading straight for them. Losing situational awareness costs passengers and flight crews their lives. The goal of communication must therefore include establishing communication patterns that serve to enhance situational awareness rather than diminish it.

Traditional command-and-control models of authority and leadership function to keep critical information away from many of the people who need it and encourage styles of interaction that may make it difficult or impossible for people to return their full attention to their tasks following interruption or to maintain situational awareness when things go awry. Patterns of communication in which commands or orders are shouted, in which authority figures fail to demonstrate respect and regard for subordinates, or which overload subordinates with unnecessary information and multiple orders increase stress levels and thus jeopardize both attention to task and situational awareness.

Many traditional-model occupational hierarchies operate on the fantasy that "true professionals" cannot be put off their game because someone screamed at them or otherwise upset them. No matter what happens, the true professional is able to return to task and to perform admirably. What we now know about how the brain works under attack or stress completely contradicts this widely held notion. When people are in "fight or flight" mode, they typically cannot, in fact, easily return their full attention to the task at hand. When they are under stress for either professional or personal reasons, their "professionalism" does *not* actually trump feelings of anxiety, fear, or sadness.[8] Nor can professionalism erase the impact of fatigue or stress resulting from excessive workloads (which we will address in detail in another chapter).

Aviation's approach to interpersonal communication and professional relationships has developed by studying how people realistically function at work (human-factors research) and through scientific research on how the brain really works under stress.[9] CRM's communications practices and team strategies build on this evidence rather than on conventional cultural beliefs about status, deference, toughness, professionalism, and the effects of these sorts of elements on desirable human capabilities. Many aspects of the CRM training that help pilots and crew keep planes where they belong could save patients' lives as well if adopted in health care.

CRM Communications training focuses on the following:

- Making introductions and setting the stage for teamwork
- Conducting appropriate briefings
- Creating/reaffirming a shared language
- Establishing mutual understanding of decisions about operations
- Inviting participation
- Seeking information and direction from others when necessary
- Promoting appropriate assertiveness to maintain safe operations
- Examining self and group, including critiquing as appropriate

These factors are interrelated in their functions and in the ways in which they are addressed, and all apply to both communication and team building. Let's look at how these individual components relate to CRM.

MAKING INTRODUCTIONS AND SETTING THE STAGE FOR TEAMWORK

Most people are unaware of the "backstage" preparations that contribute to a successful flight. Before pilots and flight attendants walk through the locked doors to the jetway to begin their various duties, they commence a process that sets out and articulates plans, details, and specifics for the upcoming flight. This routine—the preflight crew briefing—serves to communicate directly the observations and expectations of the captain, and to set the tone for opening lines of communication for the entire crew. The crew briefing is the first step in building an effective team on the spot—and it begins with the simple act of making introductions. The pilots, who may never have met before, introduce themselves to one another, as well as to the flight attendants and any other crew members. As Chesley Sullenberger describes it in his book *Highest Duty*, when he began the first leg of a four-leg trip—one he had no idea would end so dramatically in the Hudson River—the first thing he did was introduce himself to his copilot, Jeffrey Skiles, and the flight attendants, Sheila Dail, Donna Dent, and Doreen Welsh: "[Jeff Skiles] and I had never met before, so we introduced ourselves. Along with Sheila, Donna, and Doreen, we'd be a team for the next four days."[10]

Any crew briefing will start off with introductions. *The importance of introductions cannot be overstated*: research has indicated conclusively that the act of simply exchanging names has a measurable positive impact on team building and communication (and interestingly, also on *job satisfaction*). Patrick has noted that if a flight attendant was unable to attend the briefing, he or she will frequently drop in on the cockpit before the flight just to say, "Hi, my name is . . ." and "get a visual" on who the rest of the crew is. He states, "We all know the full names of the other crew members from the 'Crew Orders' briefing sheet. Then at the actual briefing we go around the room and make introductions by first names. It seems like a small thing, but when you start out with the crew knowing each other on a first-name basis, it really improves 'approachability' for everyone."

Introductions are so important to the coming together and effective functioning of a team that considerable time is spent training people in communicating such apparently simple information as name, title, and rank. Perhaps even more important than the specifics of the information are the *other cues* that communicate so much about what individuals may expect their team relationship to be: tone of voice, self-presentation and demeanor, eye contact and other body language.

Early on in CRM development, one major airline produced a training video illustrating the impact of first meetings. The video contains two versions. In the first version, affectionately referred to as the "bad captain video," only the captain knows that the simulation interaction is being videotaped. In this rendering, he shoehorns himself into the left seat, turns to the first officer and engineer, and brusquely introduces himself. His tone is cold and condescending, and his body language reinforces his sense of superiority and his lack of respect for the subordinate crew members. Nuanced body language confirms the captain's regard for the existing hierarchy, which places the second officer (SO) at the bottom of the cockpit food chain and which the captain unmistakably reinforces in his dismissive treatment of the SO. The captain starts out with, "OK, this is how it's gonna be . . . ," issues a proclamation of "how it's gonna be," and then turns his attention to the instrument panel. Once his back is turned, the engineer (unaware that the entire scene is being videotaped, you'll recall) offers his raised middle finger in collective response and commentary. Entertaining as the video was, it demonstrated the hostile environment that can be created with something as simple as a poorly executed introduction.

In the second version, known as the "good captain video," everyone is aware of the videotaping, and the introduction is scripted to reflect a much more congenial and collegial atmosphere. As the captain slides into his seat, his entire demeanor and tone have changed. With a welcoming smile and friendly affect he introduces himself. While still maintaining his command presence, he creates an environment that indicates that all present—himself included—are members of a team and that he is open to the concerns of and input from other crew members. This approach creates an entirely different atmosphere in the cockpit. One introduction will foster the coming together of a functioning team, while the other will produce sullen acquiescence at best and resentful obedience at worst.

Because they enhance safety, introductions play a key role in CRM communications and team building. The airline industry long ago figured out what brain science is now documenting: although we are constantly admonished not to judge a book by its cover, the human brain works by doing precisely that. With huge amounts of information to process, to get through the day our brains continually take shortcuts. One of those involves reacting immediately to initial signals. If the captain sends out the kinds of signals the "bad captain" broadcast loud and clear, the immediate gut response will be to feel intimidated or antagonized, and the brain will be on alert to look out for this guy. The crew members will not be inclined to stop to wonder whether he's just had a bad day or otherwise give him the benefit of the doubt. In these circumstances it is entirely possible that they will withhold valuable information at a critical time, believing the captain will not welcome their contributions and may even respond punitively.

CONDUCTING APPROPRIATE BRIEFINGS

The portrayal of bad and good captains in the instructional videos also refers to the critical issue of briefings to promote teamwork and safety. The purpose of briefings is to impart, share, and clarify information among crew members to promote more effective operation. "In aviation," Helmreich and Musson write, "briefings by the captain to other cockpit crew have become standard. Intended course, any expectations of delay or bad weather, specific crewmember roles as well as expected norms of behavior are all communicated before each flight. . . . Furthermore, specifics of the intended flight plan are communicated and each crewmember should be asked to verify their understanding of those plans. This is generally referred to as establishing a 'shared mental model.'"[11]

Briefings are a critical communication venue and format for teams and teamwork. The initial briefing provides the captain the opportunity to establish a team environment that is conducive to safety by emphasizing the importance of interactive decision making and participation. In it the captain addresses pertinent safety and operational issues and identifies potential problems, such as weather and abnormal system operations. He or she also provides guidelines for crew actions, including standard operating procedures, distribution of crew workload,

> **What Briefings Should Be**
>
> • **Brief**
> • Concise
> • Ten points maximum
> • Inclusive (include all parties)

and any anticipated deviations from normal procedures. For example, if the weather forecast is reporting turbulence thirty to sixty minutes into a long flight, the captain might ask the flight attendants to delay the meal service until he or she has determined that the flight is in sufficiently clear air to safely pull out the heavy meal carts. In this briefing, the captain confirms his or her commitment to the well-being of the crew as well as to following company policies and lays out the expectation that all crew members will do likewise.

When United and other airlines began to videotape crew communication during simulator training in the 1980s, they brought in the cameras precisely because a lot of crew members insisted that they didn't need extra communications and team-building training. They believed that they were not only proficient aviators but also skilled communicators. The company installed the cameras in the simulators, where in the pressures of the environment they were quickly forgotten by the working crews. During the postevent debriefs, when confronted with video proof, crews were literally shocked at their own behaviors. They realized that they often unconsciously adopted behaviors that silenced fellow crew members. This created the "aha moment" that is often a prerequisite of change. It wasn't that the captain was telling the first officer or flight attendant to "shut up and hop to it" in so many words. It was the effects of body language, tone of voice, the stray remark, a casual dismissal of a crew member's concern or comment—all captured on video—that conveyed the message that subordinates (any noncaptains, that is to say) were nonpersons when it came to flying.

Good briefings are addressed to the specific and appropriate audiences—those who will be involved directly in the matters to be discussed. They don't happen just once but continue throughout the various phases of the flight, as necessary to further enhance communication, minimize confusion, establish and maintain expectations, and elicit optimal participation from the crew. Because the timing of a briefing is as important as its content, it should be conducted when the crew is not distracted by other duties. The takeoff-departure briefing is done close to the time that the aircraft will be taking the runway, at a time when it can be stopped and the brakes set so that there are no other distractions. The crew preflight briefing is ideally accomplished prior to boarding the aircraft. Because the realities of today's fast-paced operational tempo usually preclude an off-site briefing (e.g., a private room in the airport), the second choice will generally be in the jetway before the crew actually boards the aircraft. Should that not be possible, the briefing will be in the cabin (prior to passenger boarding) with the captain addressing the entire group, including the cockpit crew and flight attendants.

The first onboard briefing of a flight generally involves a discussion among the cockpit crew during the flight-planning process. If the pilots are meeting for the first time, they exchange introductions, including currency and their own background as professional aviators.[12] Then there is discussion about flight-specific information, delegation of duties, maintenance issues, weather, and security as they may apply. Duties are appointed according to who is designated as the pilot flying (PF) and who is the pilot monitoring (PM). Every commercial aircraft has two sets of controls and two pilots at those controls: the captain, who is ultimately responsible and accountable for every operational decision, and the copilot, or first officer, who's essentially second in command of the aircraft in the event that the captain becomes incapacitated for any reason. The actual flying duties are split evenly between the captain and copilot, who generally alternate actual control of the aircraft on each flight leg. The pilot who is at the controls and flying the aircraft is designated as the PF. The pilot who is not flying must be equally engaged, as the PM. The PM is usually responsible for all communications duties and backs up the PF's every action by monitoring the aircraft status. This redundancy is essential at all times but is particularly important with the increased reliance on automation. The PF will initiate an automated action, but both the PF and PM will verify that the aircraft is actually responding as instructed. *At appropriate times*, the pilots, who are each doing their assigned jobs, must update each other. For example, in the case of an emergency or abnormal procedure, the PM needs to update the PF on the status of the abnormal problem, what can be expected, flight limitations, and similar matters; likewise, the PF will update the PM on such things as the last air traffic control (ATC) assignments and aircraft status. This coordinated teamwork is as essential to basic operations as it is to accident prevention and safety.

Briefings, as the word implies, should be brief. By definition this should not be a ten-minute dissertation. In CRM training, captains learn how to give pertinent information briefly, and the rest of the crew learns how to similarly exchange important points. *None of this comes naturally.* Conducting communicative conversations—not just critical ones in times of conflict, disagreement, or stress—is a proficiency-based skill that gets better with practice. Like all performance-essential skills, it also needs to be rehearsed formally—in a learning-refresher setting on a regular basis.

One essential aspect of communication is ensuring the appropriate level of detail. So a captain will learn not only not to go on forever but also to avoid being too brief, as in "If anything happens before V1, we'll abort!"[13] This statement is noncommunicative because it doesn't specify *what* you are planning to abort for. "If 'anything' happens" is pretty ambiguous. The statement lacks any of specific details that really need to be shared *prior* to the event in order for other relevant crew members to have a shared expectation. An effective takeoff briefing would sound something like: "VFR takeoff, 'close-in community' departure, cleared to 6,000 feet, heading 220 to intercept the ABC 260-degree radial. Contact departure control at 2,000 feet and transition altitude is 3,000 feet. We'll abort for any malfunction below 80 knots. We'll 'load-shed' between 80 and V1 and consider taking off as opposed to aborting for minor issues.[14] Any questions?" This briefing—given in "pilot-speak" as appropriate to the audience—tells the other pilot precisely what he or she can expect for the first few critical moments of the flight. Most important, if there is a conflict or misunderstanding about what the pilot has planned to do, the decision process has been considered on the ground before the brakes are ever released.

Flight attendants also brief one another. Michelle Quintas, a flight attendant for United Airlines, explains,

> As flight attendants, we come together for the first FA briefing in our [own] domicile, our office place where we check in together before the flight. Usually, at the same time, the pilots meet together: they get weather report, information about plane, fuel levels, past or currently needed maintenance, wind and altitudes, routing so they know how much fuel to put on. Then they brief us. They'll tell us stuff that could ultimately affect our work. Say we're heading for Chicago, they might tell us it's very busy in Chicago and we only have enough fuel to circle once so be ready to divert. They tell us if any federal air marshal is on board—usually they're there to randomly check the flight, or a threat level has increased. For example, if the flight is going to London, there might be higher coverage going in and out of London because London is determined to be a higher risk. That type of stuff might also come up with a customer service rep who briefs the purser, if, for example, someone is sick, angry, drunk. They might tell us they did a background check and yes, they can get on the plane, but just watch out.

CREATING/REAFFIRMING A SHARED LANGUAGE

In both routine and nonroutine situations, the team has to behave predictably. Predictable behavior is a constant rehearsal for managing the unpredictable. Teams can't behave predictably, however, if people don't understand each other. Flight is difficult enough when you're moving across national borders and languages. But if—as is most common—the cockpit, cabin, and ground crew speak the same national language—say, English or Japanese—but different occupational languages, they can still misunderstand one another.

In aviation, teammates are taught to share the same language, which will include specialized terms, abbreviations, occupational shorthand names and phrases, and so forth. Operational cockpit communications use standard aviation terminology (recall the example of pilot-speak in the briefing above). Checklist responses are standardized so that any deviations will be immediately recognized and flagged for clarification; operational terminology is also clearly defined by SOPs.

Take the essential issue of aircraft orientation as an example. When someone says, "left" and you are facing them, your left and theirs are actually in opposite directions. So in the service of clear communication aviation crews are trained to state "aircraft left" or "aircraft right" so that they are using the same frame of reference:

> **"Secure the Building!"**
>
> When we make a statement, its interpretation is subject to the context and point of reference of the receiver. In the military, service members often joke about how the same words can have a very different meaning to members of different services. Take, for example, the expression "Secure the building!"
>
> An *army* soldier would order a tank platoon, surround the building, set up an assault, and take the building by storm of overwhelming force;
>
> A *marine* would interpret the order by building a twelve-foot-high perimeter fence, topped with barbed wire, installing a gate, and manning it with armed guards;
>
> An *airman* would approach the building's owner and negotiate a two-year lease with an option to buy;
>
> A *sailor* would simply empty the trash, turn out the lights, and lock the doors on the way out.

1. All references to right and left, or forward and back, are given *from the perspective of a person standing in the center of the aircraft, facing forward* (toward the cockpit). Even if you are facing the back of the aircraft and talking about the wing on your left side, you refer to it as "aircraft right." (Given that most flight attendant jump seats face aft, the importance of using these references correctly cannot be overstated.)
2. Engines are numbered from aircraft left to aircraft right. Typically, three- and four-engine aircraft refer to engine numbers (one, two, three, four, numbered in sequence from aircraft left to aircraft right). Two-engine aircraft can either be numbered engines or referred to as left and right engines.
3. Up and down—in commercial aviation, that's understood to be aircraft up and aircraft down. In military aviation, one may need to be a little more specific.

Because clear communication with everyone who is a party to the conversation is critical, established, standard phraseology is used at all times. For example, when a pilot is concerned about having enough fuel to manage a landing delay at a busy airport, he or she will say, "Center, Flight 123, we can hold until 1950Z; then we'll have to proceed to our alternate, XYZ." This statement will be understandable and therefore will communicate quickly and accurately to the flight deck, cabin crew, and air traffic control. Use of everyday speech or nonstandard terms can pose dangers—and in fact has caused disaster. On January 25, 1990, Avianca Flight 52 ran out of fuel and crashed near JFK Airport. Use of nonstandard phraseology was a major contributing cause. When they were nearly out of gas, the Avianca copilot stated to air traffic control that they were "low on fuel," a phrase that has no official meaning in the professional FAA controller system of reference. Had the pilots declared "emergency fuel," their meaning would instantly have been clear, and they would have been given priority handling to get the aircraft on the ground. In this case, the misunderstanding caused enough of a delay that the aircraft ran out of fuel and crashed fifteen miles from the airport.[15]

Conceptual clarity—understanding key concepts and ideas in the same ways—is also part of a common language and is as essential to successful communication as precision of terminology. Therefore, crew briefings clarify any concepts or issues that could be ambiguous. For example, the universally recognized "sterile cockpit" rule in commercial aviation refers to the operation of the aircraft between the ground and ten thousand feet of altitude. FAA regulations require that there be no nonessential conversation during the periods from the initiation of the preflight checklist through climb-out to ten thousand feet and again during descent from ten thousand feet to completion of the final parking checklist. "Nonessential" communication includes calls from the cabin crew for matters that can wait, such as checking the weather at destination and flight time. It is possible, though, that some flight attendants may take this prohibition *too* literally and feel constrained from calling the cockpit with essential information related to security (e.g., a disruptive passenger) or safety (e.g., snow/ice accumulation detected on the wing prior to takeoff).

One captain told Suzanne that he *always* clarifies the concept of sterile cockpit to flight attendants. "It may seem far-fetched," he said, "but some flight attendants may take the concept so literally that they wouldn't violate the sterile cockpit rule even if they observed that an engine was on fire!" So he tells flight attendants, "Sterile cockpit isn't a stop sign, it's a yield sign. In other words, tell me if you think something really serious is going on. *Please!!!*"

Good communication in briefings saves time on needless conflicts because captains and crew are on the same page about operations large and small. Michelle Quintas gives the example of setting parameters for cabin crew contacts with the cockpit: "He'll say, for instance, 'All calls should go to the purser.' During the flight, then, the captain will call the purser, say, if there's a delay. He'll tell the purser 'there will be such and such a delay; would you like to tell the passengers?' . . . [Then we can] tell the passengers [about the delay, and that] they can get out their cell phones and we'll give them some water."[16]

Clear and inclusive communication at appropriate times is essential in assuring that the team doesn't fracture into its constituent parts in an emergency. In high-tempo/high-stress situations—for example, while dealing with emergency or abnormal procedures—crew members from cockpit to cabin can become so involved in their own individual duties that they can lose track of what the others are doing—in other words, each begins essentially to operate solo. In unanticipated circumstances pilots need to keep the flight attendants in the loop as the situation progresses so that they may prepare appropriately. Flight attendants also have to communicate with each other and with passengers, who will need to be advised of the situation and reminded that cooperation with FA instructions is essential to everyone's safety. If we compare what happened in the United Flight 173 crash (Portland, 1978) with what happened with the Jet-Blue Flight 292 in 2005, we see that one of the clear differences was that the captain of Flight 173 did not brief the flight attendants. This omission established the conditions for their disorganization when the emergency situation developed. They were out of the loop and could not prepare themselves or their passengers for what was about to happen. Post-CRM, JetBlue 292's FAs were continuously kept informed and were thus able to be part of a hyperorganized crew that helped create a safe outcome.

Crew Resource Management can be effective only if all crew members are communicating about ongoing operational decisions. This means that the pilot in command (PIC) has established minimum acceptable standards (or bottom lines) for safe operation and has communicated these, along with their related expectations, to all relevant parties.

INVITING PARTICIPATION

It's not enough for team leaders to communicate unidirectionally with crew members: inquiries are invited, and orders, commands, and advice are constantly repeated to demonstrate that they have been properly received and understood. If those on the receiving end of a message do not acknowledge having received it, then something may be very wrong. Team leaders must encourage crew members to express their concerns, ask for clarification in an ambiguous situation, offer information, and issue a challenge when they believe that someone of a higher rank is about to make a mistake. "The best-case scenario," says Michelle Quintas, "is the captain briefs us all and asks for our perspective. He'll ask us if we have any concerns, and for feedback."

Because traditional imbalances of power and status may make people feel awkward about certain kinds and directions (up or down the hierarchy) of communication, in CRM training captains are taught not only to do briefings but how to do briefings. The good-captain/bad-captain videos we cited above are one example. In many airlines, captains are given a reference card to keep in their flight bag that gives them guidance about how to talk to crew members. On a flight from Amsterdam to Boston, Suzanne sat next to the captain who worked flying cargo. As they talked about CRM, the captain, John

How to Create Effective Communication

- Be clear—avoid ambiguous terms
- Be specific—avoid the "hint and hope"
- Be concise—say only enough to convey the message
- Be timely—say it now if it needs saying

Griffiths, pulled out his CRM toolkit five-by-seven card and handed it to her. It read:

There is also a section entitled "Recognize red flags, like not talking/listening, rushing, ambiguity/confusion," reminding captains to be aware of the individual and collective states of crew members that might adversely affect communication or teamwork success.

SEEKING INFORMATION AND DIRECTION FROM OTHERS

A particularly useful idea in ambivalent or conflict situations is CRM's radical proposition that a captain or other team member ask another, "What would you be comfortable with?" Captain Griffiths told Suzanne he uses that one a lot and then described a typical incident:

> The other day, we were flying cargo from Dubai to Paris and my copilot was concerned that we didn't have enough fuel on board. I thought we had plenty, but instead of saying, 'Hey, I'm the captain, suck it up kid,' I asked him what he wanted to do. We couldn't take on any more fuel, and if we had to stop and refuel in Munich or Frankfurt it would cost $10,000 and delay us by an hour, which would have meant the cargo would have missed some connections, which would also cost. After we talked about all of this, I asked, 'What would you feel comfortable with?' We agreed to keep very close track of the fuel and if it looked like we needed to, we'd stop to refuel. That was fine with him. He got to be part of the decision-making process and he knew I meant it when I said we'd stop if he felt it was necessary. He didn't want to take over or be the captain—all he wanted was to be heard. This training has helped. It's a desire to be right, to be correct, to have it your own way that gets you into trouble. Sometimes you need help to just let that go.

Griffiths said that his copilot had formulated his concerns in a way that maintained the relationship but simultaneously conveyed the urgency of his worries. This did not simply happen because the first officer was born with the gift of expressing himself with confidence. The first officer, like other members of the team, was taught that he was expected to play a role in the mission—whether it was verifying a landing clearance, contributing system knowledge in solving a problem, or expressing his concerns about adequate fuel levels.

USING THE APPROPRIATE LEVEL OF ASSERTIVENESS TO GET THE JOB DONE

In the pre-CRM era, as we have learned, crew members were reluctant to assert, persist, or state matters of concern with sufficient urgency even, on occasion, at the cost of their own lives. There's a world of difference between a first officer who says, "I think I see a land mass out there in front of us," and one who says, "We are flying into a mountain, Pull UP! Now!!" Or between the flight attendant who observes ice accumulation on the wings and fails to act for fear of violating the sterile cockpit rule and one who picks up the interphone and immediately relays his urgent concerns to the cockpit.

CRM training teaches people to provide clear, direct information and to do so with the degree of urgency that befits the situation, no matter what their role or rank. To do this, they're taught a few simple rules:

1. State critical information with appropriate level of persistence—*talk.*
2. Learn to sense another crew member's concern—*listen.*
3. Make your position known when safety is in question—*be assertive.*
4. Make sure your message is received and understood—*review.*
5. Don't hint and hope—*be direct.*

Even in seemingly routine operations, clarity, directness, and timeliness in expressing concerns are critical to prevent the routine from *becoming* critical. Consider this operational example. Typically, commercial flights are dispatched with enough fuel reserves to allow a diversion to at least one alternate airport should weather conditions at the destination force a change in plans. Yet there are numerous examples of flights where crews accepted delays at their destination for so long that they burned too far into their reserve fuel and had no remaining option to divert to an alternate airport. Avianca 52 (JFK, 1990) is a case in point. Another is United 173 (Portland, 1978), which eventually flamed out on approach and crashed in the forest.

The hallmark of appropriate assertiveness is an "action statement" that clearly expresses the concerns of a crew member and suggests a specific solution. Stated together with a confirming question that requires an answer—"Don't you agree?"—the action statement communicates, and may even set into motion, a specific plan. Take the example of a flight that has been dispatched from Airport A to Airport B, with an alternate destination of Airport C. Destination Airport B is experiencing significant arrival delays due to the weather and a closed runway. Arriving flights are being placed in holding patterns for as long as a half hour. The first officer, Jim, knows the aircraft has enough fuel to hold for fifteen minutes, at which time it will need to proceed to alternate destination C in order to ensure that the plane has enough fuel to get there.

The plane has now been holding for ten minutes; the crew has five minutes remaining before a divert decision *must* be made. The captain, Fred, a seasoned old coot, hasn't said a word about his intentions. First officer Jim is getting concerned about getting backed into a corner. So how does he proceed? What does he say? An action statement with a confirming question would go something like this: "Fred, we have five minutes of fuel remaining before we either divert to C or become committed to landing at B. I suggest that we tell ATC that we will be departing holding for our alternate, C, in five minutes, unless an immediate approach clearance for destination B can be granted. *Don't you agree?"*

In reality, Fred may agree with Jim's recommended course of action, and Jim has communicated his concern in a respectful manner and offered a clear solution. He has opened the door to a discussion of alternatives, and even if Fred doesn't agree with his suggestion, he is compelled to respond to it with some sort of alternative solution—perhaps getting an updated forecast and then make a decision based on the update.

Jim's action statement, like so much in CRM, may seem obvious on its face; it is not so obvious in practice. In fact, most people use only part of it—omitting the confirming question—and consequently achieve only partial results. The purpose of the action statement is to achieve a specific result or solution to a specific problem or issue—to get closure. CRM teaches crew members precisely how to do it effectively using the following protocol.

The first element of the action statement is *naming names*. Crew members are taught to ask themselves the following: Who are you addressing? If you are trying to communicate with a specific person, then address that person by name or title (e.g., Fred or Captain). This makes it clear which person you are addressing; you capture his or her attention *and* you attach a certain level of importance or urgency to the statement that is about to follow. Think about it when you're in a normal conversation. To emphasize a particular point, we often say the name of the person we're talking to. Not only does naming names add urgency to the conversation, but it also reinforces team building. To say the person's name, you have to know it.

Then comes part two: the *problem* you're addressing. What's called for here is not a dissertation on the problem but in the spirit of the "brief" briefing, a concise articulation stating explicitly just the facts, along with why you consider this to be of concern.

Next comes part three: the *solution. Your role as team member is not to just complain about the problem but to assist in solving it.* What exactly are you recommending? If you are enough of a professional to recognize the problem, you should be able to at least *propose* a solution—even if it isn't the one that gets used. By doing this, you have opened the door to an alternative plan of action.

And then comes the final step, which is too often neglected: Seek *agreement* by posing a challenge or a confirming question. This can be as simple as the question, "Don't you agree?" The agreement statement obligates the other person to formulate some sort of response. It provides closure to the action statement, just as using the other person's name at the beginning provides an opening that arouses that person's attention. This technique may sound similar to the SBAR (situation, background, assessment, recommendation) tool that has become increasingly utilized in health care facilities. This simple tool, which was developed by physician Michael Leonard and his colleagues at Kaiser Permanente of Colorado, is a good first step toward better communication.[17]

One of the major goals of the action statement is to avoid the huge and potentially fatal communication pitfall of hinting and hoping. A lot of us are taught that it is not polite to confront another person by directly stating a problem, opinion, or disagreement. Hinting and hoping is a communication strategy that courteous people are tempted to use to avoid confrontation, to preserve someone else's sense of dignity or status, or to protect themselves from criticism and rejection. People hint and hope every day. Patrick jokes that his wife may ask him, "Are you going to wear those socks with those shoes?" when what she really means is, "Your socks don't match." He usually takes the hint, but what if he didn't and what if the hint was intended to draw attention to something really serious?

Imagine what could happen if a PM on approach told the PF, "You're a little low." The statement could actually mean that the PF is a few feet low, or it could mean that the aircraft is actually a few *hundred* feet low. Big difference! When you are flying a five hundred thousand-pound airplane at 195 miles per hour close to the ground, accurately defining "a little low" could literally spell the difference between life and death. Is this worth it just to avoid hurting the other person's feelings or risking a reprimand?

To get around the tricky issue of status, hurt feelings, face-saving, and so forth, CRM places the emphasis on *what* is right, not *who* is right. To sidestep the "who" discussion and get immediately to the "what," crew members are taught to

- *Challenge, but with respect*: Remember, this is not about who is right. Everyone on the crew has a role to play and everyone deserves to maintain his or her own dignity and respect.
- *Have a constructive intent*: If there is no point to a challenge, save it for the debrief. In other words, if the challenge serves no constructive purpose at the time that it is initiated, you are just nagging (and you may be deflecting attention from important operational matters).
- *Be specific*: Hinting and hoping is ineffective. "You're a little low" is a hint with the hope that the PF will respond. "You're a steady one dot low—Pull up!" lets the PF know precisely what the facts are and that he or she either needs to get back up on the glide slope *right now* or go around![18]
- *Be timely*: Don't wait until the situation gets worse—for example, until the PF has descended from one dot to two dots below the glide slope—before you speak up.
- *Use questions*: In aviation there are many ways to accomplish tasks. If you walk into the cockpit after a break and don't understand why a fuel pump is off, ask. Chances are there is a good explanation, but maybe your partner actually forgot to restart the pump when attempting to balance fuel. Mistakes happen.
- *Actively seek information*: Timely challenges with respect that are constructive in nature and specific in intent work the best. Some challengers may use the

Specific Phrases to Use When Challenging Another Team Member

- "I'm uncomfortable with . . ."
- "I'm concerned about . . ."
- "Are you ready for . . .?"
- "Shouldn't we be . . .?"
- "What heading/altitude did he assign us . . .?"
- "I thought he gave us . . ."

These are all phrases that capture attention and can serve to communicate a level of concern that should be taken into consideration by others.

inquisitive approach. Don't wait until after the fact or until it's too late to do anything about the problem.

- *Question ambiguous or difficult situations until there is understanding*: If in doubt, ask questions to clarify. If you are uneasy about something, don't discount that feeling. Chances are good that somebody else on the crew feels the same way.
- *Take nothing for granted*: Traditional training in this area did an adequate job in training crew members to challenge or speak up when something

seemed unsafe or unwise. However, to challenge something, one must first detect it, and detection requires effective monitoring.

EXAMINATION AND CRITIQUE OF SELF AND GROUP

In commercial aviation there are two distinct avenues for identifying and addressing problems as they arise. One is a fairly robust and very effective reporting system (discussed in detail in chapter 8). The other is at a more immediate operational level and deals with issues in a more real-time fashion.

Self-examination is part of a larger process that is devoted to making sure the same mistakes don't happen over and over again. Situations can also be discussed directly among the people involved through what is known as a debrief. A debrief—a subject we will return to in subsequent chapters—is the "after" part of the communication cycle. As Helmreich and others have described, it is the cornerstone of creating a high-reliability environment; it is never about pointing fingers or assigning blame. The process of debriefing and self-assessment is

> the vehicle used to ensure an open and honest dialog for the primary goal of improving individual and team performance. Adopting and fostering a learning mentality shows a commitment to truly learn from shared experiences. The very fact that teams take the time to participate in the debrief and self-assessment process demonstrates this resolve. . . . [D]emonstrating professional maturity is critical in conducting team-centered debriefs. Being able to admit your weaknesses and shortcomings to others requires a great deal of courage and integrity.[19]

In practice, rather than stopping the action or hijacking critical communication during a task, conflict, emergency, or other tense situation, crew members are specifically trained to stay on task and defer discussion of the problem—if possible—until the task at hand has been accomplished safely. "Defer"—not ignore, bury, or neglect—is the operative word here. If an issue arises during the course of accomplishing a task and dealing with that specific problem would take attention away from the task, crew members learn that there is a time and place for dealing with that issue. The time to deal with this is during debriefs—a time *after* the work session in which people discuss what happened and constructively self-critique. Not only are crew members taught that they should hold debriefs, but they are also taught *how* to do so. A debrief is not a venting or blaming session. It is devoted to and analyzing problems and coming up with solutions—collectively.

If a crew member feels that something that happened could lead to improvement, he or she would say—*after* the plane has safely landed—"We could have—or should have—done this differently" and, ideally, suggest alternatives. In this case, the intent *must* be constructive. In aviation there may be a hundred ways to get to the same result, all of which are right and subject to the personal preference of the operator. As Patrick puts it,

> [I]f I truly believed that I had a better way, or more importantly, a mistake was made and not acknowledged by the other crew member, I might explain, "I've found at this airport, the controllers tend to rush us on the approach and that if I drive the situation a little more aggressively with ATC, we have a better outcome."
>
> If I had been the one who had messed up (and I was aware of it), I would acknowledge it and probably state what I would have done differently. As professionals, there would be little point in belaboring the issue. Problem identified, problem acknowledged, and solution provided—end of story. However, given the same situation, if I failed to say anything, one of the other pilots might take the initiative and talk about what happened and what should be done next time.

In instances where things are very tense—for example, the other pilot did something wrong or even uncomfortable and didn't realize or acknowledge it, or if there is a conflict relating to the operation—CRM teaches people that these kinds of things need to be debriefed rather than avoided and that the debrief should be conducted according to the following communication rules:

- Describe what happened from your point of view to start a discussion.
- Ask for reactions and perceptions.
- Ask what, if anything, could be done to make the outcome more acceptable.

PUTTING THEORY INTO PRACTICE

Thus far we've explained the theories and skills needed to create the kind of communication upon which teamwork and safety depend. Now let's look at how this communication theory is put into practice. Helen Zienkievicz was manager of health, safety, and security, onboard services, at United Airlines before she retired in 2000. She worked at United for twenty-nine years and held her position in health and safety for four. In aviation, Zienkievicz explains, enormous effort is given to helping flight attendants, as low people on the totem pole, learn how to be assertive and to communicate effectively in a hierarchical environment. She offers a typical example that FAs commonly face. They are flying at thirty-six thousand feet and they smell an odor in the back of the plane. Before CRM, she explains, they would call the captain and say,

> "I smell a funny odor in the back of the airplane. I noticed that the floor is a little bit warm and it's hot back here." If the captain has a preconceived idea that the air conditioning unit isn't working well, he may conclude that that's the problem. He'll tell the flight attendant, "There's nothing to worry about. We had this on the previous flight and it's nothing." But in a worst-case scenario, it turns out to be a cargo fire. She is right to worry. And although she is still worrying, she says to herself, "I guess he knows better. He's . . . the captain." She doesn't persist, and then you could have thick black smoke with cargo fires and don't know what's going on and it can get way out of control.

With CRM, Zienkievicz says, the flight attendant has been trained not to let her status override her experience, professional knowledge, and concerns:

> We will have trained her to deal with the captain's response by being more specific and to describe what she is seeing and smelling. She would call the captain and say the following:
> "I'm calling from door two right. I want to report to you that over the last five minutes, I've detected a burning odor that smells almost like burning wire. I smell it stronger near the aft galley. At present, I don't see any smoke. I've checked the ovens and coffeemakers and I don't see any malfunctions at this time. I've notified the purser, and we do have oven firefighting equipment ready in the event that we need it."
> She's painted a picture for the captain of what she is seeing and smelling, and what she has done and is doing about it.

If, after she explains all this to the captain, he still tells her not to worry, Zienkievicz continues, that's not the end of it. She will call again a few minutes later and say, "Captain, I need to let you know that I still smell this odor. In fact, it's worse and smells electrical and the circuit breakers are beginning to pop." With that kind of input—and given that pilots are also trained in CRM to listen—the chances that this will be dealt with before it becomes a catastrophe are high.

The captains, first officers, and flight attendants who have spoken here have demonstrated that in aviation, CRM training about good communication is not a matter of lip service. It is a constant operational reality, the object of mandatory, ongoing, recurrent training. Communication is central to the next CPI, team building.

Chapter 3

Case Study

MAIMONIDES MEDICAL CENTER

Many hospitals have launched patient safety initiatives. We have chosen this particular one as a case study because it includes so many of the elements that have made CRM successful in the airlines industry. Not simply parts of a top-down initiative led by management champions, the projects described below include frontline staff in the planning, implementation, and evaluation of patient safety programs. Unions have also been involved from the inception of these projects. Work organization has been integrated into patient safety initiatives, and trainings have included some recurrent efforts to make sure messages remain current and are constantly revisited. At considerable cost, the hospital has financed these programs. This means they are not susceptible to the typical fate of initiatives supported by foundation or government grants, in which success may be rewarded by failure to refund projects that have good outcomes. In such cases, many hospitals do not continue to finance these projects themselves once grant money has run out, and thus successful projects that could enhance patient safety vanish.

WALKING THE WALK

In spring 2010 a nurse educator at Maimonides Hospital in Brooklyn, New York, was in the operating room, mentoring a new graduate who'd just joined the nursing staff. The operation was a tense one. The patient had suffered from a life-threatening abdominal aortic aneurysm. A weakened wall in the largest artery in the abdomen, the aorta, had ruptured, and if it wasn't quickly repaired, the patient could bleed to death. The hospital has developed safety protocols to make sure that in their rush to repair this kind of problem, surgeons don't inadvertently leave foreign objects—like sponges, pads, or towels (among other things)—inside the wound. In surgeries like this one, surgeons will often put a towel directly into the gaping abdominal cavity to push away the intestines so they can access the aorta. It is thus possible to actually leave a towel inside the patient. To prevent that, Maimonides requires surgeons to use special towels—in this case white—that have radiopaque tags and radio frequency (RF) chips affixed to them. Before closing the wound, a surgeon can wave a special RF wand over the surgical area to make sure nothing has been left inside the patient, and the tags allow an X-ray to identify the presence of a potentially retained towel as well. Other towels that are not X-ray-sensitive are of different colors—at Maimonides, green or blue.

The surgeon asked for a blue towel, and the new nurse assisting reached for the non-radiopaque towel. The nurse educator caught the mistake and said, "No, we need to use a white towel." The surgeon balked. The new nurse, who might otherwise have been intimidated by his rank, was urged by her educator to give him the white towel, not the blue. The surgeon again refused. As a very seasoned nurse, the educator calmly asked the surgeon three times to take the white towel. He dug in his heels. At this point she left the room and put in calls to Dr. David Feldman, then vice president of patient safety, and Pam Mestel, RN, executive director of perioperative services. After making the calls, she returned to the operating room to make sure that all the surgical counts were correct and that nothing—towels, sponges, or other foreign objects—had been left inside the patient. The patient left the OR and recovered without a hitch.

The nurse educator talked again with Feldman. Although the patient did not come to harm, she knew that he could have. Feldman agreed that this is "the kind of operation where you don't want something you can't see or detect inside the patient," and he understood why the educator was so persistent.

Feldman talked with both the nurse educator and the surgeon, but the conversation did not go well. So he decided to move to the next step. Had the patient been harmed, a root-cause analysis would have been required by the state of New York. Although a near miss like this did not require any further exploration on the part of the hospital, Feldman and his safety team decided to conduct a critical incident review. The presentation included the director of risk management, the medical director, the chairman of the department of surgery and Feldman and Mestel. As Mestel recounts, "As the educator stood by, a new nurse gave a forty-minute presentation on the history of how we've progressed at Maimonides to keep patients safe with our count policies, retained foreign bodies, and so forth. She came with a pillowcase full of sponges, pads, and towels as well as the RF wand. No one interrupted her: there was not a peep around the room."

The session was not about assigning blame but about advancing institutional learning. It also helped to build the kind of psychological safety that CRM has created in the airline industry and that we will explore later.[1] "The moral of the story," Mestel recalls, "is that the nurse showed them that in a respectful way, we can disagree with the surgeon, who historically is the captain of the ship. The entire institutional hierarchy supported her."

In fact, Mestel added, David Feldman sent the nurse a handwritten note to let her know how much he appreciated her efforts to maintain patient safety. "I was very proud and pleased that this nurse stood her ground and that we as an institution stood with her," says Tom Smith, Maimonides senior VP and chief nursing officer.

This incident at Maimonides was part of an ongoing evolution in institutional transformation. Through a series of multilayered initiatives that embody many of the principles we have seen in CRM, Maimonides Medical Center has been working to transform a culture based on a traditional steep hierarchy into one that respects not only the players at the top of the health care ladder but those at every rung. Maimonides thus serves as a case study of how an existing culture can begin the kind of much-needed transformation that has taken place in the aviation industry.

Maimonides, which celebrated its centennial in 2011, is a 710-bed tertiary care hospital that is located in the Bay Ridge Section of Brooklyn—one of the most ethnically diverse in the borough. Today the hospital employs 6,500 workers, including 1,500 nurses. Four unions represent its staff. These are 1199/SEIU (Service Employees International Union) United Healthcare Workers East, which represents nonnursing staff; New York State Nurses Association (NYSNA), which represents registered nurses; and the Committee of Interns and Residents (CIR) affiliated with 1199/SEIU, which represents medical house staff.

At a hospital this size, patient safety efforts are ongoing, and initiatives to deliver safer care take place in too many venues to enumerate. To illustrate the ways in which teamwork and communication have become central to patient safety at Maimonides we will focus on two primary examples: the Maimonides Strategic Alliance and the Code of Mutual Respect. Although these were started as two distinct entities, their goals are overlapping and they embody the kind of principles and mechanisms that have made safety a reality in the airline industry. Like CRM, these safety initiatives are notable for their inclusion of rank-and-file workers and the unions that are major players in the hospital.

THE STRATEGIC ALLIANCE

The Strategic Alliance (SA) at Maimonides grew out of a 1994 citywide labor negotiation between the League of Voluntary Hospitals and Nursing Homes in New York City and 1199/ SEIU United Healthcare Workers East (1199). The CEOs of all these hospitals agreed to expand their Job Security Fund and Training and Upgrading Fund to include a "labor management project." In 1996 Maimonides began serious work on this project. As Pamela Brier—its current CEO, who was then its chief operating officer—says, "I have long felt that everyone in the hospital—at all levels of the organization—should have the wherewithal to contribute to making the hospital better by having their voices heard. Of course the best way to do that was to create teamwork with management working with the various unions that represent workers in the institution."

Brier and her colleagues in both unions and management determined to create "a vehicle," Brier says, "to oversee and structure the organizational process of fostering mutual respect, trust, effective communication, and the active participation of staff at all levels in department and unit decision making." Sondra Olendorf, senior vice president and at the time chief nursing officer, also strongly supported this approach.

In 1997 the New York State Nurses Association joined the effort. Michael Chacon of NYSNA at Maimonides recalls that patient safety and worker satisfaction in the patient safety process went hand in hand: "We felt that management sometimes made decisions and then tried to promote them with the staff. People didn't feel invested in that kind of initiative. Frontline staff needed to come together because, in many instances, they had solutions to the problems that higher-level management was trying to address."

In 1997 the hospital formed a labor management council (LMC) to oversee the work of creating effective participation in decision making. This council includes senior management, and union representatives. Various units have created departmental labor management committees (DLMCs) that deal with both patient satisfaction and workplace issues. The SA has worked with both external and internal consultants. Peter Lazes and his colleagues at the Cornell University School of Industrial and Labor Relations were hired to train SA members in problem solving, team building, and work redesign. Internal consultants, or "developers"—one from each union and one from management—work full-time for the alliance to assure that critical issues are raised. They are paid for by the hospital but were hired through a joint process that included the unions and management. Pierre Devaud is the management staff developer, Paul Stuart the staff developer for 1199/SEIU, and Cicely Wilkinson the developer for NYSNA. CIR, which joined the alliance in 2004, has its own developer. At this writing there are thirteen DLMCs operating on Maimonides units, with plans to expand them to all hospital units.

What makes this experiment different from other, more traditional labor-management cooperation initiatives is its serious effort to engage frontline workers not only in problem solving around patient safety but in decisions about all aspects of care, including the hiring of managerial staff. "At Maimonides, managers are not just hired and then brought in to meet the group of workers they will be supervising," Brier explains. "Groups are convened with workers and managers to agree what kind of candidates we are looking for, to interview the candidates, and to finally select those who will work here. Honestly," Brier adds, "we have never been in a situation where we did not agree."

This kind of commitment to joint work has been applied to some very serious patient safety problems. One example was the work of the Strategic Alliance on cardiology units after a patient death due to failure to respond to alarms. Another had to do with hospital cleanliness.

Problems in the Cardiology Units

In 2006 a patient died on the cardiology service. Root-cause analyses revealed that the cause of death was the failure to respond in a timely manner to monitors and alarms alerting staff that the patient was in trouble and needed immediate assistance. When a cardiac alarm goes off, seconds—quite literally—count. Nurses and doctors have a minute or less to respond. But in this case, and others that did not result in death, response time fluctuated between 2.5 and 8 minutes.

At many hospitals, when something bad happens to a patient, the initial impulse is often to blame nurses or other staff for their failure to respond quickly. "That was the default position," says Veronica Richardson, a medical/surgical RN and local bargaining unit (LBU) executive committee chairperson for NYSNA at Maimonides. Finding an individual to blame and then disciplining that person rather than looking at the systemic issues that made all the slices in the Swiss cheese line up so that patients could easily fall through has generally been hardwired into management thinking. At Maimonides, however, that particular circuit was being rewired, and a new way of thinking about error and improving care had rerouted managerial and staff and union responses.

The cardiac unit DLMC, which was made up of twenty staff members—including registered nurses, patient care technicians, information specialists, physician assistants, nurse practitioners, nurse managers, physicians, and nurse educators—was both the vehicle and the forum for this new way of thinking. Performance-improvement specialists and a resident met weekly for five months to conduct an in-depth analysis of what had led to this death. Staff from departments like Patient Transport, Radiology Health Information Technology (HIT), and Materials Information Systems (MIS) also attended when needed. Cornell's Peter Lazes was also on hand to help guide the process.

To ascertain how to prevent further patient problems, the DLMC group began by charting patients' journeys into and out of the hospital. This detailed analysis illuminated a number of serious problems, which could lead to what is known in hospital safety parlance as "failure to rescue"—which is precisely what happened to the patient who had died. The term was coined by the physician Jeffrey Silber and his colleagues at the University of Pennsylvania Medical School. Silber and his team of researchers looked at hospital mortality in different institutions and discovered that—as might be expected—certain patients are just too sick to make it through their hospital stay.[2] Nurse researchers like University of Pennsylvania's Linda Aiken and Sean Clarke further elaborated on the concept to consider factors that impacted rescue.[3] No matter how many nurses, doctors, and aides surrounded these patients, their conditions defied rescue. When, however, patients died from preventable complications, institutional factors were always involved. These included not having enough staff—usually RN staff—to monitor patients so that their educated eyes could detect a problem before it became a catastrophe. It also included being unable to mobilize institutional resources to act to rescue the patient. Although failure to rescue is not a concept used in aviation, it is definitely embodied in pre-CRM conditions. The educated eyes of a flight attendant or first officer caught a problem before it became a disaster, but the FA or FO was unable to mobilize resources—say, the captain's attention or consideration—to rescue the aircraft and its passengers.

What the cardiology DLMC discovered was a classic case of failure to rescue on a unit/system level that involved equally classic problems in teamwork and communication. The unit, it turned out, had no clear and common understanding of patient acuity (how severely ill a patient is). Without this understanding the correct number of educated eyes (i.e., RNs and nursing assistants) were not assigned to care for and monitor patients.

Because transporters were also involved in the DLMC, the group was better able to identify failure-to-rescue problems with patient transport. Like other hospital patients, cardiac patients are constantly being transported across the institution for X-rays or tests. Because they are highly unstable, they may seem all right when they leave a unit but suddenly develop problems requiring instant action as they are being moved through hospital corridors. The group discovered that patients were not transferred to other departments with a knowledgeable licensed staff member accompanying them. If a patient's condition deteriorated, people were not always equipped to help them.

Nurses in the DLMC also identified what they considered an interlinked failure in accountability for responding to alarms. "The nurses felt that they bore the entire burden of responding to alarms," says Richardson. "An alarm would go off in room two, but the nurse was with a sick patient in room four. Non-nursing personnel would be sitting at the nurses' station and look up, and the mentality would be that it was the nurse's responsibility to respond. Nobody would consider that the nurse couldn't be in two places at once. The response—particularly among physicians—was, 'Why isn't the nurse responding to that alarm?'"

Hand-offs are another well-known variable in cases of failure to rescue, and they were a problem here. When nurses changed shifts, they did not always effectively relay information about a patient's condition to the next people who would be caring for that patient. Without critical information, nurses and managers could not effectively coordinate care. Finally, the DLMC discovered that nurses weren't the only ones who had problems dealing with monitors and alarms. Staff did not know how to make minor adjustments to medical equipment, which meant that minor problems would often sideline a piece of equipment.

Because frontline employees from all shifts participated in discussions that also included attending physicians and nurse practitioners, workers felt far more comfortable expressing their real concerns and making suggestions. "The committee created a safe place so that people could brainstorm without feeling they couldn't say certain things," Richardson comments. The nurses, NYSNA representatives explain, realized that the DLMC was taking unit accountability for the problems uncovered and not just placing blame on any one group.

The group was therefore able to get an accurate picture of the problem and propose solutions. These solutions however, required serious management commitment not only because they involved changes in protocols or policies but because they involved changes in practice. It would require significant financial resources to successfully implement and sustain them over the long term. Because management agreed to this investment, the solutions could move from words on paper to actual hospital practice. The solutions—on which all disciplines and occupational groups agreed—included

- establishing new clinical protocols to correctly define patient acuity;
- making sure all patient acuity was assessed at least on a daily basis, if not more frequently;
- communicating acuity assessments in daily rounds with all staff, including physicians, to ensure accurate staffing levels;
- providing information on acuity in shift-to-shift reports on patients and making sure that acuity information was in the patient's chart;
- establishing a new procedure to ensure that patients would be accompanied by a licensed practitioner when they left the unit for tests and involving patient transport in the implementation of the procedure;
- creating the same standard for individualized alarm settings, checking them at the start of a new shift, and using them on all four units;
- providing more training on equipment to make sure it operated properly;
- retraining nurses in how to set alarms and suspend a monitor without disabling others;
- creating a logging system for tracking equipment failure and repairs, as well as tracking when patients left and returned to their floor.

Most of these solutions—once they'd been agreed upon—required training and education, and management put money into implementing them.

"People sat down and listened to the staff. Staff identified that everyone involved in patient care needed to be educated. It wasn't only management that became engaged—physicians did too," Richardson explains. "They made the commitment to engage and communicate with staff and be part of the hand-off process." Once these solutions were agreed on, DLMC members and nurse educators trained all staff, including physicians, on new procedures and protocols, and the group designated an RN and nursing assistant to monitor the implementation of all changes to make sure all solutions were implemented and sustained.

The main business of the cardiology DLMC appeared to be finished once the recommended changes had been implemented and all staff training conducted. Like the safety advocates in the airline industry, however, cardiology DLMC members understand that sustainable safety and quality measures cannot be a one-shot affair and must be consistently monitored, evaluated, and revisited. To do this over the long term, the cardiology DLMC has continued to hold monthly meetings and collect data on response times to alarms. When these data reveal any problems in meeting the appropriate response time or dealing with any of the problems the group identified, the DLMC considers the problem and suggests a solution. As a result of the multidisciplinary and all-encompassing work of the cardiac staff, the response time to monitors is now less than one minute on all four cardiology units and has remained at this level.

Since launching work on alarm time, the cardiology DLMC has also done work on other issues that have led to improvements for both patients and staff. A larger group meets monthly, and a smaller one meets beforehand to prepare for the larger meeting. Meetings are always held on the same day at the same time. In addition, staff members are paid to attend, and if they come in to participate on a day off, they are paid for their attendance. "Management," Sondra Olendorf explains, "provides extra staff to take on the patient or workload of nurses or other staff so that their minds, not just their time, have been freed up."

"Early on," Olendorf continues, "when we questioned staff about their concerns about participating in these initiatives, their biggest one was that they had no one to take on their patients or their work. If they attended the DLMC meetings, they would return to their jobs only to find they were way behind." This proved to be a major barrier to attendance, one that would not be solved, she says, just by having another RN watch over a nurse's patient or another aide keep an eye out on things for the absent aide. "We bring in relief staff for different categories of workers so that they can attend meetings without worrying about how far behind they'll be when the meeting is over. This is a big commitment but one that has really made a difference."

The next project that the cardiology DLMC will undertake is to put every person who works on the unit—regardless of job category or shift—through the training that accompanies the unit or department roll-out of the Maimonides Code of Mutual Respect.

Hospital Cleanliness

What Florence Nightingale recognized over 150 years ago remains as true today as it was in the nineteenth century. When it comes to patient and staff safety in a hospital, cleanliness is, in fact, a matter of life and death. To prevent infections in all patients—but particularly in those who are older and thus have weaker immune systems—requires a two-step process. Step one is cleaning—physically removing germs by wiping or scrubbing. Step two is disinfecting—using products that will kill any remaining germs after a surface is clean. In hospitals both cleaning and disinfecting are necessary for every surface—floors, beds, rails, tubes, lines, monitors, and more. The last step in the chain of cleanliness and disinfection involves carefully removing all hazardous waste and sharps so they can be appropriately disposed of and will not present a danger to patients, staff, or the surrounding community. Keeping workers who clean hospitals safe so they do not become patients themselves is often overlooked in efforts to enhance patient safety.

While Maimonides executives and staff were certainly cognizant of the two-step process that assures safety, the hospital was not as clean as it could have been, something CEO Pamela Brier recognized when she suffered from a major auto accident and became a patient in her own hospital.

Again the approach could have been one of shame and blame—an easy one to take since hospital cleanliness is the purview of housekeeping staff, who are traditionally the lowest on the medical totem pole. But again the hospital eschewed this approach. Rather than berating hospital cleaners, the support service vice president and managers discussed the issue and in several large group meetings invited housekeepers to play a role in figuring out how to make the hospital cleaner. To do this, they formed what was called the study action team. Five staff members (four cleaners and one supervisor) were relieved of their regular duties and assigned to work on this team. For four months their full-time job was to interview staff, analyze work processes on all three shifts, and visit other hospitals to check on their procedures and equipment. They also engaged nursing staff, physicians, unit coordinators, and various administrators throughout the hospital to gather their ideas and concerns about unit and hospital-wide cleanliness.

The fact that the group was made up of cleaners, not just managers, allowed members to enter backstage and private spaces and to really understand the work processes and concerns of those whose job it is to keep the hospital clean. "Everyone on this team had equal input and equal responsibility," says RN Paulette Cirillo, who was then executive director of nursing for the Departments of Medicine and Surgery. "Everyone had equal input as we tried to develop an approach to keep the hospital clean."

What the study action team discovered when it looked at the problems of the environmental services departments was that staff lacked the requisite equipment and supplies because the inventory system that should have made sufficient supplies available didn't function effectively. For example, not all supplies were available at the beginning of shifts for employees. There also wasn't enough cleaning staff—particularly on the graveyard shift, which in turn created problems for workers on day and afternoon shifts. As a result, morning or afternoon staff would come into a room or corridor and discover that garbage hadn't been removed, as it should have been on a previous shift. The group also identified another important issue.

Even though many workers had been employed as hospital cleaners for a number of years, some weren't adequately trained in how to keep the hospital clean. As a result, cleaning staff weren't really sure whether a room was clean, and they couldn't turn rooms around quickly enough for new patients. Moreover, housekeeping and nursing staff didn't communicate well with each other. Thus housekeepers often didn't know which rooms needed to be cleaned urgently and which didn't.

To assess the impact of cleanliness on patient satisfaction, the hospital did not rely solely on standard hospital satisfaction surveys, like Press-Ganey scores (Press-Ganey is a for-profit organization that surveys patients). The study action team developed its own survey instrument to determine whether patient rooms as well as all public areas and nursing stations were cleaned in a timely fashion. Members of the team were responsible for making sure that staff had the appropriate training not only in housekeeping skills but also in infection control and dealing with bodily fluids and chemical hazards. The team was also responsible for helping to establish a new process for purchasing cleaning equipment and supplies and for negotiating with management, particularly around staffing on the graveyard shift. It also worked on developing more effective communication between nursing and housekeeping staff. "This effort wasn't just about making sure people picked up pieces of paper in a hallway or mopped a floor correctly. We also wanted to make sure everything was in its proper place, like for example a code cart," Cirillo explains. "We even developed an acronym that helped people if they went on a unit and discovered that something was not clean."

As a result of these activities, Maimonides is now a cleaner and safer hospital. Moreover, these joint efforts did not end with cleanliness and changes on the cardiology units but continue to target a variety of patient safety problems. The decision to involve frontline staff and unions on an ongoing basis produced not only a genuine group of allies but also an ongoing ability to strategize about crucial patient safety and worker safety issues. It uncovered not only problems and solutions but also aspects of work organization that needed to be changed to sustain safety over the long term.

THE CODE OF MUTUAL RESPECT

Health care administrators, professionals, and safety advocates now recognize that teamwork and communication are central to patient care. Since teamwork means that all members of the team, no matter where they are positioned, must feel free to speak up, psychological safety—the sense that people will not be blown off, humiliated, belittled, made fun of, or simply ignored when they raise critical issues or express their views and perspectives—is key. In health care, belittling, shaming, blaming, and even abusive behavior is all too prevalent not only between occupations of higher status and those that are considered subordinate but also within professions and occupations. To create an environment where people feel safe to speak up and are supported when they actually *do* speak up, Maimonides developed not only the Strategic Alliance but also what is known as the Code of Mutual Respect. The latter involves not only on-the-book policies but actual rubber-hits-the-road practices.

The Code of Mutual Respect was born after Sondra Olendorf attended a conference on trust in health care held at the Harvard School of Public Health in 2002. Olendorf was convinced that physicians needed to hear this message. She invited David Feldman, vice president of perioperative services, and Warren Wexelman, a cardiologist and former president of the medical staff, to go with her when the conference was held the following year. Feldman had long been concerned about relationships in health care. Over his career he'd heard plenty of physicians complaining that there were so many people telling them what to do and so many restrictions. Maybe it's our own damn fault, he thought. Maybe we haven't taken the steps to say what's right and what isn't right.

When they came back from the conference, both Feldman and Olendorf recognized that the traditional way physicians and nurses related not only negatively impacted patient care but also provided poor behavioral models for other staff— regardless of the discipline or occupation. So they both began to work their respective sides of the institutional street, with Feldman taking the lead on next steps.

Olendorf, who knew that nurses were held in high esteem by the public, felt members of her staff needed to build on that trust and help doctors understand that they were far more than angels of mercy, that they had real knowledge that was critical to everyone's ability to care for patients. Both Feldman and Olendorf were convinced that targeting physician-nurse behavior was a way to change the traditional physician command-and-control approach to the health care team. Both knew they had to help physicians understand why these traditional approaches were destructive rather than constructive. Once physicians understood this, they could play a key role in adopting behaviors that encouraged people to participate on what would become a team in actual practice rather than in name only. This in turn, Olendorf explains, "would help patients feel really secure since all members of the team would be on the same page, and the team in its entirety could be trusted."

Convinced that physicians at Maimonides had to take a leading institutional role in creating an environment in which it was safe for people to resolve conflicts equitably, without favoring one group of high-status players over all others, Feldman began writing what was to become the Code of Mutual Respect (see appendix for the full code). "I thought about calling it the Code of Behavior," he recalls. "But that sounded too punitive, so it became the Code of Mutual Respect."

To encourage genuine mutual respect, Feldman, Wexelman, and other medical staff leaders sent the document to other senior physicians, department chairs, nursing staff members, and administrators for their comments and suggestions. Initially, says Brier, there was a lot of resistance to the code. People said they didn't need it because "we already do it." It took a lot of behind-the-scenes effort on the part of the executive office to encourage medical staff leaders to adopt the code, which they did In June of 2004, when they formally adopted it and decided to make the entire medical staff accountable for its principles. From the beginning neither physicians nor administrators wanted the code to be a rod that would be mobilized to discipline the spoiled child. Although they wanted it to be rigorously adhered to and knew it had to have teeth, they understood that disrespect isn't caused by nasty people who wake up in the morning determined to make those they work with miserable. It's instead a result of socialization, workplace stress, and lack of training in communication, teamwork, and conflict resolution as well as glitches in workplace organization.

While Feldman and the physician leadership were working on writing and re-fining the code, Olendorf began doing work with nurses and nursing leadership to help them change some of their dysfunctional patterns of behavior. "Nurses have been socialized to be deferential," Olendorf explains. "Doctors have been trained to give out orders and take total responsibility, to be the heroes. Nurses, on the other hand, have been trained to take on more subservient roles—and then com-plain about it. They'll act deferential and then bemoan the fact that the doctor doesn't understand what they do or thinks the nurse is just there to change a dressing and nothing more."

Olendorf understood that if nurses and doctors were to function respectfully on a team and model respectful behavior for others, "doctors would have to come down a peg and nurses would have to elevate themselves in their own eyes so that both professions could understand that nurses can't do it without doctors and doc-tors can't do it without nurses." Olendorf spent two years working with her nurs-ing staff, giving a series of PowerPoint presentations and holding discussions to help nurses prepare themselves to function as full members of the health care team—members who, Olendorf says, are different but equal in their impact on patient care.

As their work converged, Feldman, Olendorf, Wexelman, and other hospital leaders were not entirely sure how to proceed once the code was written and ad-opted and their preparatory work was done. That's where Kathryn Kaplan, the chief learning officer, came in. In 2005 Maimonides hired Kaplan, who had begun her career as a psychiatric occupational therapist until she got a doctorate in man-agement and organization. Kaplan recognized that turning the code from a "piece of paper to actual practice" would take a multifaceted, long-term approach.[4]

She was impressed with a study conducted by the American Association of Critical Care Nurses and Vital Smarts entitled *Silence Kills*.[5] It documented the kinds of problems disrespectful behavior and lack of teamwork create in hospitals across the United States. Hospital leaders such as Feldman, Olendorf, and Wexelman already knew that a culture of silence does indeed kill any inclination to raise safety issues, particularly if the incident involves someone of higher status. "The message not only made sense," says Feldman, "but for the purpose of making the larger argument in the institution, we now had the data to show that it actually is true. I found it very powerful and it helped us in making the claim that if nurses and other staff are constantly being yelled at by doctors, they're not going to call them until it's too late. The same thing can happen with residents. I know this after having been a resident for many years. It socializes you to be silent, to accept silence from those of lower status, and to create a culture of silence."

To begin to erode that culture, Feldman, Kaplan, and twenty-three hospital staff members spent two eight-hour sessions being trained in the "crucial conversations" methodology. This group included representatives from 1199 and the NYSNA, as well as other members of the NYSNA. They returned to the institution and distilled the ten lessons of crucial conversations into ten forty-five minute sessions that they piloted with perioperative staff. They chose the operating room because surgeons comprise one of the most hierarchical groups in medicine, and the operating room can be the locus of one of its most toxic hierarchies. After perioperative services was chosen for the first training, Mestel and Feldman held a meeting of all the staff at which Brier promised full support from the president's office. She explains that she told the group that "no doctor or other person would be exempt from following the code, no matter how important they were to the hospital. "Subsequently," she adds, "on two separate occasions managers who could not follow the principles of the code and thus created a hostile workplace were asked to leave the institution."

Twenty people from several different departments—including pediatric, emergency, and psychiatry—were also trained as crucial conversations trainers. Staff in *numerous* departments have been trained in the program itself. This kind of training is part of the five-pronged program Kaplan designed. The five components are

- pilot leadership;
- mediated conversations;
- tracking of operational systems issues;
- skills training;
- measurement.

The most important phase in the Maimonides culture transformation began after the launch of crucial conversations workshops. This is what Kaplan, Mestel, and Feldman refer to as the "accountability phase." The code includes a five-step progressive discipline process for physicians, which mirrors the process used for all other employees. At most hospitals, when someone reports a physician for a behavioral problem, a medical director, who may or may not be trained in dealing with such problems, is usually the one who addresses the issue. At Maimonides, the vice president of human resources, Mark Leff, and Kaplan trained twenty-five physicians to investigate reports of code violations. Any staff member or physician can report a suspected code violation by picking up the phone and calling the code hotline .

When a complaint is made, a physician who does not work in the same department as the physician whose behavior has been questioned is notified, and this begins the process of talking to all the parties involved, any witnesses, and other interested parties. A report is then written and submitted to the three physician leaders of what is known as the medical staff subcommittee on respect, which is part of the medical staff peer review committee. "Once an investigation has been completed," Feldman explains,

> we meet with the physician. We meet with them regardless of whether or not somebody thought they violated the code or not. We ask investigators to answer three questions when they do an investigation: (1) did the physician violate our code; (2) did anybody else; and (3) were there systems' issues that should be addressed? Whether or not the physician investigator thinks they were disrespectful, we meet with the physician and we talk. Now, if it turns out the investigator did think they were disrespectful, what happens next depends how often the physician has done it. If it's the first time, it's just a talk. Nothing gets written down. We don't call anybody about it, unless it's a resident. Then we call the program director because residents are here for a limited period of time.
>
> We have an obligation to intervene any time there's an issue. But for an attending physician, nobody hears about it, unless they heard about it some other way. I don't call anybody the first time. The second time, there's a letter that goes in their file. And we meet with them along with the chair, or the chair's designee. The third time, the medical director gets involved. There's another letter and it's a final warning. The fourth time we recommend—we don't have power to do this, and we only recommend—that the executive medical council suspend the doctor. And the last time, we recommend they be terminated. Thankfully, we haven't gotten past the third step. We had one doctor after the third step leave because we said to him, "You know what? Maybe you really ought to work somewhere else." And he needed to leave.

When physicians or other workers have difficulties adhering to the code, the hospital offers mediated conversations that are used to help uncover what actually happened. In this case physicians, supervisors, or others trained to mediate get the parties together to try to help them understand one another. "The goal," Feldman explains, "is to make sure they can air their differences and at least understand each other, which doesn't mean that they have to be friends, but they have to be able to work with each other so they need to be respectful."

Maimonides also offers psychological and psychiatric services to staff as well as coaching. Feldman explains, however, that whatever services are utilized,

"You're still going to be held to the same standard as everybody else. So, you've got to figure out a way, if you can't figure out a way to be respectful, how you can help yourself or we'll help you."

In each mediated conversation, Kaplan elaborates, there is not only a mediator but also an advocate who represents the parties involved. If a person in a different occupation or discipline has a problem with someone in another, or of another rank, each person involved can call upon someone with whom he or she feels safe and who he or she feels shares the same point of view. "We want to make it safe for each person to have a difficult conversation and to have someone with them to support them and translate their perspective," Kaplan explains.

> For example, I recently conducted a mediated conversation with an attending physician and a physician assistant (PA). The advocate for the attending was a long-term faculty member who the physician felt could help represent her interests. The PA, who was new to the hospital as well as young, was accompanied by her supervisor. If it's someone like a nurse or a technician who is in a union, then he or she might call upon a union representative to be an advocate. But this would not be a traditional grievance meeting.

In order to, as Kaplan terms it, "embed the code into the institution," hospital staff members like him who are involved in promoting the code recognize that it is critical to train other staff to act as mediators.

The Maimonides Code of Mutual Respect is also unique in that it recognizes the system issues involved in behavior by addressing those created through work organization. For example, the operating rooms created what is known as a "GLITCH Book," an acronym for Gathering Little Things That Can Help. Anyone in the OR can use the book to identify issues that get people frustrated so that they can be addressed before a confrontation results. Investigators try to find out if problems that occurred between individuals were a result not of personalities, bad moods, or bad socialization but of unresolved workplace problems that need to be addressed. As Feldman describes it, the question is,

> Was someone disrespectful, was anybody else, and were there systems issues involved that we can fix? We have a whole list of them, many of which we've fixed. Some are not so easy to fix. If somebody gets frustrated about parking, that's a pretty tough one to fix. Many doctors are frustrated with the Medicare fee schedule. I don't think we're going to be fixing that, at least not here at Maimonides. But here is an example of something that could have been and was eventually fixed.
>
> A doctor tried to call a floor to find out about a patient. The person who works on the floor at the phone was at lunch and there was nobody answering the phone. So he's calling and calling and calling. And finally some poor nurse answered. And what do you think he did? He went crazy.
>
> So, number one, he shouldn't be screaming at anybody. That's not going to help him. Number two, we ought to have somebody answering the phone. So we

talked to the nurse manager, a few others, and they now have somebody covering the phone when the person who covers the phone is at lunch. That's a simple fix and it's worth fixing those things. But the message still has to be, OK, we'll fix this frustration, but if something else gets you frustrated, you have to start being responsible for your actions and how you respond to frustration.

Because safety leaders at Maimonides, like those in aviation, recognize that a one-time introduction of concepts like how to create teamwork and deal with conflict is not enough, Kaplan and other code leaders have developed what they call a "sustainability system." "Sustainability sessions," are offered five times a year for people in the departments who have already been exposed to the crucial conversations workshops. Though not as long as those workshops, these one-and-a-half-hour sessions help introduce new employees to the principles of the code and conflict resolution skills. The sessions are also offered to anyone else in the department who feels he or she needs a refresher. Every time new employees come on to one of the units that have been trained in crucial conversations, the VP of perioperative services, chief learning officer, and executive director of perioperative services now meet with them. Similar collaborative initiatives are being conducted throughout the hospital.

In the airline industry, CRM began to produce not only a different kind of pilot but a different process through which airlines selected pilots. Today airlines are no longer interested in employing aviators solely on the basis of their technical skills. They deliberately select people who can and want to work with others. The process is not perfect, but it has helped to change the kind of person in the cockpit. At Maimonides, in all clinical departments, the evaluation and competency assessment of physicians now include the expectation of compliance with the code, as well as teamwork and safety. "It's something that the medical staff endorses," Feldman says. "Any medical staff member that comes to Maimonides at the time of credentialing or recredentialing gets a copy of the code and has to sign a statement saying they've read it and agreed to abide. Working together respectfully, sharing information, and working out problems, whether big or small, is something with which people now must comply, just as they must comply with other codes the hospital has."

Chapter 4

Team Building

GAINING THE COURAGE TO SPEAK UP

Robin Scott began his career as a pilot in 2002, when at age twenty-four he landed his dream job with a commuter airline. During his initial flight training and then in his orientation at the commuter, Scott says he learned a great deal about teamwork in a variety of CRM courses. "In our three month new-hire course, we read and heard a great deal about how CRM and collaboration had helped avert disaster. We did simulated scenarios with a captain who would ignore us, shut us down, or try to intimidate us," Scott recalls.

> We learned how to deal with that. When I got out and started "flying the line," I definitely felt this helped me, empowered me. You're on probation for almost a year and you don't want to ruffle any feathers. You don't want any captain to blacklist you or start spreading the rumor that you're one of those big mouths who thinks he knows it all. You want to get along. So I was concerned about where to draw the line with safety. What to do if it was a gray area. But CRM taught us, "No, you have to speak up, this isn't a one man show."

Scott remembers his teamwork training as a high point in a sometimes tedious career path on a commuter airline. "When I think back on it, I keep getting flashbacks of smiling faces. You meet a new crew each trip. You do about four trips a month. With each captain you meet, there seemed to be a script they would go through which took up everything to expect on the trip. But mostly what they would reiterate was that the door is open, feel free, speak up. It was a very positive, upbeat approach." What Robin Scott describes is the creation of an atmosphere of "psychological safety"—a phenomenon that the Harvard Business School professor Amy Edmondson identifies as key to allowing team members to express their concerns about safety.[1]

In aviation, it is now clearly understood that *the whole*—the *team*—is much more effective than the sum of its individual parts, and team building has become one of the cornerstones of effective CRM and is one of the four CPIs. As we outline the team-building CPI, you'll notice that the information on teamwork is not implemented in isolation. Team building significantly affects—and is affected by—both successful communication and workload management. For example, we discuss conflict management as a function of team building and team leadership, yet conflict management is also a part of communication. Because conflict also produces stress, it affects workload management. So you'll find stress management in the workload section and some mention of conflict management there too. CRM is characterized by deliberate redundancy for two reasons: (1) we know that to change their behavior people need to hear and practice things over and over again if they're going to develop the mental musculature that makes teamwork possible; and (2) all aspects of CRM interact with and influence each other.

THE THEORY BEHIND THE PRACTICE

If you were sitting in on a CRM session on teamwork or acting as a fly on the wall in a line-oriented flight training (LOFT) event (also known as line-oriented simulation) in a cockpit simulator, what would perhaps strike you is the practical focus of the lessons of CRM. Of course, there are plenty of charts and graphs that catalog the research and rationale for teamwork. But this isn't just some theoretical lecture. It's a series of practical lessons; some might seem to be little more than common sense. In fact, there is an enormous amount of theory behind this practice, and it's worth briefly illuminating how one has informed the other.

In the CRM CPI on teamwork, perhaps the most important theoretical underpinnings come from studies of what teams are and how they work most effectively. CRM helps crew members develop what we've called team intelligence because they've learned to understand the qualities that constitute a team and requirements for effective team functioning. The researchers and scholars who have influenced the evolution of teamwork in aviation have helped aviators and airline companies understand that a team is more than a group of individuals engaged in the same project at the same time. Just having a bunch of people assigned to the same activity (flying a plane, taking care of a patient) or occupying the same space (a cockpit, cabin, or operating room) does not create a team. A team is not a group of intimate strangers engaged in "parallel play" in a particular workplace setting.[2]

The team concept has become quite popular in many businesses in recent years. We see teams everywhere, or at least that's what we are often led to believe.

Check out any hospital website, and there will be something about the "health care team." Go into Whole Foods or Wal-Mart, and you will be introduced to "team members." So . . . are all these teams really teams? Not necessarily. A true team is something very particular. It consists of a trained aggregate of persons with

- a specific individual and interactive role;
- adistributed set of necessary skills;
- shared and explicit purposes, information, goals, plans, protocols, and feedback mechanisms.

If a group of individuals meets this description and works cohesively in this fashion, it may be said to be a team. As Robert C. Ginnett observes, "Good teamwork is sometimes on a different plane (no pun intended) than good individual work."[3] The whole point of a team is that the team's "performance will exceed that of any individual in any group."[4]

This is also the thrust of the work of one of the people whose theories have heavily influenced CRM—the Harvard sociologist J. Richard Hackman, who has spent decades observing, describing, and analyzing teams (including aviation teams). Hackman articulates five conditions of successful teamwork. "The team must be a real team, rather than a team in name only; it has a compelling direction for its work; it has an enabling structure that facilitates teamwork; it operates within a supportive organizational context; and it has expert teamwork coaching."[5] In their complex analysis in *Interprofessional Teamwork for Health and Social Care*, Scott Reeves and his coauthors identify six key dimensions of teamwork: "effective patient/client care, shared team identity, shared commitment, clear team roles and responsibilities, interdependence between team members, and integration between work practices."[6]

Simply accomplishing a particular task or set of tasks—performing an activity or activities—is not enough, Hackman cautions, to qualify as a successful team. To be effective, a team must satisfy three other requirements:

> **Five Conditions for Successful Teams (Hackman)**
>
> - A real team vs. team in name only
> - Compelling direction for work
> - An enabling structure
> - Supportive organizational context
> - Expert coaching

1. It must produce an output that "meets the standards of quantity, quality, and timeliness of the people who receive, review, and/or use that output."
2. The process through which that output is produced must enhance "the capability of members to work together interdependently in the future."
3. The process through which the team or group works must contribute "to the growth and personal well-being of team members."[7]

Before CRM, there was little to no effort devoted to creating a true team environment in aviation. If captains believed the other pilots staffing the flight deck had little to contribute to their decision making, they would hardly have considered flight attendants and other airline personnel as having valuable information and legitimate concerns. Indeed, the autocratic captain would even have considered himself exempt from working or collaborating with other persons or occupations of "lower status." Each person on, or connected to, the airplane might have thought he or she had a compelling direction for their work, but few shared their view of that direction with the people they worked near. They certainly did not consider it important to create shared goals and mental models. With no real vision of a team and teamwork there could be no enabling structure for a team, nor could there be organizational support for teams. As to coaching, kings do not normally coach commoners: they command, dominate, punish—even chop off the occasional head.

As we have seen, Hackman's other qualifications for successful teamwork were also missions improbable pre-CRM. Failures caused by unrecognized human factors were not producing quality outcomes. On the contrary, they were producing horrifying accidents and an enormous and unpublicized number of near misses. Too many people who were expected to be working together were—like the disorganized crew of United Flight 173—unable to form cohesive teams that would be able to come together in crisis situations. More to the point, some of the more autocratic captains were producing a lot of anxious subordinates who were very often too intimidated to do anything proactive; they simply went down with the ship. So when CRM began in aviation, it provided a textbook case of moving from collections of individuals carrying out separate tasks to the kind of teamwork Hackman has outlined.[8]

CRM is based on the theoretical understanding of what a team is and how best to create effective teamwork. Its aim is to identify and create many teams on many levels and make sure they can integrate to produce safe circumstances for all aspects of flight. This means bringing teamwork to the cockpit crew, the cabin crew, the ground crew, maintenance, security—even the air traffic control system. In each arena, there are numerous elements. The key to effective teamwork is to first recognize and identify who is on your team and then to develop the skills to utilize all team members to their full extent.

THE COMMERCIAL AIRLINE CRM TEAM

A great deal of discussion here has been devoted to the crucial role of leadership in team development. But who is the actual CRM team? The answer: it's complicated. The CRM team—several teams, actually—is a fairly large and diverse group. The cockpit crew is a team within itself. The flight attendants are a separate team as

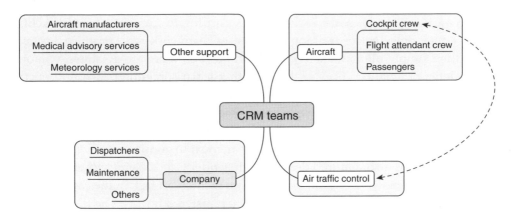

Figure 4.1. CRM team relationships

well. Air crews now even consider the passengers a part of the larger aircraft team, as they would perform critical functions in an evacuation or security situation. Combined, they make up the larger aircraft crew team.

The air crew has at its disposal numerous support organizations—some obvious, such as air traffic Control, and some that are less so, such as medical advisory services.

The way to bring individuals together into teams is by helping them gain both the technical knowledge and the skills required to fly and operate—or to support the flight and operation of—an aircraft and the cognitive and interpersonal skills needed to manage the flight and its myriad of potential contingencies within an organized, complex system. As Hutchins describes it, most human endeavors involve *distributed cognition*. Two kinds of cognition are involved: "the cognition that is the task and the cognition that governs the coordination of elements of the task. In such a case, the group performing the cognitive task may have cognitive properties that differ from the cognitive properties of any individual."[9]

These cognitive skills and their appropriate distribution are essential elements of team intelligence. They involve the mental processes used for gaining and maintaining situational awareness, for solving problems, and for making decisions. When it comes to pilots and flight attendants, one of the things CRM training does is maximize the good and neutralize the not-so-good manifestations of the so-called right stuff. Thus, for pilots, CRM focuses on their job, their pride in their work, and their tendency toward maximizing technical proficiency. It does this while minimizing traits that could impede teamwork and safety—like the self-perception of invulnerability ("That might happen to the other guy but not to me") or the belief that their decision making remains unimpaired by in-flight emergencies or that a true professional can leave behind personal problems on entering the flight deck ("Hey, I'm not at all bothered by the fact that my wife just told me she's leaving me for some rock star"). According to Captain Larry Rockcliff, Airbus's vice president of training, the goal of teamwork is to produce *aviators* rather than simply pilots: "There are pilots and then there are aviators. Aviators are students of aviation. They're the ones that learn something each and every time they go out, and it doesn't matter if they have a brand-new officer who is new on the airplane or if they are flying with someone with lots of experience. They know they are going to learn something and they share that information. Pilots, on the other hand, are the ones who think they are next to godliness."

Teamwork has also required dealing with gender issues. Long ago, all flight attendants—then known as stewardesses—were women. In fact, in the early days of commercial aviation, they were required to be registered nurses. The RN stewardess killed two birds with one stone, Drew Whitelegg writes in *Working the Skies: The Fast-Paced Disorienting World of the Flight Attendant.* As women they gave male passengers something pleasing to "look at," and as nurses, they assuaged passenger fears of this new mode of transport.[10]

For years, the safety role of the flight attendant took a backseat to her more domestic functions. Stewardesses, for example, were not allowed to be married; then when marriage was allowed, they were not allowed to be divorced, and they were forced to adhere to strict weight and age requirements. Because airlines did not compete on price, competition in the industry centered on service. Taking advantage of the sexual revolution of the 1960s and 1970s, in 1971, National Airlines led the pack when it launched its "Fly Me" campaign featuring ads with smiling stewardesses telling passengers, "Hi, I'm Cheryl—Fly Me," or "Fly Eileen from the easy gateway of Miami." Stewardesses were clad in miniskirts and skin-tight tops. International airlines quickly advanced the trend. In 1972, Asian airlines, like Singapore International, followed suit with the "Singapore Girl,"—a stewardess who promised a mix of Asian charm, passive female service, and mysterious Asian sexuality,[11] while Air Jamaica promised, "We make you feel good all over," and Air France asked passengers, "Have you ever done it the French way?"[12]

These kinds of ads, not surprisingly, made sexual harassment, from the cockpit as well as the passengers, a huge problem for flight attendants. Because the ads coincided with the second wave of the feminist movement, this all-female workforce began to fight back with what became known as the "Stewardesses' Rebellion," creating groups like Stewardesses for Women's Rights, whose slogan was "Fly Me? Go Fly Yourself."

With the passage of Title VII of the Civil Rights Act of 1964, job discrimination on the basis of gender was outlawed. Using Title VII, stewardesses began the transformation into flight attendants and formed their own unions. Interestingly, what was to become the major flight attendants union, the Association of Flight Attendants (AFA), began with the financial and moral support of the Airline Pilots Association (ALPA), and AFA was initially a part of ALPA They fought to end restrictions limiting employment to an upper age of thirty-five and successfully got rid of restrictions against married and divorced staff. That rebellion also led to the entrance of male flight attendants into the occupation and the gradual acceptance of homosexuals as flight attendants. It also targeted sexual harassment of cockpit crew. Pilots are still overwhelmingly male, with between 5 and 7 percent female.[13] While the number of male flight attendants continues to climb, as of 2007 about 75 percent were still women.

This lopsidedness has traditionally prompted many of them to retreat when assertiveness was called for. Even though stewardesses were redefined in the 1970s as flight attendants, socialization to degrees of status was (and is) still alive and well in the airline industry as well as in the culture at large. For this reason, safety depends on resocializing not only pilots but also flight attendants and other airline personnel. This is why teamwork training involves learning not only how to be a team leader but how to be an effective team member as well.

ELEMENTS OF EFFECTIVE TEAM BUILDING

Team building starts with appropriate leadership, which involves applying team intelligence to the exercise of authority. One of the most important and innovative aspects of CRM is the attention it devotes to helping those in command of an aircraft exercise authority in a way that elicits followership in members of the aviation team. If crews and ground personnel are to be able to work together in both routine and crisis situations, they need to learn how to lead as well as how to follow. They need to learn how to make decisions, state needs and concerns, manage conflicts, and bring the team together in stressful situations.

One key to this kind of successful teamwork is a leader who views himself or herself as a contributor to group accomplishment rather than as a solo performer or star. This view is captured in the Airbus CRM training's definition of the job of the team leader: "To help team members execute their jobs efficiently and effectively." Accomplishing this goal requires mastering a number of significant lessons. First of all, it entails recognition that getting an airplane safely to its destination involves a *group* of people, each of whom has a job to do that is distinct from that of the captain. One of the ways of getting this point across in CRM is by actually charting out the rhythms of the work of all the people on the aircraft so that they know what is happening when. According to Steve Predmore, vice president of safety at JetBlue:

> Pilots have been trained to believe that they shoulder the ultimate responsibility for the aircraft and that everything depends on their knowledge and expertise. In fact, other people in the company have knowledge and expertise that can serve as a resource for the captain and can enhance decision making. To help captains and other pilots to understand this, JetBlue would actually escort them around the airport to meet other personnel and observe them at work. In this manner, they were able to see what skills various staff have and how they can serve as resources.

But perhaps the most important way to foster a sense of group participation is by helping both captain and crew understand what leadership involves, how it differs from command, and how a good leader should exercise the authority that is embedded in the position of commander.

According to Webster's dictionary, authority is "the power or right to command, act, enforce obedience, or make final decisions."[14] But "authority" comes from the Latin *augere*—"to cause to grow, to increase," and it is in this sense of growing and increasing (the roles and voices of others) that authority functions in the true team. In many occupations and areas of life, authority seems to be granted because an individual has inherited a particular position or been given it by virtue of his or her class or status or because (as is the case in aviation and health care, where good technical skills *presumptively* also make one a good leader or manager) he or she has demonstrated ability in one particular skill or craft. Authority in these cases is entirely a matter of individual action, skill, competence, or excellence.

In aviation there is no question about the captain's right to exercise authority. According to Federal Aviation Regulations (FARs), the captain is "directly responsible for, and is the final authority as to, the operation of that aircraft."[15] The cockpit is not a democracy, and the captain *always* makes the final decision. When two captains occupy the flight deck, the pilot whose name is on the flight plan as pilot in command is the responsible party from a legal standpoint. Thus it is the PIC who bears the legal responsibility for the safe operation of the aircraft.

The question for CRM is not simply the exercise of authority granted by a captain's formal position but the "effectiveness of that authority," which "is influenced by peers' and coworkers' respect for that authority."[16] Although CRM training insists on the recognition of the captain's authority, it is concerned with the safe and effective exercise of authority—authority that is secure rather than insecure.

SECURE AUTHORITY

The exercise of authority need not be "authoritarian" ("favoring or enforcing strict obedience . . . at the expense of personal freedom")[17] or autocratic ("taking no account of other people's wishes or opinions; domineering").[18] In order to "de-authoritarianize" expressions of authority, CRM changed what we call the "dynamics of cool" in the airline industry. The pre-CRM captain typically exercised his authority according to the following two rules, which—although they have been lightheartedly posted on bumper stickers, in briefing rooms, and even in cockpits throughout the world—nevertheless have the ring of truth:

> **The Two Rules of Commercial Aviation**
>
> - Rule 1: The captain is ALWAYS right
> - Rule 2: See Rule 1

These rules almost ensure that those in positions of power can become so preoccupied with their right and responsibility to exercise authority that they forget about the need to exercise it *correctly*. Or as CRM would rephrase it, they focus too much on *who* is right and not enough on *what* is right. To readjust this focus, in CRM the word "authority" no longer stands on its own but is often accompanied by one of two other words—"insecure" and "secure." Someone who exhibits *secure authority*

- exhibits good leadership skills;
- doesn't merely invite but requires participation by others;
- empowers others to assume certain leadership roles;
- invites feedback from others.

On the other hand, an individual demonstrates *insecure authority* by

- jealous guarding of his or her authority;
- autocratic behavior;
- resistance to, or discouragement of, input from others;
- refusal to allow others to assume certain leadership roles.

Teaching captains how to exercise secure authority in CRM begins by distinguishing between leadership and command. "Command" has been defined as "the power to control or dominate by position."[19] Controlling or dominating by position, as aviation learned decades ago, does not necessarily promote a safe environment. *Leadership* involves appropriately shared control and responsibility and a focus on the *what* rather than the *who* of right decisions and actions. When command is coupled with a clear understanding of leadership, then authority is less likely to be exercised in an autocratic or authoritarian fashion.

LEADERSHIP

In both initial and recurrent training in CRM, a great deal of time is spent teaching captains to be leaders. To lead involves more than a focus on the individual: it involves a concentration on the group. "Leadership," Ginnett writes, "is not about leaders in a vacuum—it is about leaders in relation to followers in a particular setting. Is there such a thing as leadership without followers? The fact is leadership is a group phenomenon."[20] In other words, you are not a leader if no one follows you, but you can be in a leadership role even if you have only one follower in a group, even if that group has only two people in it.[21] As the CRM *Leadership/Followership Recurrent Training*

Contrasting Command and Leadership

Command:

- Is designated by the organization
- Cannot be shared

Leadership:

- Is shared among crew members
- Involves both leadership and followership skill; focuses on "what is right," not "who is right"

Instructor Manual defines it, leadership is "A general systematic and relational process that emphasizes the ability to exercise skill in the movement toward goal attainment. From this perspective, leadership is proactive rather than reactive, and necessarily takes into account other members of the group."[22]

Leadership involves using influence, helping people envision their goal and plan how to attain it. It involves making decisions with the input of the crew and knowing how to elicit that input, as well as knowing how to convey decisions to the crew. It involves understanding what people need to get *their* jobs done, fostering situational awareness, and encouraging cross-monitoring. To do all this requires the use of group processes and effective interpersonal skills, including conflict resolution and stress management.

In their studies of highly effective (HI-E) captains, Ginnett and his colleagues considered the range of behaviors that were possible in the cockpit. On one end of the spectrum was the laissez-faire captain, on the other the autocratic captain, and in between the democratic/participatory captain. Not surprisingly, HI-E captains were in that golden middle. "Three methods were used to build an effective leader-team relationship: (1) establish competence, (2) disavow perfection, and (3) engage the crew."[23]

The HI-E captain begins to build his or her team at the very beginning of the flight by putting leadership principles emphasized in CRM into practice. These captains display competence by providing purpose, direction, and motivation; explaining the reason for a task; defining crew-member responsibilities; setting good examples; giving and receiving feedback; and maintaining focus. From the first briefing, Ginnett explains, a captain will—or will not—establish credibility by displaying that he or she has "given some thought to the work they [are] about to engage in" and presenting it in an organized manner. Simply taking the time and effort to thoroughly brief the crew on the flight details and the captain's expectations, emphasizing the items that are of most concern to the crew, opens the way for a depth of rapport that is invaluable in establishing teams. The researchers also found that HI-E captains

Admiral Paul Sullivan's Advice on Command and Leadership

- Lead by personal example—fair standards for all, equally applied
- Know and recognize your limitations
- Always share the credit
- Be truthful to all—in particular, yourself
- Communicate effectively: it's paramount
- Treat people with dignity and compassion
- Let juniors be stakeholders and permit initiative
- Praise in public, reprimand in private, except when witnessing unacceptable behavior
- Be loyal up and down the chain of command
- Do the right thing, no matter how difficult and painful it is
- With authority, one must accept responsibility
- Know your mission and keep focused on it
- Continue to grow professionally
- Team members want to come to work to contribute; take advantage of it
- Promise only what you can deliver, both the good and the bad; actions speak louder than words
- Be yourself!
- ***Be technically competent***

worked both in the briefing and at other opportunistic times to explain the relevant team boundary and to make the boundary more permeable. They always talked about "we" in terms of the total flight crew, as opposed to some of the LO-E (low-effective) captains who referred to the cockpit crew as "we" and the flight attendants as "you." [. . . HI-E captains] took pains to include (at least psychologically) gate personnel, maintenance, and air traffic controllers as part of the group trying to help them—not as an outside hostile group trying to thwart their objectives.

One of the remarkable outcomes of the CRM movement is that effective leaders have realized their humanity and have learned to express their vulnerability. By admitting to their crew—and especially to themselves—that they are as subject to human imperfections as anyone else, captains establish more effective team building while at the same time engaging the crew's participation and input. Thus a particularly HI-E captain might say the kind of thing that Ginnett heard from one captain in a simulator exercise: "I just want you guys to understand that they assign the seats in this airplane based on seniority, not on the basis of competence. So anything you can see or do that will help out, I'd sure appreciate hearing about it."[24]

This is true not only for captains but for leaders of the flight attendant team, known as pursers. Madonna Reid has spent her thirty-two-year career working for a major airline. In her role as purser, Reid says she has learned that "it's really critical to be there to acknowledge what's going on in the moment with a person. With that we have stronger connection and cohesion. We're not robots doing this job. When things are not working well with flight attendants, I will take five minutes and sit down in the jump seat and talk to them: 'Are you okay? You don't seem yourself today; is there anything I can do to help?' It is so important to be there to acknowledge what's going on with people."

As mentioned in chapter 2, the first briefing a captain does—whether with cabin or cockpit crews—sets the tone for the entire flight. This is why CRM training spends a lot of time focusing on *first impressions*. In the "good captain"/"bad captain" videos (discussed in chapter 2) the contrast between the two approaches is as profound in effect as it is obvious to the senses. The bad captain is what Ginnett would term a LO-E captain, while the good captain is HI-E. His well-thought-out introduction invites participation, is sincere and personable, and is addressed the specific people and circumstances involved in *this particular flight*. HI-E leaders don't do canned briefings.[25]

Other characteristics of the HI-E captain will include not being too "directive" with the group. In a crew briefing, the HI-E captain will actually spend as much time listening as talking. These captains encourage crews to speak in briefings and debriefings, and they provide feedback mechanisms to correct problems in a way that is nonblaming and nonjudgmental.[26] Good leaders also establish norms and define roles and boundaries without being so concerned that someone will overstep them that they create an unsafe interpersonal climate.

Cross-monitoring is perhaps one of the most essential elements of teamwork. It starts with the captain telling members of his crew that he wants their input—even when that input suggests that he has made or is about to make a mistake. Cross-monitoring applies to all members of a team, who observe others team members so as to catch potential errors or omissions in the carrying out of their roles and responsibilities. This is not a way of playing "gotcha" but is a team-wide backup safety system. In flight operations, cross-monitoring provides constant backup. It is frequently specified procedurally in regulations and SOPs, but it is also an integral part of every aspect of flight operations.

An example of procedural (specified) cross-monitoring involves "callouts" of altitude changes. This may seem like overkill to an outside observer, but it is both effective and necessary, considering the consequences of an inadvertent altitude deviation when so many aircraft share limited airspace. When assigned an altitude change by ATC, the PM repeats the altitude (ATC: "ABC 123, climb to and maintain flight level 250 [25,000 feet]." PM: "ABC 123, Two-Five-Oh.") The appropriate pilot (PM or PF, depending on the mode of flight—autopilot or manual) sets the assigned altitude in the altitude warning indicator (AWI), repeats the assignment aloud to the other pilot, and points to the AWI. The other pilot responds, "Two-Five-Oh." One thousand feet prior to reaching the assigned altitude, one pilot will state to the other, "Twenty-Four for Twenty-Five," or "One to go." The other pilot will then confirm and verbally acknowledge the alert by repeating the callout.

Most procedures are cross-monitored by very specific guidelines defined in SOPs or regulations. But every other non-specified task is cross-monitored as well. Continual monitoring in the cockpit is essential to a safe flight. The PM observes every action by the PF and understands what the PF is doing at every turn. If the PM does not understand this, he is required to ask for clarification until there is common agreement and understanding. His query, which prior to CRM might have been considered "insubordinate," has been reframed as an expected part of the job of a team member.

All this training has paid off. Data from audits of countless airplane flights consistently confirm that when captains articulated a vision for the flight, the first officers would initiate a response to an operational problem without further direction. When captains exhibited good conduct and high standards, first officers exhibited similar behavior. When captains were receptive to suggestions and input, first officers displayed a willingness to offer these.

On the other hand, if captains were inflexible, did not articulate a clear vision for the crew, failed to meet company standards, or did not obtain commitment from crew members, neither first officers nor captains were likely to exhibit good leadership or followership skills when there was a problem. This was especially evident during a serious crisis. In fact, the more severe an abnormal situation, the less effective the crew was in exhibiting teamwork skills. These ratings were not dependent on status, role, or time together as a crew.

These skills are also taught to flight attendants in their leadership role as pursers. At her airline, for example, Madonna Reid describes attending purser training for a week:

> The company brought in British trainers. We had lessons on how to manage people, to managing crews, to conflict resolution. We did personality testing, because the procedure that would work best for you might not work for another person. They put us in role-play situations. They videoed us. It was an entire week, with one-to-one, small-group, and large-group learning situations. You had to demonstrate writing skills—we write a lot of reports—demonstrate readable, intelligent spelling; you had to be able to communicate one to one; they would give you a conflict—you were on the airplane and you had to resolve it.

DECISION MAKING

> The frontiers are not east or west, north or south, but wherever a man confronts a fact.
>
> —*Henry David Thoreau*

One of the primary functions of the team leader is to make decisions. The central goal of CRM is to ensure that high-quality decisions are made across the whole spectrum of flight operations. Decision making is one of the most complex areas of leadership in teams as well as one of the most important for team members. Indeed, the measure of a high-functioning team is how decisions are made and implemented. Individuals functioning in the same space or around the same set of activities cohere as a team when decisions are made with the input of all involved, when those decisions are clearly communicated and understood, and when the decisions of the team leader are accepted by team members.

Team cohesion can be judged as well by the ways in which members contribute to decision making and how comfortable they feel with any decision a team leader makes. In groups that are teams in name only, decision making becomes a potentially competitive activity that can generate more resentment than commitment. In such groups, individuals typically complain that they had little or no input in decision making, that their concerns were ignored or dismissed at best or trivialized or belittled at worst. For them the decision-making process is often the locus of both shame and blame. They may feel shamed or humiliated when they try to express their concerns and are brushed off. As a result, when they discuss a particular decision that their superior has made, they tend focus on *who* rather than *what* and may question the authority of the decision maker rather than the process through which he or she came to a particular decision.

When people who are supposed to *lead* actually only command, they may perceive efforts of subordinates to participate in decision making as insubordination or view them in competitive rather than collaborative terms ("She's trying to wear the pants in the family" or "He's trying to take over"). They may erroneously assume that they are being challenged when they are not. In response to a climate of perceived disrespect, individuals who are supposed to function as team members may respond in ways that actually subvert teamwork and set individuals on the defensive against one another.

To assure that team leaders will make their decisions using all the available information and resources, CRM training both describes the optimal decision-making practice and gives team leaders the practical skills they need to arrive at decisions inclusively and effectively. The decision-making process involves the following:

Identifying the problem

- Communicate the problem.
- Solicit input from other sources.
- Think beyond the obvious alternatives.

Obtaining commitment

- All crew members are responsible for contributing to the decision-making process.
- Consider relevant SOPs and FARs.

Stating the plan

- Make plan known to crew, customers, and others as appropriate.
- Clearly communicate decisions to reduce confusion and misunderstanding.[27]

The range of decisions that pilots are called upon to make in the course of virtually any flight highlights just how much judgment goes into so-called standardized activities and how many people are actually involved in—and potentially suffer the consequences of—these decisions.

While checklists and other aviation activities have been standardized, flight, like medical treatment, is highly unpredictable and involves dozens of decisions that are both

---

Some Critical Decisions That Could Be Faced in Any Flight

- Weather not as forecast: divert or continue?
- What to do in fuel-critical situations
- Takeoff decision when conditions are deteriorating
- How to manage system malfunctions
- How to cope effectively with mechanical malfunctions
- What to do with passenger or crew medical emergencies

technical and relational: choosing where to divert after a system malfunction or when fuel is short and the weather is deteriorating; determining how to cope with a passenger's medical emergency; evaluating whether to take off with a deferred maintenance item (given past experience with the projected weather and traffic at the destination); deciding whether an exhausted flight attendant should be working or should get some rest; contending with a first officer who might have overstepped his authority; figuring out how to deal with an emergency that arose from something that technology was supposed to have banished forever; and so on ad infinitum.[28]

Decision-making skills are critical for team leaders in every aspect of crew activities. In Madonna Reid's purser class, "We did scenarios that forced us to make very quick decisions. For example, you know you're going to crash on an island: you have to get together as a group and very quickly decide what five things will you take, what five things will you do first once you've crashed. What kind of communication do you use to get people moving and agreeing? We learned a lot, like the fact that . . . what you hear isn't always what was said."

Identifying a problem, team leaders learn, is hardly simple. Consider the issue of whether to divert because of a mechanical difficulty or whether a first officer has exceeded his authority or what to do about a flight attendant and a passenger in a conflict. The first step is to identify whether something actually constitutes a problem that demands action. For example, a flight attendant calls because she has heard a strange noise in an engine. Does this noise indicate a potentially serious problem? Is someone imagining it or overreacting to sounds within the normal range? Post-9/11 security concerns make an investigation by one of the pilots in the form of a personal visit to the cabin problematic if not impossible. Resolving the noise report will take a little more imagination and inquiry and will tap into the pilots' communication skills; it also requires a substantial level of trust in the cabin crew's ability to observe and accurately communicate what they see. In this example, the pilots will ask the FA for additional information: How long have you been hearing the noise? Have you ever heard this before? Did passengers notice? Did other FAs notice? And so on. Combining this information with observations of engine instruments, they will begin to develop a mental model of the situation and determine (1) whether there is a need for concern and (2) if so, what the plan should be (divert? emergency landing? evacuation?) so that the cabin crew can start to make plans accordingly. In addition, if it is determined that there is a valid concern, the cockpit will immediately get company dispatch and maintenance departments into the loop.

In another example, a crew is awaiting push-back from the gate, but the captain has not yet arrived on board—he was delayed and is racing to get on the aircraft. The first officer takes it upon himself to review the flight plan, brief the cabin crew, and make the initial call to the passengers—duties normally handled by the captain. The captain arrives and finds out the first officer has done his job for him.

Has the first officer exceeded his authority or stepped on the captain's toes? Should this matter be discussed? Is it a one-off action or part of a pattern? Although many decisions are clear-cut, the captain's judgment is most critical when conditions are ambiguous and no clear guidance is provided in manuals, checklists, or company policy. These difficulties are always exacerbated in time-pressured situations.

It is always important to find out the facts so that decisions can be made on the basis of information rather than assumptions. In the *Leadership/Followership Recurrent Training Instructor Manual* a number of scenarios help captains hone their decision-making skills. In the preceding scenario of the perhaps overzealous first officer, the instructors might ask the captain, "What tasks (listed below) would you wish the first officer to complete in preparation for the flight while waiting for you?"

- Pull the weather information packet.
- Have the paperwork required for the flight to proceed waiting for the captain in the cockpit.
- Greet and brief the flight attendants.
- Perform first officer preflight duties.
- Perform captain preflight duties.
- Make a preliminary fuel-load decision based on release and weather.
- Make a final fuel-load decision.
- Greet the passengers through the initial public address system call.
- Discuss a potential maintenance discrepancy with a mechanic (e.g., questionable tire).
- Write up a maintenance discrepancy and have it addressed.
- Receive the ATC clearance, having it available for when the captain arrives.
- Greet gate agent, be certain he or she is informed, and discuss potential delay.
- List any other steps you would likely take/like to see taken.

Facilitators further ask these questions:

- What factors might influence whether the first officer chooses to perform a task (e.g., familiarity with the captain, previous similar experience, etc.)?
- Are there "rules" that define what it is appropriate for the first officer to do? Are these written, unwritten, cultural, or otherwise?
- What if the first officer were the late-arriving crew member? Would you, as captain, get the ship totally set to go (including carrying out the first officer's tasks)?
- Would you, as the first officer, expect the captain to perform some of the first-officer, role-specific duties?

The idea here is "to investigate authority relationships and boundaries across cockpit roles. The facilitator should encourage the Captain and First Officer to discuss the balance between situational leadership, authority boundaries, and role-specific duties." The answers to these questions and others will determine the decision the captain makes.[29]

Here is another scenario. A passenger suddenly becomes very sick, with vomiting and severe diarrhea, and is not able to get up and get to the lavatory. The flight is totally full. There is a physician on board who, after examining the passenger, says that the situation is not critical and the passenger is medically stable enough to travel to the flight's final destination, two hours ahead. However, the immediate environment surrounding the passenger is soiled and very unpleasant. In deciding how to respond to this turn of events, the captain has to balance a series of factors that include the well-being of the ill passenger, the immediate comfort of other passengers nearby, the ability of the cabin crew to do their jobs, and the considerable inconvenience and cost a diversion could cause.

MEMBERSHIP AND FOLLOWERSHIP

We have generally been socialized to view leadership as a linear, one-way, top-down function whose primary aim is getting things done. CRM has considerably redefined that view. As the role of the modern cockpit crew changes, the skills required of the crew members change also. We are now aware that leadership is an activity that involves both leaders *and followers* as they interact to accomplish goals. Followership skills are as important as leadership skills to the safe and efficient performance of flight crews and to effective teamwork in any setting.

Although there is an enormous amount of literature and discussion within management circles about the importance and how-to's of leadership, there tends to be little discussion of the equally important corollary of followership. But Ginnett reminds us, "[Y]ou are not a leader if you have no followers." For the purposes of marketing, it may be great to advertise "an army of one"; for the purposes of fighting a war, there could be nothing worse.[30]

The process of moving from a dysfunctional toxic hierarchy to true teamwork is not necessarily smooth. Learning new role parameters and behaviors takes practice, and trust is built up through a period of trial and error. For those who have been socialized not to speak up, what does it mean to suddenly be asked to express their concerns and challenge authority when necessary? Robin Scott, whom we met at the beginning of this chapter, described his concerns that speaking up might mean being blacklisted. A previously subordinate group that is suddenly told that they can be assertive may also inappropriately confuse assertion with aggression. In her work with nurses, Suzanne has often seen RNs who think they

Inquire, Advocate, and Assert: Northwest Airlines Flight 288, October 21, 2009

When Northwest Airlines Flight 188 was scheduled to land at Minneapolis on October 21, 2009, flight attendants noticed that as the scheduled arrival time approached, the aircraft had not started its descent from cruise altitude. The lead flight attendant exercised her prerogative to inquire about the delay, sensing something that didn't seem quite right.

The FA contacted the flight deck on the intercom to inquire whether the flight would be arriving late. The precise details are at this point largely unclear, but the actions of the flight attendant made the pilots suddenly aware that they had failed to begin their arrival as planned. Had the lead FA not taken the initiative and inquired, the outcome of this event—a perfect although delayed landing—might have been quite different (for example, anything from being forced to land at another airport to running out of fuel).

are being assertive when they have actually crossed into being aggressive ("I am going to teach that intern/resident/attending a thing or two!").

Understanding the complexity of this dynamic, CRM focuses significant attention on defining what it is to be a good team member or follower and conveying the skills that assure that people can be heard without being misunderstood, so that they can participate in the creation of a psychologically safe work environment. The three most crucial activities that make an effective team member are

- inquiry;
- advocacy; and
- assertion.

INQUIRY

It is not blind obedience one wants from followers in teamwork. Particularly where safety is concerned, it is input, cross-monitoring, thoughtfulness, and contributions to situational awareness and clarity. Deference, we'll recall, led to crashes. Step one in skilled followership is inquiry. For example, if someone does not understand an order or an action taken in flight, he or she is supposed to question it—not sarcastically or aggressively ("What the hell are you trying to do?" "What can you possibly be thinking?" "Are you trying to crash this plane?") but firmly and clearly. Questions could include "Can you clarify that captain?" "I am not clear about this"; "Can you explain your rationale?" "Can you help me better understand?"

ADVOCACY

The term "advocacy" comes from the noun "advocate," which is defined as "one whose job was to plead cases in a court of law."[31] Advocacy always suggests stating a position, pleading, supporting, recommending, making an argument, defending something or someone. In this case, the obligation of a first officer, flight attendant, or other member of an airline crew is to advocate for their concerns.

If we go back to the example of the passenger who was suddenly and uncontrollably sick, the captain's decision will be made in part based on whether the flight attendant has been skillful in advocating for a position (e.g., land now or press on). The FA's description of the problem is critical to a captain who is locked in the flight deck. If she simply says, "It's messy back here," she is both unclear and unassertive.

But suppose she says, "The passenger's clothes and the seat are soiled, and the surrounding rug is soaked all the way across and forward and aft several rows. This part of the cabin is unpleasant, unsanitary, and unsafe. I think that it would be wrong to continue the flight. Because of the health hazard, I suggest we land as soon as possible to deal with this situation."[32] Here the flight attendant is much more descriptive and assertive and has advocated for a particular solution, based upon the information available.

ASSERTION

In the cases described above, going through steps one and two resolved the issue. That isn't always the case, which makes step three–assertion—essential. We cannot overstate the fact that during the thirty-year evolution of CRM, the captain has maintained the ultimate authority over and responsibility for his aircraft. Yet CRM encourages the FOs and FAs to be as assertive as required to assure the safe outcome of the flight. For a first officer, this ultimately could even involve taking control of the aircraft from the captain. The question of where to cross that line is a complex and challenging one at best, and such an extreme action is never taken lightly. For this reason, policies on appropriate assertiveness must be clearly stated and clearly understood by all parties.

PEOPLE SKILLS

> "As much as anything, aviation character is the triumph of humility and common sense over arrogance and overconfidence."
> —Captain Don Keating, Crew Resource Management LLC

It takes a lot of work to assure that humility and common sense will triumph over arrogance and overconfidence. This is done by mobilizing the people skills that will create the right emotional climate. Everything taught in CRM is designed to create that kind of climate. There is no one crew performance indicator that deals with how human beings interrelate. The field of human-factors research is grounded in the awareness that human beings aren't infallible as they interact with machines and with each other. As we saw in the communication CPI, people need to learn how to communicate effectively—without pushing each other's buttons, without reacting defensively, and without retreating into what has been called "malicious obedience." Every CRM team CPI thus includes something like the Short Course in Human Relations summarized below. The focus on human beings interacting permeates

A Short Course in Human Relations: Getting along in a Complex World and Demanding Environment

The six most important words you can say:
"I admit I made a mistake."

The five most important words you can say:
"You did a good job."

The four most important words you can say:
"What is your opinion?"

The three most important words you can say:
"If you please."

The two most important words you can say:
"Thank you."

The least important word you can say:
"I."

every aspect of the CRM activities. Today people skills—nowadays often called emotional intelligence—are all the rage in management circles. People skills are, of course, important when working on teams. The problem is that in too many cases, management courses and consultants disconnect emotions and the people who are supposed to master them from work organization, stressors, power relationships, and status hierarchies in the workplace or professional culture. CRM, by contrast, teaches people skills to support *team* intelligence in the context of workplace realities.

CONFLICT RESOLUTION

One of those workplace realities is conflict, which is moderated through the application of conflict resolution skills. A favorite video clip sometimes used in CRM courses to show conflict—followed by a less than appropriate resolution—is a scene from the 1950s-era film *The High and the Mighty*. In the scene, John Wayne (the FO) and Robert Stack (the captain) experience a serious operational disagreement. John Wayne resolves it in a manner that suits his character well but is ill advised: he reaches over and slaps Robert Stack silly to advocate for his point of view. All too often those are the social lessons we learn about resolving conflict ("Might makes right," or "I win."). However, resorting to fisticuffs at thirty-six thousand feet is obviously not a great idea.

But what do you do when conflict arises in the flight deck or cabin because of operational or interpersonal issues? CRM accepts that conflict is normal and inevitable. Good teams usually go through a process of development in which a certain amount of tension and conflict simply cannot be avoided; in fact, when well managed and openly discussed, they actually contribute to the establishment of accepted ground rules and consolidation of a group identity. Getting the most out of a group means consideration of often-contradictory values, perspectives, and opinions. Decisions that have the potential for ambiguity or prolonged disagreement should be resolved by company policies and procedures if at all possible, thereby making further debate unnecessary within the team and removing unnecessary sources of friction.

The entire focus of both communication and teamwork training in CRM is to help people cope not only with complicated machines but also with the complex and challenging interpersonal differences that can be unmanageable when people fail to respect and adapt to different backgrounds and belief systems and establish the critical commonalities–like safety and survival—that help build an effective team environment.

In the aviation context this is particularly critical because conflicts that occur as a result of interpersonal problems, disagreements about an operational decision, passenger disruptions, and a host of other issues usually happen many thousands of feet up in the air and sometimes during difficult weather or when other problems are also occurring. It is a watchword of problem solving in the aviation world that "It is better to be down here discussing how we are going to get up there than to be up there trying to figure out how we are going to get down here!" Policies and procedures are designed to ensure that as much has been covered before flight as possible, but

> **Operational and Interpersonal Conflict**
>
> **Operational conflict** is often a result of operational challenges where two (or more) individuals have difficulty coming to a common conclusion or course of action. It may be caused by a wide variety of factors, which may include weather, mechanical anomalies, fatigue, and any number of stressors associated with the business of getting the aircraft from one place to another.
>
> **Interpersonal conflict** is more typically caused by personality differences, differing political views, philosophies, and so on. By respecting different ideas and opinions, we can obtain a broader understanding of the nature of the problem and get more alternatives from which to select the best solution. Although this is an essential part of team building, the final arbiter must be the team leader—the captain. Strong leadership is essential. Although the captain must consider all reasonable inputs as time allows, he or she must ultimately make the final decision.

they cannot cover every possible situation. Because of the often time-critical nature of the aviation environment, it is imperative to identify, talk through, and resolve conflicts on the ground as best we can *before* we encounter them in flight—but we must also have the tools and the skills to reach resolution at any altitude.

To deal with the tensions that inevitably arise between human beings, even in the best of situations, both team leaders and members are given training in conflict management and resolution. Captain John Griffiths, a pilot with Federal Express, handed Suzanne a five-by-seven card from his flight bag. On its tab were the words "CRM Toolkit." On both sides were condensed instructions for how to relate to others—with sections such as "Crew Support Process—Relay Information, Express Concern, Make an Emergency Statement"; "The Five-Step Assertion Model"; and "Conflict Management." Here is the advice to captains regarding conflict management:

- Ask three questions: What do I expect? What do others expect? Why do I expect what I expect?
- Make three statements: Make an "I" statement of concern. Clearly state the problem. Propose a solution.
- Do three things: Stop talking and listen. Abandon your idea if the other is better. Be assertive if required.

Although this is simply Conflict Management 101, it is noteworthy that every CRM recurrent training program contains similar guidance in one form or another.

This kind of guidance can be crucial, as the following incident illustrates. One flight attendant, who requested that her name not be used, described an incident in which acting assertively likely saved an aircraft, passengers, and crew from certain catastrophe:

> I had been flying for fifteen years. I was based in Dallas/Fort Worth and we were flying an all-night turn to Los Angeles. It was one of those really rare wintry nights in Dallas when an ice storm was blowing in, and we pushed back and got in a long line to take off, and must have waited for at least forty-five minutes. The pressure was on to get going. We were on a MD-88, and I was one of two flight attendants on the far aft jump seat, which is situated between the two aft engines with no windows; you are in a black hole back there. When they began their take-off roll, they started to crank the engines, and there was a high-pitched screeching sound that was ear-splitting and unlike any sound we had EVER heard on an aircraft of any kind. . . . I immediately picked up the interphone and gave the emergency ring to the cockpit and without waiting for them to pick up, knowing that they usually monitor the calls anyway, started saying "abort." The pilots cut power, and we were able to abort. The captain called back and asked what was wrong and I told him—and he was quite angry that I had advised him to abort because I heard "something funny," and he told me he would taxi around and go again.
>
> I had just enough seniority by then to have the nerve to stand up to him, and I told him I knew this was being recorded and I was advising not to go, to return to the gate. He told me that if we returned to the gate he was "putting me off the plane for good." I was scared but more scared to fly that plane so I told him that was fine. He did not expect that, and said again that we were going anyway. I told him if he started the takeoff roll, I would open the aft service door. He then had no choice but to go back to the gate, where he was going to leave me.
>
> When we arrived back at the gate, the mechanics inspected the engine, only to find that ice chunks had been sucked up into the engine as it fired up and completely stripped it clean. The noise was the metal disintegrating. There were no more blades in the engine, and we surely would have crashed.
>
> The captain never said a word to me, but he didn't put me off the plane either. I hope he quietly learned that we learn to fly by sound in the back of the plane, and that is a huge part of what CRM is all about. We may not know how to fly the plane, but we can recognize the smallest of aberrations in the sound or pitch of the aircraft after years of flying in the back of the plane, and that is priceless info to factor in.

The FA was never reprimanded by the company for this incident, as her actions may have saved the aircraft and all on board. Nor was she ever acknowledged. She was eventually gratified to learn that the company later used this incident to help teach CRM in recurrent training.

That CRM training has helped crews work as a team to maintain safety was spotlighted in March 2012 when a JetBlue aircraft on a flight from New York to Las Vegas had to make an emergency landing. The first officer refused to let the emotionally distraught and threatening captain back into the cockpit once he had left to go the bathroom, and then passengers had to subdue him until the plane made an emergency landing. The incident provoked much comment—and hopefully action—about airline screening systems. Are airlines sufficiently aware of emotional problems pilots may have? Will pilots report such problems or do they fear retaliation, particularly in a time of severe cost-cutting?[33] Although there was much gnashing of teeth about this incident, what must be remembered is *how efficiently it was handled*. The first officer assumed command of the aircraft and made sure the captain was no longer a threat. Forty years ago, he may not have taken such a proactive approach. Flight attendants who, in this incident, helped to subdue the captain, before CRM would have worried about taking such measures. Former United flight attendant Nancy Burns, who worked both pre- and post-CRM said, "If that had happened before CRM I wouldn't have had the courage to help subdue a captain, even if he was acting like a crazy person. I probably would have pushed him back into the cockpit and let the first officer deal with him, which of course would have been exactly the wrong thing to do. The crew faced a terrible situation, which would have been very hard to predict, and they acted as a team to resolve it, even by involving passengers." We hope health care personnel can get the training to do the same.

Chapter 5

Case Study

OSHER CLINICAL CENTER FOR
COMPLEMENTARY AND INTEGRATIVE
MEDICAL THERAPIES

Teamwork initiatives have been undertaken with varying degrees of success and longevity in a wide range of health care settings. We include the Osher Clinical Center (OCC) as a case study because it is unique in many respects, including both its success and its longevity, as well as its thoroughgoing commitment to a team approach to patient care. As one of the few integrative care clinics in the United States to be a fully-fledged clinical entity within a conventional academic medical center, the OCC, as well as its clinician team, has been met with considerable skepticism at every step of the way and has satisfactorily laid most of it to rest through excellent clinical outcomes and very high patient satisfaction ratings. Recent and ongoing clinical research has thus far upheld the success of the OCC's integrative, team-based treatment model and its positive patient outcomes. Presently its medical director is working with the administration of its parent hospital to position the OCC as the main portal of entry for back-pain patients coming into the academic medical center for their care.[1]

TEAM BUILDING FROM SCRATCH

Picture the following scenario. You are an invisible observer in a meeting room in the outpatient services building of a big-name academic medical center. It is late 2010. A patient case conference is under way. A dozen or so clinicians are sitting around a table glancing at the case notes while one of them presents the patient. Among these clinicians are two chiropractors; two massage and movement therapists (one also a yoga therapy instructor) from two different training paradigms; one psychiatrist (also trained in mindfulness-based stress reduction—MBSR); two nutritionists; two acupuncturists from two different practice paradigms (Chinese and Japanese); two MDs, both general internal medicine physicians; an occupational therapist; a physical therapist (also trained in craniosacral therapy, a branch of osteopathic medicine); and a practitioner of Chinese forms of both therapeutic massage and acupuncture.

The patient in question is a woman in her early forties who has terrible chronic pain that has not responded well to standard medical treatments and interventional surgeries. Her problem started after an accident that produced pain in only one location, but over time the pain has spread and become constant and now has disabled her almost completely. The clinician presenting the patient is a chiropractor who conducted her intake history and interview. All in the room are listening respectfully, thoughtfully, asking questions from time to time.

The chiropractor asks members of the clinician team what they think might be an optimal course of treatment for this unfortunate woman. She thinks one of the other clinicians should provide the first line of treatment because the woman's pain is "too hot" for her to be handled physically with techniques that involve any sort of pressure, even light massage. The clinicians suggest ways that they each might approach the patient; they suggest other members of the clinician team as best first-line providers; they ask each other for insights from their respective frames of reference. Someone proposes that the treatment begin with light-touch craniosacral therapy to abate the pain and calm the patient enough for hands-on treatments to be considered. Acupuncture would be good, they think, when the patient is able to tolerate it: what would be the approaches of the two acupuncturists, and which might be better for this particular person and situation? The psychiatrist should be involved, both in his conventional capacity as a therapist to help this woman manage her burden of pain and to teach her techniques of MBSR to help control it. A consensual treatment plan takes shape.

In many medical settings this kind of attentive, reflective, and egalitarian exchange among such a widely diverse group of caregivers and professions would be relatively rare in a patient care conference. Certainly the majority of these particular clinicians would not be represented. In the clinic where *this* case conference was held, both the diverse assemblage of clinicians and the inclusive and collegial interaction style emerged from many purposeful and interconnecting factors. They grew out of years of careful and deliberate planning and preliminary research. They required months of education and training specifically designed to create a *team* of diverse clinician-peers with a shared body of knowledge, a common language, clearly articulated common goals, and an inclusive model of communication. They were backed by thousands of hours of legal exploration and political diplomacy within the complex academic medical center in which the clinic is housed. Finally, they are the result of ongoing, recurrent practice at maintaining and enhancing a smoothly functioning, patient-centered, integrated, team approach both to patient care and to collegial interaction. Most important to this group's functioning, this is a medical setting whose founders *built the team before they built the clinic.* Teamwork of this kind is as much a firm foundation of the clinic as the building materials and structural supports upon which its physical plant rests.

Welcome to the Osher Clinical Center for Complementary and Integrative Medical Therapies at the Brigham and Women's Hospital in Chestnut Hill, Massachusetts.

WHERE IT ALL STARTED

This remarkable clinic was first conceived in the 1990s by David M. Eisenberg, MD, then director of the Center for Alternative Medicine Research and Education at Beth Israel Deaconess Medical Center and associate professor of medicine at Harvard Medical School. Through a combination of federal research grant funding and philanthropic gifts from the Bernard Osher Foundation, Dr. Eisenberg put together a planning and implementation group that worked to create this kind of clinic and integrate it into a large academic medical center.[2] The goal of the center would be to address primarily musculoskeletal pain through integrating conventional medical therapies with selected complementary/alternative medicine (CAM) approaches. This approach was meant to be replicable, testable, and financially sustainable.

In order to create this kind of integration, a group of clinicians, each of whom had individual private practices, would have to be transformed into a functioning team that shared the care of many of the same patients and communicated well about them. They would have to understand and respect each other and learn not to perceive their professional variability as representing de facto superior or inferior practices. Instead (as happened in CRM) they would have to view one another as resources, each with something of significant value to offer.

To achieve this, they would have to learn about each profession's theoretical foundations, training requirements, and clinical practices. They would have to learn how to take multiple frames of reference into account; how to ask questions without embarrassment, receive answers without skepticism, and articulate their viewpoints without argument. They would have to learn to think, learn to communicate, and learn to *learn* in brand-new ways.

The plan from the very beginning was to have medical doctors and CAM providers work together as peers and as members of a health care team that could best design care plans for individual patients through consulting together, conferring on their thoughts about treatment plans for shared patients and how best to integrate those. These clinicians would share their clinical notes through a single electronic medical record designed to accommodate input from each of their specialties with its particular ways of approaching assessment of patients and treatment of pain. The range of clinicians envisioned included conventionally trained neurologists, rheumatologists and orthopedic surgeons, along with chiropractors, acupuncturists, yoga, massage, and movement therapists, nutritionists, nurse-practitioners, and psychiatrists. This meant that any training curriculum would have to acquaint all the clinicians with one another's professions and clinical techniques, as well as create the kind of teamwork that would be essential for integrative care to function.

A curriculum planning committee (CPC) that included representatives of both conventional and CAM professions, as well as specialists in education, organizational development, clinical management, group dynamics, and social sciences, worked together over several months to develop a training curriculum. (Bonnie participated in both the curriculum planning and its implementation and documented the progress of these efforts.)

The CPC knew that its intended audience was a diverse set of skilled clinicians (about twenty-five in all) who had extensive knowledge and skill in their own fields, variable degrees of knowledge in other related fields, and perhaps no knowledge at all in still other fields represented in the clinician mix. All of them would have prior experiences, expectations, and almost certainly skepticism or even prejudice with respect to some of the represented disciplines. Disciplines within conventional medicine have typically struggled with each other over knowledge, technique, status, and turf. Between conventional medicine and CAM there has historically been not only suspicion but even outright antipathy (such as between chiropractic and conventional medicine, for example). The critical question in planning and establishing the OCC was, How can we transform these former skeptics and very independent clinicians into a trusting and smooth-functioning multidisciplinary team of colleagues?

From the outset, the model of teamwork and the goal of creating a team of peers formulating *values-based decisions and clinic operational design* informed all of the training program design. The two broad goals of the training curriculum were (1) peer-to-peer education and training—clinicians teaching each other as professional partners and equals working together to build a broad-based, shared body of knowledge; and (2) team building—creating a sense of respect and trust among the clinicians and a culture of collaboration within the group and for the planned clinic.

To realize these goals, the training program would have to accommodate a wide variety of instructional techniques and preferred learning styles that would include lectures, demonstrations, modeling, team-building exercises, role-playing, and self-reflection (as well as prospective observational studies to assess the value of the team being created). When the CPC began to discuss less formal approaches such as role-playing, team-building exercises, and reflective activities, members expressed a great deal of anxiety that "the docs won't like that" (or, in its strongest form, "We can't do that because the docs won't like it"). Many seemed to feel certain that physician resistance to these teaching and learning techniques would be an impediment to training success and team building. This reflected the fact that physicians held the traditionally highest-status titles and professions in the training pool and were accustomed to tremendous autonomy but also quite a bit of formality in their education and practice settings. What if they walked out of sessions whose instructional methods they disliked or felt confused by, or refused to "play" in the more informal or improvisational exercises?

Like many pilots in early CRM, physicians tend to be very resistant to role-playing in particular, fearing that it will make them look ridiculous or that they will fail or be "exposed" when they are out of their usual well-contained element. Its open-ended and self-revelatory nature can make role-playing feel like a personal risk rather than a learning tool. Physicians' deeply felt professional mandate to be right, responsible, and in control makes these situations very uncomfortable for a lot of docs. Only after considerable discussion was the CPC able to articulate the fact that the center's education and training tactics would in fact be *stretching comfort zones for all participants* at one time or another and that this served a valuable purpose.

After the training, participants recognized that this principle had contributed to breaking down barriers and therefore to promoting a group or team identity. During the training program, they began to grasp that—in terms of exposure to new knowledge, materials, and methods—"we're all in this together." On the first day of the training program, the facilitators announced that discomfort at various times was to be expected for all participants and that we would plan to discuss them together as part of the group identity-building process.

The final training curriculum totaled 112 instructional hours, formatted to be implemented over fourteen days of 8 hours each, one day per week for fourteen weeks. All participants were paid their regular salaries for the training days.[3] This served both as an incentive, since it guaranteed that they would not lose their clinical income for the day, and as an indicator of the importance of the training: this was *not* "time out" of regular clinical life but a central part of becoming a clinician team and of working in an integrative model of care delivery. (It was also very much the price of doing business within an academic medical center, as full-time clinicians must generate their salaries based on a combination of clinical revenues, revenues from teaching, and/or revenues from sponsored research projects, such as this one.) All participants were expected, barring unforeseen emergency, to be on time and to be actively present and participating for the full training day. Cell phones and pagers were to be *off* (not merely silenced) except during planned breaks and check-in intervals—that is, participants had to have arranged coverage so that their attention could remain focused. (This was to prove hardest to sustain as the training program progressed, particularly among the conventional medical doctors.) Participants had to commit to attending sessions for the full fourteen weeks.

A TWO-STAGE APPROACH

The training program was designed to have two general stages. The first stage concentrated on creating and deepening a shared knowledge base, creating a common language and lexicon, and fostering development of a team identity and culture. The second stage introduced a shift of *method* primarily to experiential and practicum-based learning. It shifted the *focus* to functional group dynamics and role expectations and collective production of specific work products (e.g., vision and mission statements, cross-disciplinary triage criteria, interdisciplinary medical record templates).

In stage one, representatives of each clinical discipline explained in formal didactic sessions the theories and practices of their discipline with respect to health and illness and its approaches to treating pain, with low back pain as the shared specific example. They reviewed the status of research in the discipline and its findings with respect to musculoskeletal problems and back pain, discussed the training and certification requirements for the profession, and described a "typical" clinical day in assessing and treating pain patients. Clinicians representing each discipline had been asked to contribute two research papers to the general syllabus materials: one favorable to its discipline's approach to pain, specifically back pain, and one critical of it. These papers were also discussed and critiqued in plenary group sessions. The discussions helped people acquire a preliminary understanding of each discipline and its theoretical, diagnostic, and therapeutic approaches and also highlighted differences among specialties in clinical approach and in perspectives on patients and patient-clinician relationships. Hands-on demonstrations of some of the pain-assessment techniques of the discipline in question broke up the didactic sessions and elicited questions and still more discussion.

Team-building exercises were incorporated into each training day and included physical and cognitive activities centered on name, face, and discipline recognition; interactive communication; and collective problem solving. A few of these were plenary activities, but the majority were carried out in smaller breakout groups. The training facilitators assigned participants to different groups, varying the groups' composition from one exercise to the next throughout the curriculum. This guaranteed that they would all interact directly in small group settings across the weeks. At the opening of the first day, facilitators distributed a list of ground rules for participation in the training curriculum and sought additional suggestions from participants.

The curriculum required decision making by consensus, in both small and plenary groups, with *consensus* defined as "not a 100 percent agreement on all matters but rather an agreement to go forward with a structure or plan that all parties can agree to support."[4]

OCC Clinician Team Training Ground Rules

The following is a list of reminders to all to ensure that we are able to provide an environment that is conducive to learning and respectful and enjoyable for everyone.

- Please plan to arrive in time to begin at 8:00 a.m. each day of the training and return promptly from breaks. We will close by 5:00 p.m. or before each day so that evening plans can be respected. Should you need to be absent from any session due to an unforeseen circumstance, please let [clinical administrator] know as soon as possible [cell phone number provided].
- Please put all cell phones and pagers on vibrate and respond to critical calls outside the meeting room so as not to disrupt the rest of the group. [Clinical administrator] will receive any calls for you coming to the hotel and will contact you directly.
- Realizing that we all have different and valuable contributions to make to the group's learning and working together, let's ensure that everyone can feel comfortable both to respectfully voice thoughts and opinions and to respectfully respond to those of others. "Seek first to understand."
- Since individuals perceive information and learn differently, be willing to explore alternative methods of experiencing, learning, and working as a team. Some activities we will engage in will be very familiar to you; others may be very different from any training you have experienced in the past. . . . Be willing to engage in the unknown.
- Please make a commitment to provide honest and constructive feedback on a regular basis to the team that developed this fourteen-day program; that team is committed to being as flexible and accommodating as possible to make sure that this training is a valuable use of your time and energy. All ideas to improve these sessions on an ongoing basis are heartily encouraged.
- Let's agree that IT'S PERFECTLY ACCEPTABLE TO HAVE FUN WHILE WE'RE WORKING AND LEARNING. Life is too short to have it otherwise.

Throughout the program, a large board labeled Language/Lexicon was displayed in the room as the place for participants to post sticky notes containing terms that were unknown to them or whose meanings within a particular discipline or context they did not understand. This was critical since many terms were unfamiliar to members of different disciplines, while some that *seemed* familiar were actually given different definitions by the different disciplines. In order to speak the same language people could not assume that "hot," for example, meant the same in Chinese traditional medicine as it did in conventional biomedicine. A few sample terms added to the lexicon over the weeks included the following:

- *Qi* (pronounced "chee"): *In traditional Chinese medicine*, one of the basic substances that pervade the universe; a subtle influence or vital energy that moves through the body in specific channels (meridians), that is the driver of most physiologic processes, and whose proper balance is necessary for maintaining health.[5]
- *Physician*:—*In conventional medicine*, an MD and sometimes also a DO (doctor of osteopathy), but sometimes not, depending on individual opinion of the validity of osteopathic medical education; *in chiropractic and osteopathy*, an MD, a DO, or a DC (doctor of chiropractic); all are considered, and referred to as, physicians.
- *Chakras*: *In Hindu thought and yogic tradition*, energy centers aligned along the spine and connecting with energy

available from the cosmos; generally agreed to be seven in number; important to health and to spiritual development.[6]

- *Arthrodesis*: *In conventional medicine,* a surgical procedure to fuse a joint into a fixed position; limits joint mobility but may be effective in reducing pain from the affected area.
- *Heat*: *In conventional medicine,* the quality of being warm to the touch or to the internal perception of the patient; a fever will often produce a subjective feeling of heat to the person who has it and may be felt as heat on the person's forehead or other part of the body by a caregiver; *in many health systems derived from Asian, South Asian, Arabic, Spanish-speaking, and other cultures,* an essential or humoral quality within the body and also typifying foods and beverages, medicaments, symptoms, etc. Keeping an internal balance between hot and cold elements in the body is essential to good health and is a goal of many therapeutic interventions.

This short selection reflects both terms that are discipline-specific and some that are used across disciplines but have discipline-specific meanings. From the first training day the ongoing collection and documentation of these terms formed the basis of *conscious creation of a common language* with shared meanings and identified terms with multiple meanings and therefore with the potential for introducing misunderstanding or confusion into team discussions.

Creating a commonly usable and comprehensible language is an essential feature of teambuilding and good health care delivery: the entire team membership has access to the common language, as well as a basis for understanding and becoming familiar with specialized terms used by specific member disciplines. (This is presently a major impediment to true teamwork in inpatient medical settings, where physicians and nurses use very different terminologies, both by hospital policy and occasionally by law. The use of some medical terms constitutes diagnosis, a practice reserved to physicians by most states' medical practices acts. We include a fuller discussion of this issue in chapter 10.)

Terms collected on any given training day were returned to the group on the following training day, and their meanings, contexts of use, and potential for confusion were discussed. Participants quickly learned to clarify meanings by asking for brief explanations of unfamiliar terms as well as by requesting examples of specific usages: "Do you mean 'inflammation' like in conventional medicine or 'inflammation' as understood in acupuncture?" (An illustration of this kind of multiple meaning, and of the need to be very clear about the lexicon and aware of the contexts of terminology, occurred in the present-day clinic. A patient was seen by an OCC acupuncturist, who mentioned that his "qi [was] blocked in his liver." Accordingly, he came to the office of the OCC physician and medical director Donald Levy to request a lab order for liver function tests. They had a lively discussion about origins and contexts of language related to liver pathology.

Dr. Levy explained that even if the patient's qi was very much blocked in his liver [Chinese medical interpretation], his liver function tests [biomedical blood testing by a lab] would in all likelihood be normal. The differing conceptual frameworks of the two systems of explaining causal conditions and manifestations of illness generated very different levels of abstraction and understanding of what was happening that involved the patient's liver.)

Active and recurrent discussion of language and lexicon kept the concept of creation and mastery of a common language toward the forefront of participants' awareness as a feature of team development. The group also identified a need for all its members to become increasingly conversant with medical language and terminology. The clinic's success would depend in part upon communicating and successfully sharing medical records with both primary and subspecialty physicians outside the integrative clinic, who would make referrals to the clinic and receive patients from it. At the same time, this cumulative language-making process completely legitimized anyone's asking, during any presentation or discussion, some version of "I'm not familiar with that term. What does it mean?" This in turn helped to flatten the traditional status hierarchy of the participating clinicians' disciplines, since *everyone* was hearing unfamiliar terms fairly frequently.

In addition to the language/lexicon board, there was an "issues/reactions" board present at every training day where participants could post sticky notes expressing any thoughts, issues, or reactions to things said that had occurred to them during the day. They could identify themselves if they were comfortable doing that or ask questions anonymously. Facilitators collected these notes at the end of each training day and incorporated them into discussions at the next week's training session. At that time, if the group wished to pursue an issue further, it would decide where in the remaining curriculum schedule to raise the issue for group discussion and consensus formation. This introduced an important element of flexibility into the curriculum design that allowed participants to take increasing ownership of significant portions of their own developmental training—which again strengthened group identity and supported the sense of common purpose (team building for collaborative patient care).

Here is a selection of items that appeared on the issues/reactions Board, and that reinforced the desirable outcomes just mentioned:

Training Day (TD) 1: "Why is 'touchy-feely' a term of . . . disdain, even among health professionals who must *touch* their patients and take into account (their own and) their patients' *feelings*?" (emphasis in original). "How does it feel to the chiropractors to have so much concern expressed about (and restrictions placed on) cervical manipulation?"

TD2: "For patients with acute LBP [lower back pain], will MDs mind if the patient sees the acupuncturist prior to taking meds (anti-inflammatory)?"

TD3: "Many times we use technical terms, or initials of [organizations, syndromes, symptoms] or medications, etc. Please remind folks to explain, or [not to] assume everybody knows this terminology."

TD4: "Please limit sideline conversations about things that are important for the whole group to discuss; if there are dissatisfactions, worries, great ideas, etc., they need to come out before the whole group."

TD5: "During small group discussions, there are some members who have yet to express their thoughts. In many cases, the same few members are able to lead the group and interject their thoughts in an imbalanced fashion. Perhaps the small groups can make an effort to ensure that all are heard in an organic fashion."

TD7: "It seems to be (for the most part) that it is predominantly the MDs that sometimes arrive after the start of conference and/or are often absent later in the day, which I fear may send the message that MDs are somehow unique with respect to the value of their time. What is the effect of this message in forming our nonhierarchical working relationships?" [written by an MD]

TD10: "Perhaps we need to spend some time clarifying the treatment plan creation process? I can see using a small group format to get some consensus on this process."

The curriculum was designed to incorporate *briefings* at the beginning of each training day, as well as *debriefings and reflection* at the end of each day. The language/lexicon and issues/reactions boards (which came to be known collectively as the "big boards") provided some of the content for daily debriefings (issues) or for the next day's opening briefing (both categories). As the group continued to coalesce over the weeks, group-identified priorities also were noted as "issues" or were directly presented to members of the CPC so that the curriculum content could be modified as needed to incorporate group priorities or to discuss CPC- or group-identified roadblocks. Daily opening briefings introduced carryover issues from the previous session(s) and outlined the planned activities and discussions of the day, getting all participants on the same page before the day's activities began.

On the first day, team-building exercises started with preliminary development and articulation of a shared set of values. A story of a collective journey on a sailing vessel—through fair and foul weather, safe and treacherous waters—provided the framework for this activity. Everyone had been given a preliminary list of eighteen predefined values (e.g., fairness, friendliness, equality, hard work, and so on) on a worksheet listing the terms and some proposed definitions for each. Everyone was asked to assign priority numbers to their most important values, adding additional terms they felt were needed. Then a facilitator began to tell the story of the group's travels.[7]

The fictional journey was beset by a series of calamities. At each crisis point participants had to sacrifice three to five of their values in order to "save their own lives" and continue on the journey. (For example, halfway through the narrative, one's list might contain the values fairness, creativity, self-actualization, helping others, learning, expertise, challenge, patient-centeredness, pleasure/happiness, stability/security, respect/prestige, and health. Here, in the narrative, our ship runs aground and begins to sink. To secure a place in the lifeboats, each participant must throw out three of these twelve cherished items. Which three would go?) At the journey's end—a desirable utopian paradise—each participant could have only five remaining values with which to disembark, having been obligated along the way to continually pare down the list to his or her five absolute highest priorities.

In small groups participants discussed the values they had preserved, the order in which they had sacrificed their other values, and their personal reasons for making these choices. They brought back their discoveries to the plenary for further discussion. This outcome produced several interesting results:

1. Within small groups as well as in the plenary session, people were astonished to find how *little* they agreed about which values had priority and why (one small group reported that not one single value item was common to all six members' final lists). Almost all had assumed that as voluntary participants in the creation of a novel clinic based on a peer/teamwork model of care and incorporating CAM therapies, they would agree on almost everything.

2. Participants genuinely experienced how difficult it was to forfeit or even to negotiate about values they considered indispensable. This enhanced their understanding of how important it was to learn the process of negotiating common outcomes that all team members could support.

3. Participants discovered that they each had definitions of certain values that differed from one another as well as from the definitions provided on the worksheets, and they had to collectively decide how to respond to these incongruities. *Explicit articulation of shared values—and articulation of consensual meanings—was the first step toward clear and unambiguous communication and creation of a shared mental model, two necessary elements of teamwork.*

Discoveries and outcomes of the values exercise were later integrated into the team's work in formulating a values statement to underpin vision and mission statements for the future clinic and to serve as a touchstone for subsequent team decisions and actions ("Is this consistent with our stated values?").

The second phase of the curriculum shifted toward enhanced understanding of each discipline's techniques and practices, creation of an interdisciplinary patient assessment/referral/treatment model, and creation of specific work products, including beginning work on templates for each discipline to be incorporated into a single electronic medical record. The primary teaching and learning mode for this phase of the curriculum was experiential, with open-ended discussion and Q/A sessions. Over these weeks, participating clinicians were invited to experience one another's assessment and intervention techniques. Anyone might ask to experience any technique in the team's collective repertoire. Participation was voluntary; no one was pressed to submit to any therapeutic technique about which he or she had trepidations (as our participating neurologist observed at the time, "I'm sure nobody wants to volunteer to get a burr hole.").[8]

All choices to try or not to try a particular technique were respected, and observation and discussion of a colleague's experiences with the varied techniques encouraged others to try many of these over time. Personal experience of colleagues' specialized skills and techniques—for example, an MD experiencing acupuncture or craniosacral therapy for the first time or an acupuncturist experiencing a first-time chiropractic adjustment—also helped to

> **Values Statement**
>
> The mission and vision Statements of the [then tentatively named] Osher Integrative Care Center of [partner hospital at that time unknown] Hospital rest on a set of shared values which are reflected in our research, education, clinical structure, and everyday operations. Foremost among these are the following:
>
> • Balance in health, work, and life
> • Caring
> • Collaboration
> • Communication
> • Ethnic and cultural sensitivity
> • Evidence
> • Holism
> • Integrity
> • Joy in work and the workplace
> • Learning, adaptation, self-correction
> • Mindfulness
> • Mutual respect
> • Open-mindedness
> • Pluralism
> • Practitioners as healing instruments
> • Relationship (patients, colleagues, community)
> • Safe, effective, and comprehensive patient care
> • Self-care
> • Shared responsibility (patients, colleagues)

deepen respect for others' professional knowledge and skills and again to enhance the sense of team identity as clinicians began to formulate conceptions of how their colleagues might contribute to the management of shared patients.

At the same time (and with Institutional Review Board approval and formal consent procedures) clinicians began to identify patients in their individual practices whom they would like to invite to participate in the training sessions as "volunteer patients" to further the education of the clinician team and to contribute to the experiential/experimental development of a multidisciplinary assessment protocol and a set of recommendations for triage in the planned clinic. Over the final six weeks of the program, roughly half of each training day was devoted to meeting the volunteer patients and testing a variety of approaches to patient assessment.

Initially, for example, a volunteer chronic-back-pain patient, referred from the private practice of one of the participating clinicians, experienced a series of assessment and diagnostic encounters with each of three clinicians (each from a different clinical profession) in a "fishbowl" setting, in which all the remaining clinicians were observers. Following these assessments, the patient was escorted into another room while the clinicians discussed and reflected upon what they had observed and what they had thought about this patient and his problems and possible courses of treatment. These discussions included all the *multiple frames of reference* represented in the clinician mix and challenged and enlarged the thinking patterns of all participants. Following the wide-ranging clinician discussion period, the patient rejoined the group and the discussion and was invited to select two or three trial treatments he might like to try from among the disciplines present. Clinicians observed and discussed with the patient the sensations and effects of the trial treatments—often to their own amazement at his or her responses.

The precise formats of the volunteer patient sessions varied from meeting to meeting so that a range of possible approaches to patient assessment and treatment planning could be explored. These sessions always included a review of feedback and suggestions from all clinicians present as well as from the volunteer patients. Through these repeated and varied *simulations* of actual clinical experiences with actual pain patients who had real, typically chronic pain, the clinician team developed and refined a consensual ideal protocol and set of triage guidelines and role expectations for working together to assess and treat patients in the future clinic. They also began to lay the groundwork for future clinical research to test the multidisciplinary, integrative therapeutic approach to patient care.

About halfway through the curriculum, as the group's team identity and team intelligence increasingly began to coalesce and people moved collectively toward the more experiential phase of the program, a few of the physician (MD) participants began to express anxiety that in the new team-driven clinic, they would actually have very little to do and/or have very little importance. Their role, they began to feel, would be reduced to screening clinic patients for red flags such as signs of malignancy or other dangerous medical conditions, while the "real work" (and the "interesting work") of treating patients' pain would all be done by the CAM clinicians. This was a very important and valuable moment in the progress of the training and a crucial one to the success of the team model.

It is entirely understandable (in fact, to be expected) that participants who previously have held the highest status and professional autonomy will come to feel uncertain—even skeptical or distressed—about "who they will actually be" once a new model of collaboration and equivalence of status has been implemented. Physicians have been used to being the ones who make the decisions. But now, in crucial decision making, they would have a very different role. No wonder they worried about being valued—and about having a role they themselves could still value—in this new environment.

This is what often happens when a group—no matter what the setting or endeavor—begins to move toward greater role equality. Those who have enjoyed the highest status in the old way of doing things will be likely at some point to experience themselves as in some way becoming disadvantaged (literally "de-advantaged"), as having the most to lose in the new model. Rather than dismissing or discounting these fears, team creation requires that colleagues reassure *all* team members of their value *to* and *in* the team as a whole. Uneasy participants need to be supported so that they can discover and experience the contours and value of their emerging roles within a team—which will, by definition, be unfamiliar. The integrative clinician training curriculum therefore incorporated team-building exercises throughout its duration, from first day to last. These exercises were increasingly complex and clearly required the knowledge and input of all of us for a successful outcome.

WHAT HAPPENED NEXT

The OCC clinician education and teamwork training had taken place over fourteen weeks in the fall of 2003. Funding had been anticipated for immediate design and construction of the physical clinic space. During this time the clinician team had planned to continue working on logistical matters such as creating necessary forms, designing patient flow, and working on the electronic medical record. They had also planned to work on direct contributions to the architectural design of the clinical space in order to incorporate the specific needs of each of the clinicians and their professional practices. Unexpectedly, the anticipated funding fell through, and replacement funding had to be sought from both public and private sources—a lengthy and labor-intensive process.

It is a testament to the depth of commitment of the clinician team that a strong core of the group persisted during this unanticipated dry spell, which lasted for the better part of four years. During this period these clinicians continued to meet weekly to discuss patients and treatments, to cross-train with each other, to discuss complex cases—many of which they shared even in the absence of a physical integrative care center—and to enhance their shared fund of knowledge. They developed a rich internal referral network that they referred to as "the virtual clinic," whereby they shared patients and trialed treatments they could not themselves offer through their colleagues who could.

Along the way there was naturally some attrition as family and professional lives moved on to other demands, opportunities, and locations, but a core group continued to stick together and to meet at the offices of the Osher Research Center of Harvard Medical School, where the original training curriculum had been developed. During the latter months of the third year, another philanthropic gift from the Bernard Osher Foundation made construction of the clinic site a reality.

The clinician team persisted then with growing optimism through a lengthy maze of legal, political, and real estate negotiations that eventually led to the creation of the Osher Clinical Center for Complementary and Integrative Medical Therapies, a free-standing clinical entity within the Brigham and Women's Hospital (BWH) in Chestnut Hill, Massachusetts.

All OCC clinicians are hired and credentialed by the Brigham. The clinic opened its doors in August 2007, three years and eight months after the last formal team training day in December 2003. Of the thirteen clinicians currently practicing at the clinic, twelve, including Medical Director Donald B. Levy, MD (an internist and primary care physician), were participants in the original training curriculum. They continue to meet weekly, together with clinic staff members and interested practitioner colleagues from other BWH clinical settings, and have developed a monthly rotation of focal points for team meetings:

- Continuing education sessions (many delivered by team members as they continue to deepen their understanding of each other's practices and theories)
- Case conferences in which all are invited to contribute questions and suggestions pertaining to better understanding and treating patients
- Administrative refinements and responses to changes in the broader environment of the academic medical center and the national health care environment
- Research conferences that include reviewing recent research findings, developing research capabilities, and planning and implementing clinical research[9]

A LOOK BACK

Before the training program began, Bonnie, as ethnographer of the process of creating the team and the clinic, interviewed (among others) each of the clinicians slated to participate in the training and work in the future clinic. Many of these had also participated to varying degrees in the planning stages of the clinic and some in the curriculum development. One of the questions asked of each interviewee was, "What if it fails?"

To a person, their answers were, "It can't fail." One opined that "even coming this far is an amazing success." Another summed up the general sentiment best when he said, "It's impossible for this to be a failure. Even if the clinic never opens, this [process] has changed the way I'll think about my patients forever."[10]

Chapter 6

Workload Management

UNITED AIRLINES FLIGHT 232

Either you manage the situation or the situation manages you.

—*Captain Al Haynes, United 232*

On July 19, 1989, Captain Al Haynes was leading his crew on a flight from Denver to Chicago and then scheduled on to Philadelphia. There were 296 souls on board United Flight 232, and it was a clear summer day. The first hour of the flight was routine. Then, an hour and seven minutes after departure, during a shallow turn at thirty-seven thousand feet, a critical engine part disintegrated. The failure not only completely disabled the center engine but ultimately resulted in a loss of all hydraulic power, which crippled the half-million-pound aircraft. The NTSB report later identified "failure of UAL maintenance personnel to detect an existing fatigue crack resulting in catastrophic failure of the No. 2 engine" to be the root cause.[1] A metal processing defect during production of the titanium compressor disk evolved into a small crack, which then led to the failure of the part and ultimately the disintegration of the affected engine.

The destruction of the engine immediately severed all of the aircraft's hydraulic lines, essential for powering the rudder, elevator, and ailerons, all crucial to maneuvering the plane. The nearest suitable airport for an emergency landing was Sioux City, Iowa. In the thirty-four minutes before crash landing just short of the airport runway, the pilots had to devise a strategy to bring the plane under control, assess damage, choose a landing site, and prepare the crew and passengers for the crash. Although they had no hydraulics—and as a result, no flight controls—they managed to get the aircraft to Sioux City and save 185 lives. This in spite of the fact that, as Captain Haynes stated, "We've all been through a single system failure or double failures [in training], but never a complete hydraulic failure." No procedure had ever been developed to fit just this scenario, but the CRM training Haynes and his crew had undergone had taught them how to form the kind of team that managed to save most of the passengers from certain disaster.

That team consisted of three pilots and eight flight attendants. It turned out that there was a fourth DC-10 pilot on board, who happened to be deadheading on the aircraft. Shortly after the engine failure, the fourth pilot—Dennis E. Fitch, a United Airlines DC-10 instructor pilot and check airman—became aware of a mechanical "concern" and sent a note to the cockpit advising the captain of his presence and qualifications and offering assistance if needed. On behalf of a crew that was running short of ideas and options, Captain Haynes accepted Fitch's help and expertise. Haynes then led his pilot crew of (now) four to their new destination of Sioux City. One of the first actions he took after making sure that the aircraft was stable was to call the purser up to the cockpit to advise her of the situation and ask her to prepare the cabin for a crash landing. When Haynes describes the events of United 232, he gives great credit to the purser and her flight attendant crew for initially keeping the passengers calm and under control. This preparation allowed 185 people to survive a situation that by all accounts should have been deadly for everyone.

Orchestrating the actions of a crew in an unusual or emergency situation is a finely honed skill. Minute-by-minute analysis of the cockpit conversation revealed a group that became hyperorganized during this crisis. Their conversations contained a series of intense interactions—averaging thirty-one communications per minute (one per second at its peak). During these conversations, junior crew members freely suggested alternatives and the captain responded by welcoming that input. Bursts of social conversation provided emotional relief and support, enabling the crew to cope with what must have been extreme stress and to save the lives of 185 of the 296 people on board.

CRM training allowed the captain to deal with the emergent problem rather having to respond to the crisis *and* fly the airplane. Human-factors studies and NTSB accident reports confirm that this assures that a captain will make better decisions. Because he was not "task saturated," Haynes was able to maintain an awareness of the big picture; gather and process information, both cognitively and verbally; and utilize his experience and expertise as well as other people's suggestions. This accident was a classic case of communication and teambuilding in action. Captain Haynes clearly credits CRM training and creation of an effective team environment, in both the cockpit and the cabin, with avoiding disaster. As Haynes said later,

> The preparation that paid off for the crew was something that United started in 1980 called Cockpit Resource Management, or Command Leadership Resource

Training (CLR), or any number of things that you want to call it. I think we called it CLR to start with. All the other airlines are now using it. Up until 1980, we kind of worked on the concept that the captain was THE authority on the aircraft. What he said, goes. And we lost a few airplanes because of that. Sometimes the captain isn't as smart as we thought he was. And we would listen to him, and do what he said, and we wouldn't know what he's talking about. . . . We had 103 years of flying experience there in the cockpit, trying to get that airplane on the ground, not one minute of which we had actually practiced, any one of us. So why would I know more about getting that airplane on the ground under those conditions than the other three? So if I hadn't used CLR, if we had not let everybody put their input in, it's a cinch we wouldn't have made it.[2]

Although Haynes and his colleagues clearly put their communication and team-building skills to work, they also mobilized another CPI—workload management. During this thirty-four-minute emergency, someone had to fly the damaged plane and talk with air traffic control, the company, and flight attendants—who in turn had to talk to and calm passengers—as well as handle dozens of other tasks. If those communications and activities had not been well managed and if all involved had not been able to assess, strategize, prioritize, implement, and perform their work under the most trying circumstances, Haynes and his crew could not have succeeded as they did.

WHAT IS WORKLOAD MANAGEMENT?

Workload management is the implementation of a strategy to balance the amount of work with the appropriate time and resources available (right number of people—staffing). It includes making sure those people are alert and vigilant (preventing fatigue); figuring out who does what (delegation); teaching people how to manage interruptions (and to limit interruptions at critical moments); prioritizing tasks and avoiding task oversaturation; and avoiding pitfalls such as continuing a project, flight, or activity even when it's becoming clearer and clearer that it is dangerous to do so. Workload management in high-reliability industries also means doing all of the above *under stress*.

If we return for a moment to the United flight, imagine what would have happened if the captain had rejected the help of the deadheading pilot and the suggestions of subordinates, if Haynes had not briefed the flight attendants, if people had been too tired to think straight, or if there hadn't been enough people to pool their creative talents and ideas *or subordinates had been afraid to offer them.* (These patterns continue to occur in health care settings). CRM is meant to take full advantage of *all* individuals in the team, but it can do that only if tasks are effectively distributed. This means not leaving anything or anyone out but also not overloading people with conflicting signals, messages, orders, and duties.

THE GLASS COCKPIT MYTH

Getting a plane from here to there *always* involves workload management, but with steadily increasing reliance on automation since the early 1980s, workload management is more important than ever before. As airplane cockpits rely more and more on digital electronic instruments, LCD screens have replaced the traditional analog dials and gauges displayed on instrument panels—thus the name "glass cockpit."

American Airlines Flight 965, Cali, Colombia, December 20, 1995

This accident was a great example of how automation caused crew members to make a huge error very precisely. During the approach to the Cali, Colombia area, the crew received a clearance to fly directly to a navigational fix named ROZO. One of the pilots programmed the flight management system (FMS) to fly the aircraft directly to that fix. Unfortunately, the pilot put in the first letter of the fix—R—and like the texting feature on your cell phone, the computer automatically filled in the rest of the letters of the fix, based upon the aircraft's proximity to all fixes that started with the letter R.

As fate would have it, they were closer to a navigational fix named ROMEO than to ROZO, so the top choice on the FMS selection display was ROMEO, not ROZO, as the pilot had probably assumed. He apparently accepted the FMS's top choice without noticing the error, and the aircraft started an immediate turn to the left—directly toward ROMEO. Unfortunately, there was a mountain directly in their path, and the aircraft plowed into it minutes later while the pilots were trying to figure out what was going on.

From a workload management perspective, there were many lessons to be learned from Flight 965. Factors included distraction, fatigue, and stress, as well as improper automation management, which resulted in a very precise path to the wrong place.

A lot of people—including the creators of the concept of the glass cockpit—thought that the introduction of such automation would *reduce* the pilots' workload. The two-person cockpit eventually replaced the standard three-person crew, eliminating the flight engineer or second officer position. In fact, however, one of the more alarming unintended consequences of the introduction of the glass cockpit is that workload has arguably *increased* with these new technologies. Incorrectly managing workloads in critical situations can lead to catastrophe. Speaking on the topic of cockpit automation, Earl Wiener, PhD, a former Air Force Pilot turned human-factors researcher, states, "[A]utomated airplanes with the highest technologies do not eliminate errors. They change the nature of the errors that are made. For example, in terms of navigational errors, automation enables pilots to make huge navigational errors very precisely."[3]

When the second officer position was eliminated, designers and analysts also discovered that there were *more conflicts* between members of the new two-person crew than anyone had ever experienced in the traditional older aircraft. Initially no one could figure out why. Further investigation revealed that when this automated technology was first delivered, operators did not provide a "philosophy of automation" to go with it. Absent such guidance, an operational vacuum was created, which was then filled by individual bias and preferences for working in the new environment. On delivery of their first glass items, some operators assumed that the pilots would automatically utilize the new equipment to its maximum potential—meaning pretty much from takeoff to touchdown. In actual fact, many pilots came to fear "hand-flying" the aircraft—even though there are clearly many situations where turning the "magic" off would be the most appropriate mode of operation. (The pilots on Qantas flight QF-32 did this when they ignored confusing automated warning messages.) Other pilots—probably not so comfortable with computer technology—chose to do the opposite, reverting to flying the old-fashioned way, ignoring the automation in all but the most basic circumstances. Conflicts ensued over these variable responses. To deal with this, companies developed automation philosophies that were incorporated into their SOPs, along with clear definitions of who was expected to do what in specified circumstances.

When operating outside the strict parameters of the SOP or checklist—during an actual emergency—proper workload management is crucial. And this requires real team leadership. The team leader must do just what Captain Haynes did: take into account crew members' individual experience, abilities, and current workload when delegating duties. CRM training in routine situations also allows team members to prioritize tasks and manage their workloads in emergencies so that there is a successful outcome. In the course of hundreds if not thousands of routine flights, they have mastered the elements of workload management, together with communication and teamwork, and thus have largely avoided the kind of disorganization that characterized so many tragic accidents in the 1970s and 1980s.

ELEMENTS OF EFFECTIVE WORKLOAD MANAGEMENT

What is the linchpin of workload management? It is understanding how the brain works, what the job of the aviator and crew involves, and how the technology interacts with the human brain and aviation work environment. This allows the kind of regulations that make sure none of the above has a negative impact on safety.

Regulation

In health care, much energy is spent trying to ensure safety through a variety of voluntary measures. Various groups interested in safety—from the prestigious Institute of Medicine to the Joint Commission (TJC) and the Institute for Health Care Improvement (IHCI)—propose a number of such measures, many of which make sense and *some* of which are implemented by institutions and administrators of goodwill. The operative word here is "some." Most of these measures are not mandatory. One of the reasons why an estimated ninety-eight thousand people die each year in the United States because of medical errors and injuries is that when it comes to teamwork, workload, and hours, there is little regulation in health care and too much left up to individual or institutional whim. In aviation, leaving things up to individual whim, status, judgment, or perception was long ago recognized to be sheer folly. This is why, at the most basic level, workload management is implemented through regulation. Staffing levels, for instance, are clearly defined in the Federal Aviation Regulations for pilots and flight attendants.

Take the job of the flight attendant. Passengers mistakenly assume that the flight attendants' function is to serve them food and beverages; in fact, the cabin crew's primary function is to assure safety. (This is why the first flight attendants were required to be registered nurses.) The food and beverage service that flight attendants provide is strictly secondary to their duty of keeping passengers safe. Keeping people safe at thirty-six thousand feet is not easy—not when some of them have boarded after having a few too many and insist on having more in flight, when an altercation breaks out between two passengers, or when someone becomes very, very sick. Suzanne once witnessed a female passenger begin to get quite aggressive and abusive with the person in front of her on a packed flight. Suzanne was deeply impressed with the skills of the flight attendant, who managed to calm her down, move the irate passenger to a different seat, and make sure the woman didn't repeat her performance with her next seatmates.

Maintaining adequate staffing is crucial to allowing flight attendants to utilize their hard-earned skills effectively. A minimum of one flight attendant is required for every fifty passenger seats on an aircraft to assist passengers in the event of an emergency. This is not up to companies to determine but is mandated by the FAA. As one flight attendant at a major airline told Suzanne, "By regulation, we're required to have four flight attendants on this aircraft, because of the number of seats. The company used to have six. Over the past couple of years, it's gone down to four (the minimum), and I can assure you if it was up to the company and if there were no regulations, we'd have only one or two."

Pilot staffing is driven by similar constraints. Modern cockpits have two positions, captain and first officer (pilot and copilot). During critical phases of flight, it takes at least two people to accomplish tasks such as takeoff, departure, arrival, approach, and landing. Should both of the pilots become incapacitated, the plane will not land itself.

Fatigue Management

Fatigue is a constant challenge in this industry (and in this era of American work culture). Mitigating the negative impact of fatigue is the goal of requirements for respite between flights and numerous other work-hours regulations. Pilots and flight attendants, by the nature of their jobs, are working away from home, seeking adequate sleep in often unfamiliar sur- roundings, and regularly crisscrossing time zones on both national and inter- national flights. This is why fatigue management is critical to effective workload management in aviation. What airlines and unions representing airline personnel have recognized is what sleep researchers have been docu- menting over the past two decades: the fact that the fatigued individual is often the last to know—or realize—the ex- tent of his or her incapacity to perform at optimum levels. Fatigue, which re- sults from the combination of sleep loss and disruption of circadian rhythms, is insidious. Before they know it, consci- entious individuals may have dozed off. This is why fatigue has been estab- lished as a contributing cause in count- less aviation accidents. Colgan Air Flight 3407 (February 12, 2009) is a great example of a tragedy in which fatigue turned out to be a major factor.

Charles A. Lindberg made history in 1927 when, at age twenty-five, he became the first person to successfully com- plete a nonstop flight across the Atlantic. Determined to make the 33½-hour jour-

> ### Colgan Air Flight 3407
>
> All too often, people who are tired do not recognize just how exhausted they are or how fatigue is having a negative impact on their judgment and performance. This is what happened on February 12, 2009, when Colgan Air Flight 3407 crashed near Buffalo, New York, killing a total of fifty passengers and crew, as well as a person on the ground. The NTSB investigation determined that, among numerous causal factors, the "pilots' performance was likely impaired by fatigue."
>
> This determination was made after the NTSB discovered that the copilot had commuted in from her home on the West Coast earlier in the day, flying throughout most of the previous night. If she had gotten any sleep at all in the twenty-four hours prior to reporting to work, it was either in one of the aircraft jump seats or in the airline crew room, neither of which is conducive to normal rest. It was also estimated that the captain had been up for at least fifteen hours prior to their 9:20 p.m. departure from Newark, New Jersey.
>
> Apparently neither pilot realized the extent of their sleep deficit or the impact that it would ultimately have on their judgment and performance. Although the company had a written fatigue policy that allows crew members to essentially call in sick because of fatigue, both pilots chose to report to work, with dire consequences.

ney by himself, he refused to take a copilot. Without the benefit of an autopilot (a technology that had yet to be invented), Lindberg had to stay awake for the entire crossing or risk certain death by flying, unconscious, into the Atlantic Ocean below. Fatigue was ultimately Lindberg's greatest challenge. He writes, "My mind clicks on and off . . . I try letting one eyelid close at a time when I prop the other open with my will. But the effort's too much. Sleep is winning. My whole body argues dully that nothing, nothing life can attain is quite so desirable as sleep. My mind is losing resolution and control."[4] The famous Spirit of Saint Louis story had a positive out- come in the end, but Lindberg confessed that it was only luck that brought him through.

Our knowledge of the impact of lack of sleep has improved immensely since Lindbergh's famous flight. Research on the impact of sleep on brain function has produced literally hundreds of studies on what happens to the brain without adequate rest (typically defined as seven or eight hours of sleep per night).[5] A lot of fatigue research has been conducted for, or applied to, efforts to increase the safety of hospitalized patients by restricting the hours of the doctors-in-training who take care of them in teaching hospitals. To apply a quantifiable perspective to sleep deprivation, in 1997 the Australian sleep researchers Drew Dawson and Kathryn Reid compared the performance impairment resulting from fatigue with that caused by alcohol consumption.[6] They found that after a person has been awake for eighteen hours, mental and physical performance on many tasks is as impaired as if he or she had a blood-alcohol content (BAC) of 0.05. After being awake for twenty-three continuous hours, people perform as badly as those having a BAC of 0.12. Given that legal impairment for driving a motor vehicle in most jurisdictions is a BAC of 0.08 (some less—0.05 in Europe!), the detrimental effect of fatigue on performance could not be more evident.

In commercial aviation—and most other workplaces—just *reporting* for work under the influence of alcohol will result in certain termination of employment and probable regulatory action, including loss of license. Yet people in this and other safety-critical industries report for work without full rest as a matter of routine. Admittedly, this situation is difficult to avoid in aviation (as it is in medicine) under certain circumstances—such as international and "back side of the clock" operations.[7] Still, it is essential that we recognize the circumstances and presence of this threat and if it is ultimately unavoidable, that we limit the risk to the greatest extent possible.

Individuals bear the primary responsibility for managing fatigue. If a pilot or FA is scheduled for a late-night departure, he or she is supposed to ensure that he or she is well rested for the flight. Crew members are encouraged to communicate with their teammates if they aren't well rested (e.g., "I didn't sleep well last night, so please keep an eye out for me"). Regulations prohibit pilots from sleeping during the flight, even in low workload situations.[8] Regulations also limit work hours for pilots and flight attendants so that companies cannot put them in them in situations where they inadvertently cause harm. FARs delineate duty limits for flight attendants and pilots, depending upon the type of flying and other factors. For example, flight attendants may not be *scheduled* for duty to exceed fourteen hours in any twenty-four-hour period. FARs also require that if a flight is scheduled to last more than eight hours, a relief pilot must be provided.[9] If the flight will last more than twelve hours, two relief pilots must be on board to allow each crew member adequate rest. Such flights are required to provide adequate rest facilities for the off-duty crew members. Most "long-haul" aircraft have special compartments where off-duty crews can sleep.

At first, some passengers may be surprised to learn that part of their crew is napping on the job. Consider that they are not being paid to nap but rather to refuel their brains with rest so that when they resume their responsibilities, they can do so effectively and safely. The airline industry has been forced to face the reality that a central part of its machinery is human and therefore subject to human limitations. Just as fuel is required to propel an aircraft, sleep is required to propel human alertness. Rather than risking the possibility that fatigue may eventually disrupt a crew's alertness, regulators have faced the facts and mandated a solution.

Avoiding Continuation Bias

One of the characteristics that defines "professionals" who aspire to high-reliability/critical-outcome occupations is that they are goal-oriented. In other words, they are driven to complete their tasks. Sometimes they become so intent on finishing the job or getting where they're going that they fail to heed cues that suggest caution or modification—even abandonment—of the original mission. This result is what is described as continuation bias. Aviation accident archives are filled with situations where pilots pressed on under circumstances that screamed for them to stop. They continued, ignoring the cues, so hyperfocused that they failed to recognize the impending peril. The result was disaster.

For this reason, pilots and flight attendants are emphatically trained to identify continuation bias. Every pilot, early in his or her career, learns about a concept that we have all experienced in one form or another: the "get-home-itis" phenomenon. This sense of urgency was a major factor in the worst disaster in aviation history, the KLM/Pan Am crash in Tenerife. Get-home-itis is aptly named so that pilots and other crew members can recognize the condition and try to avoid it. You don't have to be a pilot to recognize continuation bias. We have all experienced situations where in spite of our better judgment, we trudge forward, driving when exhausted or through a blinding snowstorm, just because we want to get home. We may have really good reasons to persist—getting home to see a loved one, not disappointing a friend with whom we've made plans, meeting deeply felt work imperatives, or wanting to help out a colleague who has to take care of a sick child. Pilots are taught early on to base their planning decisions on rational, logical criteria rather than on that urgent desire to just get home.

Following Standard Operating Procedures

We've talked a lot about SOPs throughout this book. They are an essential supporting element in workload management. SOPs standardize the approach to specific procedures, eliminating the danger of ambiguity and personal preferences regarding how a task is to be performed. Aircraft manufacturers publish operating manuals that provide the same or a similar function, but they are more generic in nature and limitations are based upon certification criteria, which may be far outside the operational capabilities, scope, or desires of the individual operating company.

Recall the prior discussion of technology and automation. It was not until operators designed a clear and focused automation *philosophy* followed by an effective SOP that the real benefits of this new technology were finally realized. SOPs delineate tasks by position: captain, copilot, pilot flying, pilot monitoring, and relief pilot (RP), if one is assigned. For automation management, tasks are further broken down by whether the PF has the autopilot on or off. This could be confusing, except that the SOPs are designed around the company's automation philosophy, which is clearly written to make intuitive sense to its flight crews.

One primary aim of SOPs is to make sure someone is always flying the airplane. This may seem to be so obvious that it isn't even worth mentioning, yet we've seen (think back to Eastern Flight 401 in the Everglades) how easily pre-CRM pilots sometimes forgot the simplest tasks during an emergency. Other pilots may be monitoring or handling various other parts of the emergency. The purser and flight attendant will have their own duties. But the SOP will clearly define who is responsible for what in each role, and duties are further allocated according to the level of automation in use. For example, when a pilot is hand-flying (low to no level of automation) the aircraft, the PM will set assigned headings, altitudes, and airspeeds into the flight management system (FMS). The PF backs up these actions and then concentrates on flying the aircraft to the assigned parameters. However, when the PF has turned "control" of the aircraft over to the automation, he or she is now in control of the FMS.

Following Checklists

The airline checklist has become the best-publicized component of the aviation safety process to be transferred into health care. In 2009 the New York surgeon and writer Atul Gawande popularized the concept of checklists in his best-selling book, *The Checklist Manifesto*. The book describes the use of airline-like checklists in hospitals.[10] One of the heroes of the book was Peter Pronovost, an intensive care physician at the Johns Hopkins School of Medicine. In

---

Northwest Airlines Flight 255, August 16, 1987

On August 16, 1987, Northwest Airlines Flight 255, a McDonnell Douglas MD-82, roared down the runway at Detroit Metro Airport toward its planned destination of Phoenix, Arizona. The aircraft carried 149 passengers and a crew of six. After rotation at approximately 170 knots, the aircraft rolled inexplicably from side to side, suddenly stalled, rolled 40 degrees to the left, and struck a light pole on the departure end of the runway, tearing off part of the wing and igniting a full load of fuel. The aircraft crashed inverted on Middlebelt Road, killing two motorists and all but one of the passengers and crew on board the aircraft. The only survivor was a four-year-old girl who lost her entire family in the crash.

The NTSB probable cause statement included the following: "The National Transportation Safety Board determines that the probable cause of the accident was the flightcrew's failure to use the taxi checklist to ensure the flaps and slats were extended for takeoff."

2010 Pronovost wrote his own rendition of the story in his book *Safe Patients, Smart Hospitals: How One Doctor's Checklist Can Help Us Change Health Care from the Inside Out*.[11] Although these books are very important, if they are to produce actual teamwork, it will be crucial that they not become part of the kind of heroic medical narrative we will discuss further in a later chapter. It would be really tragic were these books to transform the lone heroic physician who used to battle disease and death into the lone heroic physician engaged in a battle against unsafe care. In order to assure that this doesn't happen and that physicians and hospitals do not voluntarily pick and choose what aspects of the aviation safety movement they might find useful and convenient to follow and neglect or discard the rest, we pause here a moment and consider how checklists are used in aviation.

In contemporary aviation people live by checklists and die without them. It's that simple. In fact, it is because a number of people *did* die that checklists were pioneered in the 1930s. On October 30, 1935, at Wright Field in Dayton, Ohio, three aircraft companies, Boeing, Martin, and Douglass, were competing for a contract for long-range bombers. With its Model 299, Boeing seemed to be the leader of the pack and was convinced it would receive an order of up to 220 airplanes—if, that is, it successfully demonstrated its plane's superiority in a test flight. Five people were in the plane as it took off that day. Two of them were army pilots, Major Ployer Hill in the left seat and copilot Donald Putt. Boeing's chief test pilot, Leslie Tower; a Boeing mechanic; and a representative of the engine manufacturer were also in the plane. Although the taxi and takeoff went well, the plane suddenly stalled, veered over on one wing, and then plummeted, exploding in flames as it hit the ground. The pilots and passengers were badly burned, and two, including Hill, later died.

The investigation of the accident revealed that Hill was unfamiliar with that particular plane, never having flown in one before, and hadn't released the elevator lock before taking off, as he should have. Tower tried to release the handle, but by then it was too late, and the aircraft crashed. It appeared that the Model 299 was now dead, but Boeing's pilots and engineers were certain their design was superior to their competitors':

> The pilots sat down and put their heads together. What was needed was some way of making sure that everything was done; that nothing was overlooked. What resulted was a pilot's checklist. Actually, four checklists were developed—takeoff, flight, before landing, and after landing. The Model 299 was not "too much airplane for one man to fly," it was simply too complex for any one man's memory. These checklists for the pilot and co-pilot made sure that nothing was forgotten. With the checklists, careful planning, and rigorous training, the twelve aircraft managed to fly 1.8 million miles without a serious accident. The U.S. Army accepted the Model 299, and eventually ordered 12,731 of the aircraft they dubbed the B-17.[12]

More than seventy years later, checklists are *not* a choice in aviation. Going through the various checklists at the appropriate phases of a flight is nonnegotiable. In the climate for teamwork the role of the captain is running the checklists and helping others run theirs. Adhering to checklists and making sure others—including the captain—also adhere to them is also a duty of each team member. If a team member—a first officer or FA—realizes that checklists have not been adhered to, it is part of the IAA (inquiry, advocacy, assertion) mandate to inquire why not and to advocate for and assert the necessity of fulfilling that particular SOP. This is not voluntary but required by regulation.

On the face of it, nothing could be more commonsensical than a checklist. Even in normal, day-to-day flight operations, the number of tasks required by each crew member—to be performed in a specific sequence—is truly astounding. Checklists are the only way to ensure that the critical items are done. And this is just in the normal course of a routine flight.

Now consider what happens when things go wrong. Crews are trained that even in spite of their instincts or the pressure of the emergency, they absolutely *must* follow the checklist and follow it in the exact order in which it is written to make certain that they properly address the emergency. Many organizations use certain "memory items" that crews are expected to know in response to time-critical situations. One major airline had a fairly simple emergency checklist philosophy: recognizing that any emergency would raise the stress level as well as the potential for making a bad situation worse by rushing into a solution, the airline's policy was that the first step in any crisis was to first fly the airplane and then assess the situation. Pilots jokingly rendered the first step in the Emergency Checklist ("Step 1: Fly the Airplane.") as "Don't just do something—sit there!" They had only one memory item checklist; everything else was to be dealt with after consulting the expanded written checklist.

Some instructors will advise students that the first step in any emergency is to simply "start the clock"—meaning start the timer or stopwatch, an integral part of every cockpit. By doing this, they are able to satisfy that initial instinctive impulse to DO SOMETHING! Starting the clock is also a very practical way to proceed during a period when the sense of time may be influenced greatly by one's adrenal response.

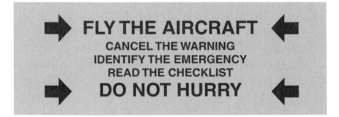

Figure 6.1. Example memory checklist

DESCENT	
PM	**PM**
Altimeters . . . . **(BOTH)** ____, **xckd**	
■ **Radio/baro minimums** . . . . **(BOTH)** ____, **xckd**	
■ V_{APP} . . . . **(BOTH)** ____, **xckd**	
■ **Approach briefing** . . . . **complete**	
■ **Autobrakes** . . . . **as reqd**	
Seat belts sign . . . . **ON**	
Exterior lights . . . . **set**	
ECAM status . . . . **ckd**	
■ **Allowable landing weight** . . . . **ckd**	

Figure 6.2. Sample A-330 descent checklist

Experience has proven that checklists are the only way to be absolutely certain that a particular job is done. They are designed to accomplish specific tasks in a certain manner and logical sequence and to maximize the efficiency and effectiveness of the resources at hand. They are deliberately simple yet comprehensive. Seeing a typical checklist, most people would not realize the amount of planning, deliberation, assessment, and testing that lies behind it. Checklist discipline has a profound influence on checklist effectiveness. Most checklists are intended as a "challenge-response" tool executed between two people. If communication is to be effective, the checklist must have simple, consistent language, and its challenges and responses must be exact so as to reduce the chance of ambiguity or confusion.

Another procedural checklist is shown above. Checklists are always utilized in the context of the other CPIs and not as a substitute for them.

Although the use of checklists and SOPs is at the heart of CRM, there are exceptions, as in the case of Qantas Flight 32, discussed in chapter 2. In this instance, the pilots avoided tragedy by wisely deciding to ignore certain computer-generated messages and use checklists selectively and relying instead on their own judgment and understanding of the situation. Likewise, in the case of US Airways Flight 1549, Captain Chesley Sullenberger did not have time to complete all his checklists before deciding to land in the Hudson. Although it might seem to contradict the message that checklists aren't optional, in fact the airlines, the FAA, researchers, and pilots all recognize that there will be situations in which the unexpected happens and captains and their crew will need to use their best judgment, skill, and expertise and if necessary deviate from the rules to resolve a problem. Deciding when to bypass the checklist or SOP is in fact encoded in airline practice by the concept known as captain's authority.

Managing Task Saturation

One of the reasons checklists are so important in high-risk situations is that they help human beings deal with the one of the hazards of operating in a very complex environment such as aviation (or health care)—task saturation. Task saturation is defined as having too many tasks to attend to realistically at any one moment. In aviation, task saturation can lead a pilot or other crew member to miss important inputs or cues in a dynamic and rapidly evolving situation.

There are basically two causes of task saturation. The first is *information overload*. You're in the air, in an emergency, and the sheer mass of sensory inputs overwhelms the human brain's ability to sort and comprehend. The second type is slightly more complicated and occurs when we fail to adequately prioritize inputs—usually because we're in a panic. What we may do in this panicked state is unwisely—and unnecessarily—bounce between important and unimportant tasks. If we eventually recognize that this is happening, we may still tend to remedy the situation by trying to focus attention on something, sometimes anything. The problem is that when we become task-saturated we quickly lose perspective. And this "I've gotta stop messing around and do something" attitude, which is referred to as "channelized attention," may lead us to select the one thing that is the very worst thing we could be doing. This is the number one human performance factor associated with loss of situational awareness, and it can result in a breakdown of procedural discipline.

So how does one avoid task saturation and the loss of situational awareness? In a nutshell: workload management. Safety experts recognize that in such a situation it is essential to concentrate on only the *critical* tasks at any given time. The lower-priority things can be dealt with later on. It's up to the captain, who has been well briefed in the perils of task saturation, to assess what needs to be done, articulate a vision that will help crew members do it, model nonpanicked behavior, distribute tasks effectively, and consistently monitor and repeat aloud what is and is not a priority.

The importance of *timing* as it relates to workload management and task distribution cannot be overstressed. Military fighter pilots joke about their mission, lightheartedly characterized as "hours and hours of boredom, punctuated be moments of sheer terror." Similarly, the majority of risk in commercial aviation occurs during only a small portion of the flight. Fifty-one percent of accidents occur during the final approach and landing phase, which occupies only 4 percent of the total time of a given flight.[13]

It is important to remain situationally aware and to recall that certain phases of the mission are much more subject to potential task saturation than others.

Workload and task distribution are also dependent on the captain's conduct, standards, and receptiveness. We now know that the captain, like anyone else, can become overwhelmed, task-saturated, or confused or may even be just plain wrong. CRM teaches that it is OK for a subordinate who may have a better grasp on the situation to speak up—even take control if necessary. This is a very delicate situation, but a truly engaged copilot or flight attendant will be proactive in trying to restore order when a situation has become chaotic.

Stress Management

In its publication "STRESS . . . At Work," the National Institute for Occupational Safety and Health (NIOSH) distinguishes between jobs that are challenging and jobs that are stressful:

> Job stress can be defined as the harmful physical and emotional responses that occur when the requirements of the job do not match the capabilities, resources, or needs of the worker. Job stress can lead to poor health and even injury.
>
> The concept of job stress is often confused with challenge, but these concepts are not the same. Challenge energizes us psychologically and physically, and it motivates us to learn new skills and master our jobs. When a challenge is met, we feel relaxed and satisfied. Thus, challenge is an important ingredient for healthy and productive work. The importance of challenge in our work lives is probably what people are referring to when they say, "a little bit of stress is good for you." Stressful work is not.[14]

There is a direct relationship between increased challenge and increased performance. Challenges put our minds and bodies on alert and sharpen our focus. A challenge is thus something we view as an opportunity, not a threat. Stress, on the other hand—and particularly unremitting stress—is very bad for you, as Robert Sapolsky explains in his excellent book *Why Zebras Don't Get Ulcers*.[15] Unlike zebras, human beings ruminate on stress. This can lead to all sorts of mental and physical problems. Job stress, we know, increases the risk of depression, cardiovascular disease, and a lot of other unpleasant health problems, as well as suicide. And it can lead to disaster in a cockpit, because *poorly managed work stress makes it impossible to train one's full attention on managing an emergency effectively.*

One of the most dangerous problems with operational stress in the cockpit is the way it can combine with the feelings of personal invulnerability that many pilots seem to have. NASA studies have shown that, prior to CRM training, most pilots believed

- their decision making was as good in emergencies as in normal situations;
- a true professional could set aside personal problems at work;
- their performance was not affected by personal problems;
- they did not make more errors under high stress;
- fatigue didn't materially affect their decision making.

All of these have proven, through research, to be *false!*

Unfortunately, those imbued with a sense of invulnerability are less likely to feel the need for countermeasures against error and most likely to fail to value the support and input of other crew members. Perceived invulnerability may lead to a disregard for safety measures, operational procedures, and teamwork. *Moreover, this attitude is easily sensed by other crew members and creates barriers to effective communication and the important exchange of information about how to resolve operational difficulties*—all of which are *essential to the safe outcome of the flight.* This is why it's critical to help pilots recognize the effects of stress and train them to manage stress by doing the following:

- Maintain a positive emotional or "team" climate.
- Recognize symptoms of stress in themselves and others.
- Maintain checklist discipline and compliance with SOPs.
- Manage low stress times to prevent complacency or lack of attention.

FLIGHT 1549: WORKLOAD MANAGEMENT IN PRACTICE

This chapter began with a description of United Flight 232. This accident, although tragic in its loss of life, was much less tragic than it might have been, largely because of effective workload management. Flight 232 is also known as the event that indisputably legitimized the investment in time and resources that had been committed to CRM training—which was, at that point, nine years along. Perhaps the most impressive example of workload management to be produced by CRM was the ditching of US Airways flight 1549 in the Hudson. We look more closely here at how workloads were managed during this incident.

US Airways Flight 1549, discussed in the introduction, capped a thirty-year commitment that the airline industry had made to CRM training. From a workload management perspective, it showed what can be done when teams prepare, rehearse, and execute their skills to the point that dealing with a crisis becomes second nature.

The now legendary Miracle on the Hudson reinforces many of the lessons of CRM. As in the case of UA Flight 232, the successful outcome of Flight 1549 was the result of CRM, specifically its focus on effective teamwork and workload management. To recap, about a minute and a half after taking off on a scheduled flight from New York to Charlotte, North Carolina, the aircraft struck a flock of Canada geese during its initial climb-out, disabling both engines, and was forced to ditch in the Hudson River. All 155 occupants safely evacuated the airliner, which was still virtually intact—though partially submerged and slowly sinking—and were quickly rescued by nearby watercraft. In the three minutes and twenty-eight seconds between the bird strike and the landing, Captain Sullenberger and First Officer Skiles had to prioritize tasks precisely and immediately or risk losing control of the aircraft and certain disaster.

From day one, every pilot—without exception—learns the following three basic steps in order of priority:

- Aviate (fly the airplane).
- Navigate (know where you are and where you are going).
- Communicate (*only* after steps one and two are under control, *talk*).

Jet aircraft are designed, in part, around the power-plant technology available at the time they go to the drawing board. They do a really great job flying when the engines are intact and operating normally. As a glider, a commercial jet doesn't do so well. The sudden, unexpected transition from powered to nonpowered flight must have been disorienting, if not completely terrifying, for the pilots of Flight 1549. There were literally hundreds of decisions to be made and tasks to be performed in only 208 seconds—all to be done while "keeping the blue side up" (aviation jargon for keeping the airplane flying, with the sky above and the earth below).

The discipline required to keep the priorities straight (aviate, navigate, communicate) *and* do everything else—run checklists and weigh alternatives in a rapidly changing situation (landing options would be changing continuously as the airplane transitioned vertically and horizontally through space)—was impressive, to say the least. It would have been easy for the pilots to panic and become task-saturated by the sheer volume of activity.

The writer Mike Singer attended one of Sully's talks on Flight 1549 and was particularly interested in how he had dealt with task saturation:

> The question I wanted to ask Sully was this: "Was there a point during the 208 seconds before you hit the water when you were so task-saturated that your brain overloaded, you panicked, started praying, and basically just hoped for the best?" I didn't have to ask, because he obviously gets this question a lot. "My pulse shot up," he told us. "My blood pressure shot up. My perceptual field narrowed because of the stress. And I had to really actively compartmentalize and focus and force that distraction away, and just concentrate on the task at hand. So I forced calm on myself and then I imposed order on the situation."[16]

This is a very insightful explanation of how one pilot very successfully dealt with the risk of task saturation. The implications of what he said are profound: If you don't allow an overwhelming number of things into your awareness, then by definition you can't be overwhelmed. In other words, you *can* control what gets into your awareness.

This does not come about by chance. Hours upon hours of simulator training teach crews to deal with numerous and compounded emergency situations. Although pilots routinely practice for hundreds of predicaments, they can't cover them all. But equally as important as rehearsing specific critical emergencies such as "V1 cuts"—if not more so—is learning to deal with crises as a team.[17] The dynamic sequence, rhythm, and flow of the crew acting as a team are fostered and reinforced through countless hours "in the box."[18] This intensive training teaches them to work through expected and *unexpected* problems *as a team* and to manage their workload by prioritizing tasks to take care of what needs to be done first and shedding the items that are not critical, considering the time available.

Captain Sullenberger, FO Skiles, and flight attendants Doreen Welsh, Donna Dent, and Sheila Dail had never rehearsed this particular scenario and certainly didn't see this one coming. Nevertheless, they rapidly coalesced into an effective team that took a very bad situation and managed it to bring it to the best conclusion available, given what they had to work with. They managed the situation rather than letting the situation mange them!

Chapter 7

Case Study

INTERPROFESSIONAL EDUCATION AND PRACTICE AT THE UNIVERSITY OF TORONTO

Interprofessional education (IPE) and interprofessional care (IPC) have become the new mantras of health care in North America and many other parts of the world. In the United States, educational accrediting bodies like the Accreditation Council for Graduate Medical Education (ACGME) and other health care professional education organizations are requiring some form of interprofessional education. The Macy Foundation has funded over thirty projects in interprofessional education and practice in the United States. The university in which Suzanne teaches—the University of Maryland Baltimore—has just launched an ambitious IPE initiative. In Canada, as we shall see in this case study, a nationally financed health care and educational system creates more integration between interprofessional education and practice, and thus both are more advanced than in the United States. Although many Canadian universities have impressive IPE/IPC initiatives, this case study focuses on the University of Toronto.

MORE THAN LEARNING TOGETHER

For more than a century, health care professionals—like pilots—have been taught to fly solo. Nurses, doctors, pharmacists, and other professionals may not have practiced in the kind of extreme solitude experienced by the French aviator and author Antoine de Saint Exupéry when he was delivering the mails or Patrick when he was a navy jet fighter pilot. There have always been other actors on the health care stage. But though they were certainly visible, they were—at best—only virtual members of a potential health care team. In reality, as Suzanne has described them, they functioned largely as intimate strangers engaged in parallel play at the patient's bedside.

To remedy this problem, the University of Toronto, several of its educational centers, and its thirteen teaching hospitals comprising the Toronto Academic

Health Sciences Network (TAHSN) have worked to create an interprofessional education and care program to teach students the skills necessary to work in interprofessional and interoccupational teams. IPE and IPC programs in Toronto involve conducting research that helps people understand team functioning in health care; developing curriculum and teaching tools that introduce health professional students to numerous opportunities to learn with, from, and about other health care professional students. Unlike many educational programs that are trying to move their students outside of their traditional professional silos by having them learn together in a classroom, for example, real interprofessional education focuses on far more than putting students in different disciplines in the same space or asking them to master a particular subject or integrate particular information into their practice. Real interprofessional education, as Reeves and Oandasan define it, involves "occasions when two or more professions learn from and about each other to improve collaboration and the quality of care."[1] Interprofessional education also involves developing and training the kind of faculty and professional staff who can serve as mentors and role models in the health care workplace. This latter effort is perhaps most important of all, since it reinforces the lessons students have learned and encourages them to change their own behaviors, attitudes, and expectations about how they practice when they move from classroom to workplace.

HISTORY

Although many Canadian health care professionals, educators, and researchers had long been interested in promoting interprofessional education and practice, their efforts got a huge boost after the "Romanow Report on Building on Values: The Future of Health Care in Canada" was released in 2002.[2] The Commission on the Future of Health Care in Canada, led by Roy J. Romanow, considered the health of Canada's Medicare system. One of its key recommendations was the creation of initiatives that would promote interprofessional education for collaborative patient-centered practice (IECPCP). The Canadian federal government took on this challenge by setting aside millions of dollars to fund IECPCP initiatives in Canadian schools of medicine, nursing, pharmacy, dentistry, and other health professions. In Ontario the government later added to that federal effort by setting aside money—to the tune of $20 million a year for three years—to fund both interprofessional education and interprofessional practice.[3]

Educators and researchers at the University of Toronto and its affiliated teaching hospitals were particularly well placed to take advantage of this new interest in IPE/IPC. The university and several of its teaching hospitals have long had unusual extradepartmental units that work in partnership with both the university and a teaching hospital affiliated with it. Two of these are the

Centre for Interprofessional Education and the Donald R. Wilson Centre for Research in Education; the latter is directed by Brian Hodges, a psychiatrist who is also vice president for education at the University Health Network and Toronto Rehabilitation Institute, which merged in 2009. "Interprofessional education and care in Toronto has benefited from something that a lot of health professional faculties and hospitals lack," Brian Hodges explains. "That is good relationships that take advantage of and combine mutual interests. The hospitals we work with are interested in patient outcomes, quality of care, and the patient experience. The university is interested in the student experience, the quality of education, and teaching. We have brought these interests together in research at the Wilson Centre and curriculum development, innovation and professional development at the Centre for Interprofessional Education. The Centre for Faculty Development has also been involved in this effort."

Researchers at the Wilson Centre have long studied IPE and IPC, exploring such things as when, in their developmental cycle, students from different disciplines should begin working together. As Hodges explains,

> If you force students together before they have a strong professional identity or bring them together when they already have a strong identity the results are very different. You need a different approach when you bring people together early in the identify formation process rather than later and vice versa. If you don't understand this, you risk simply reinforcing the hidden curriculum. You also have to help people understand that when people communicate effectively, it's not just about being nice. It's hard work that centers around creating effective practices.

In 2009 the university established the Centre for Interprofessional Education as a partnership between the university and two of its teaching hospitals—the Toronto Rehabilitation Institute and the University Health Network (made up of Toronto General, Toronto Western, and Princess Margaret Hospitals)—with a formal mandate to work at the interface of education and care. This approach is unique when contrasted with most other IPE programs worldwide that focus solely on curriculum and not the health care sector. "A joint hospital/university center with a focus on creating new models of interprofessional teaching, learning, and care was seen as having tremendous potential to transform health education and health care, ultimately changing the experience and outcomes of patients served by collaborative teams," explains its director, Maria Tassone, who was trained as a physical therapist.

As Susan Wagner, a speech language pathologist, coordinator of clinical education and senior lecturer in the Department of Speech-Language Pathology, and Faculty Lead, Curriculum, at the university's Centre for Interprofessional Education elaborates, "Before the publication of the Romanow Report, IPE had only limited appeal to many deans and professors in health sciences faculties." Although

Wagner and a number of her colleagues had created an IPE program in the rehabilitation sciences through the late 1990s and early 2000s that drew in students
from occupational therapy (OT), physical therapy (PT), and speech language pathology, it was difficult to move what was a very successful model to other health
professional schools. Then came the Romanow Report and with it, finally, serious
interest—and more important, serious money—to fulfill a mandate to actually
promote IPE.

CURRICULUM DEVELOPMENT

A group involved in IPE at Toronto got together in 2004 after Health Canada (a
federal agency dedicated to helping Canadians maintain and improve their heath
that funds programs to enhance health status in Canada) put out its first call for
IPE grants. Lynne Sinclair, a physical therapist, assistant professor of physical
therapy at the University of Toronto, past associate director of the Centre for IPE,
and past director of, education at Toronto Rehab, recounts the process that began
after the release of the Romanow Report:

> Our dean of medicine, Catherine Whiteside, gathered a group of us to get together
> to dream about what kind of interprofessional education and care was needed for
> Canada and Toronto, and we put in a grant proposal and were awarded a $1.2 mil-
> lion grant, which is quite substantial for Canadian funding. Later we were
> awarded a number of grants from HealthForceOntario—including one large grant
> of $3.4 million and later a half-a-million-dollar grant to develop a collaborative
> change leadership program.

The original Health Canada grant was targeted at the practice setting. In order
to eventually build a curriculum, its designers needed to know what was happening in the health care workplace and in the larger Canadian health care system.
Only then could they understand how to design programs to train future professionals. "Because we got such a big grant," Sinclair comments, "it showed the university and hospitals that this is important. We need to pay more attention to this.
This provided the impetus for a serious effort at curriculum change and program
design for teaching students."

In 2006 the University of Toronto's Council of Health Sciences made up of the
deans of the various health science programs formed an Office of Interprofessional Education at the university, headed by Ivy Oandasan, a family practice
physician and international scholar in IPE. After the Health Canada grant, the
university also got a provincial Ministry of Training Colleges and Universities
grant, which helped to fund the development of an IPE curriculum. In 2007–8,
representatives from each of the ten health science programs (there are now
eleven programs) met to create a competency-based longitudinal curriculum that

is woven into the experience of students from each professional health sciences faculty. These include students in dentistry, medical radiation sciences, medicine, nursing, occupational therapy, pharmacy, physical education and health, physical therapy, physician assistant programs, social work, and speech language pathology. The curriculum centers on the development of a set of core competencies framed around three constructs, values and ethics, collaboration, and communication.

The core competencies informed the creation of the learning activities and curriculum, which consist of four core and a number of elective sessions, now numbering more than eighty. These include case studies, patient panels, and team meetings, among other activities. Teaching students in multiyear programs means that the core competencies are threaded across the different stages of the students' educational journey— first exposure (introduction), immersion (development), and competence (entry into practice) of the students' educational

Three Constructs of Core Competencies of Interprofessional Education
1. Values and ethics
• Relation-centeredness
• Diversity sensitivity
• Interdependence
• Creativity/innovation
2. Collaboration
• Interprofessional theory
• Context and culture of the health care system
• Roles and responsibilities, accountabilities, and scope of practice
• Decision making/critical thinking
• Performance as an effective team—flexibility, cooperation, contribution, organization/efficiency, team health maintenance
• Change
• Proaction
3. Communication
• Listening
• Giving and receiving feedback
• Sharing information effectively
• Common language
• Dealing with conflict

journey. As they become competent, the hope is that students entering the clinical setting will establish a solid foundation upon which to build interprofessional practice in the context of what Wagner, Tassone, and her colleagues refer to as relational-centered care (which they explain is not the same as what is commonly referred to as patient-centered care.) Wagner explains that a "family practice physician who has an excellent relationship with the patient/client but has no contact with the social worker, the nurse, the dentist, the occupational therapist, and all the other individuals the patient/client is seeing for their health may have great patient/client-centered care. She or he, however, will be missing the wealth of information that others can contribute because of a lack of communication and collaboration with these team members who are also important for the patient/client."

Tassone, Wagner, and others at the Centre for IPE are careful to explain that the term "interprofessional" is defined more broadly than it is in programs in the United States and abroad. When the Toronto program uses the term it does not signify people only in the classic health professions but anyone working in health care facilities who has the potential to impact patient care. "For example," Wagner says, "to be a member of the team it is not necessary to be a regulated health professional. Someone who empties the wastebasket in a facility may be a part of the team and have valuable information."

As they move from exposure to competence through a series of learning activities, students and curriculum are then assessed and evaluated. This is not easy, Wagner points out, because the Centre for Interprofessional Education does not in fact have any students. Students come from a variety of programs and schools, each of which has its own evaluation and grading criteria. In spite of the difficulties, the IPE curriculum has included both an assessment and evaluation arm with leads for each. Again, the group at Toronto makes a distinction between assessment and evaluation. Assessment would include something like a test that focuses on individuals, while evaluation is broader, applying to the whole program or curriculum.

All this planning has influenced the learning activities that have been carefully designed both for students and for those who will shape students' education and future practice. This means not simply academic faculty but the faculty who will teach students in the clinical environment. Starting in 2007, students in many of the health professional schools at the university began to take part in a variety of learning activities that occur throughout the multiple years of their programs. Trying to figure out which activities occur in which year has not been easy since different schools have programs of different lengths.

In addition to the introductory session, each student will get all four of the core learning activities but at different times. The term "learning activities"—rather than "IPE courses"—is a deliberate one. The IPE program would never have gotten off the ground if its developers had tried to convince eleven different schools (both undergraduate and graduate)—each with a very packed set of courses—to add yet another course, one called IPE, to its list. To get around this problem, the planning group created learning activities that are integrated into each school in a different way.

For health professional students at the University of Toronto, their first exposure to IPE occurs one month after they get to school, when all 1,250 assemble together for three hours at Convocation Hall for a session entitled "Teamwork: Your Future of Interprofessional Healthcare." A dean from one of the faculties, a vice president of education from one of the hospitals, and the Centre for IPE's director welcome them to the start of their IPE journey. A patient talks to the group about how interprofessional care, or the lack thereof, affected him or her. Faculty members perform "before" and "after" skits showing poor and improved collaborative care. And finally, someone from a community health facility—perhaps a community clinic—describes how interprofessional practice works in the real health care workplace.

Students are divided up into "buzz groups" of six interprofessional students and a facilitator who oversees one or two groups. These groups get together after each section of the day's activities and discuss some questions that have been designed to elicit further inquiry and reflection.

A second core IPE session, "Conflict in Interprofessional Life," takes place in the following year. In its original iteration, this session was only for students in nursing, social work, and medicine. In March of 2011 the three-hour session was rolled out for all eleven schools. To accommodate hundreds of students, it was held three different times in the course of two days. The session included a one-hour lecture, which also had some surprise guerrilla theater in which faculty members engaged in a conflict. Then the students watched a DVD of a discharge in which two actors, each from an unidentified profession, got into a conflict. The students had to apply what they have learned in the lecture and course work to resolve the conflict.

At yet another juncture in their education, students take part in a four-day core case-based session. For seven of the professions—medicine, dentistry, pharmacy, nursing, OT, PT, and more recently physician assistant training—this session is about pain and pain management. It had been developed and taught for six years before the IPE curriculum was implemented. Because the center's mandate was to find outstanding programs that could be incorporated into the curriculum, that's precisely what it did.

Students who cannot attend the pain session attend a palliative care case-based session. Faculty members present a case, which is related to issues of palliative care. At first students see only part of the case unfold and discuss it. Then they receive envelopes containing further information that relates to their specific profession. They then bring that information to the table for further discussion. For students taking the pain curriculum, the palliative care session is available as an elective.

Perhaps the most interesting aspect of the IPE curriculum is the core learning activity that takes place in the practice setting. There are two models of these—structured IPE placement and flexible learning activities.

The structured IPE placement grew out of the recognition that something had to be done to address the traditional student experience in the clinical setting. Students, like working professionals, arrive on a unit, whether a clinic or a rehab hospital, and work *next to or near* other professionals or students in other faculties without ever necessarily working *with* them. At the University of Toronto, most students overlap with those from other faculties for four to six weeks. The IPE curriculum developers determined that having students together at the same time in the same place caring for real patients presented an opportunity that could not be ignored.

In 2004 Lynne Sinclair and Mandy Lowe, both leaders at the Toronto Rehabilitation Institute at the time, developed a model for an interprofessional placement that, if successful, could be adapted in other health care facilities and settings. The geriatric day hospital at the Toronto Rehab, Sinclair explains, was a logical pilot site because teamwork between disciplines was often the norm. Patient satisfaction scores for the unit were high, and staff often reported that this was a unit on which they would prefer to work. Then in 2005 another placement was begun on the stroke unit.

In developing this model, leaders recognized that students would need to be coached in their IPE tutorials by faculty members who were not the supervisors in their profession-specific training program. Instead, facilitators were trained to specifically guide interprofessional groups of students through the placement—leading them in discussions and formal sessions about patient care in a way that highlighted interprofessional issues.

During the first week of their structured IPE placements the students meet for an introductory tutorial in which they talk about their different educational backgrounds, scope of practice, and how they can work together as a team. Students then meet weekly for a series of themed tutorials, which consider different issues relating to their patients. These might include topics like pain management, informed consent, or aphasia. "The discussions," Sinclair explains, "are about something to which all the students can contribute as they share what it is they are doing—say, as a nursing or OT or PT student—to alleviate a patient's pain, or help with other issues."

The final aspect of the placement is a presentation that all the students prepare together. Students may themselves come up with the subject, or it may emerge from their interaction with staff. For example, staff on one unit at the Toronto Rehab told students that they were concerned about the smooth functioning of their discharge process. They suggested that students spend some time understanding the process and searching the literature for IPE best practices around discharges. The students could come back and give staff recommendations based on their findings. On another unit the issue was rounding, in which staff visit patients and discuss their problems. Staff members were concerned that they weren't getting through the material they needed to review in the time allotted to rounding. So students got together and did a quality improvement project to help improve rounds and encourage more collaborative conversations. Once the model at Toronto Rehab was developed and successfully implemented, it became the one used and adapted for all structured IPE placements in other facilities. Funding from the Provincial Ministry of Health and Long Term Care was received to specifically develop a tool kit for others to use to develop their own IPE placements.

Because offering structured IPE placements for all 1,250 students at the university requires a huge amount of work in recruiting sites and training, not all health professional students will actually go through this program. Because the university is committed to having all students experience some formal interprofessional collaboration during their clinical rotation, those who are not in structured placements participate in what is called flexible IPE learning activities. Both the structured and flexible models are based on the IPE curriculum core competencies. The first such activity follows.

Participation in interprofessional team education

- Interprofessional lunch-and-learn sessions, journal club discussions, patient/ client team-based case discussions, and interprofessional grand rounds
- An interprofessional team education session should include:
- Involvement of two or more professions
- Significant interactivity between participants
- Opportunities to learn about, from, and with one another
- Interprofessional teaching/learning moments

Learning objectives

- Reflection
- Identification of factors that may contribute to or hinder team collaboration,
- including power and hierarchy
- Assuming diverse roles in an interprofessional group and supporting others in their roles

Before attending the session, students are given guidance about what kinds of questions to ask and issues to consider, and then they discuss this in a debriefing with their supervisors.

Wagner gives the example of a hospital that is having an interprofessional educational session on wound care. Even though there are mainly doctors and nurses in the audience, a speech language pathology student might attend that session. Before she went to the session, she would meet with her preceptor to discuss what she might be seeing and how this might apply to her field. Then they would reflect and discuss their response to the session. "One of the things the student might consider and later discuss is how the interprofessional session really was. It may not have been what the student expected, but that too is a topic of both concern and reflection. We talk a lot about interprofessional teams," Wagner says candidly, "but there are really very few groups out there that are truly interprofessional."

The second activity is shadowing and interviewing a team member. The final activity is participation in two team meetings with at least two team members involved. Team meetings can be patient rounds, discharge planning meetings, and patient/ client/family meetings. Through these meetings, students gain an understanding of interprofessional team dynamics and group processes through effective interprofessional communication.

Although this curriculum is as well thought out and as comprehensive as possible for one that is superimposed on already extant programs packed to the brim with course work and clinical placements, Tassone and her colleagues recognize how vulnerable it is to the "hidden curriculum"—implicit or explicit messages students might receive from members of the various disciplines they will encounter in the practice setting. For this reason, enormous attention has been given to developing facilitators, leaders, and faculty who will educate students in the workplaces they will enter during their clinical rotations. Facilitators who lead students on their interprofessional journey are given training and guidance.

Lowe, an occupational therapist who is now faculty lead of clinical and professional development at the center, points out why this is so important. "My first time facilitating a structured IPE placement was at the Toronto Rehab. I'm an occupational therapist and I partner with physical therapists. We had been discussing something that could help students learn about 'transfers.' A social work student was in the group. When the discussion came to an end, the social work student raised her hand and said, 'When I heard we were going to learn about transfers I thought you meant transfers from acute care to rehab.'"

Lowe was surprised and then had an aha moment. "Of course she thought that was what we meant. But because we were OTs and PTs, what we meant was transferring the patient from bed to wheelchair. So now we make sure to tell people that, as facilitators, they need to step back and think about how they use language and have an awareness about the assumptions that they make. They also have to stop and ask students if everything is clear and make sure to encourage them to ask questions even if that means interrupting the discussion."

The Centre for IPE has encouraged other hospitals to develop IPE placements for their own settings, and its faculty works with institutional leadership and staff to modify and adapt the model to the patient context in which it will be used. They term this process "cocreation." Faculty members from the center help new people at new sites consider questions like the following:

- What would an IPE structured placement or learning activity look like in practice?
- Why is it important?
- What should you consider when planning IPE?

"You can have very good people who can practice or even teach in one discipline in your setting," Lowe comments, "but that does not mean they know how to lead an interprofessional education. Which is why we have a workshop to train them to do just that." Fortunately, the provincial government funded the center to put much of the knowledge and experience it had gathered about IPE into free resources and DVDs sold at a very low cost, which are available online and help create guidelines and checklists for how to run an IPE program or placement.[4]

Because faculty and professional development is so crucial, every year the Centre for IPE runs a five-day certificate course called "Educating Health Professionals in Interprofessional Care" (EHPIC). The course has also been offered in a customized three-day version for use in both university and practice settings, locally and internationally in countries such as the United States and Denmark. "The course aims to develop leaders in interprofessional education who have the knowledge, skills, and attitudes to teach both learners and fellow colleagues the art and science of working collaboratively for patient-centered care," says Tassone. The program covers areas such as professional and collaborator roles, collaborative teams, facilitator skills, attention to process, leading change, and assessment and evaluation.

Finally, the center runs a year-long collaborative change leadership (CCL) program, whose goal is, Tassone explains, to develop systemic-change leaders who can transform their own clinical organizations and lead staff in collaborative care initiatives for quality and safety. We have very traditional ways of preparing managers and leaders, but we don't necessarily train leaders to have a collaborative, emergent, change approach and this is the purpose of the program," Tassone says. In 2009–10, the program trained fifty-four people who have leadership roles in twenty-three different health education and health care organizations across the province.

The goal of the IPE curriculum is to introduce students to a new way of practicing in a new paradigm in health care. The hope is that enough exposure will produce the kind of critical mass that will lead these new professionals not simply to expect or role-model a new approach once they graduate but to demand that the system continue to change. A speech language pathology student who graduated and is now in practice told Suzanne about the epiphany she had when doing her structured interprofessional placement. She had been trying unsuccessfully to help a patient with problems swallowing. Then she watched an OT student adjust the patient's wheelchair. Amazingly, this eased his swallowing problems. She confessed that without this hands-on interprofessional experience, she would never have thought of calling on an OT to help with a swallowing problem. Now that she has seen that other professionals and staff have resources and knowledge she had never imagined, she will never practice the same way again. Although she did not use these precise words, she said she wants to work in a practice setting that appreciates this kind of team resource management and fosters the kind of team intelligence that makes it possible.

A pharmacy student, Maria Zhang, also said that structured placement had transformed her view of what she wanted from professional practice. As she recalls, "It was eye-opening to collaborate and learn with students from other disciplines. I began to understand how they navigated their entry to practice and the roles they play in different settings." Most important, Zhang says, she learned something too few students in traditional pharmacy or other health care programs understand—that teamwork and collaboration really add something to professional practice and patient care.

Zhang pointed to the work she and her teammates did with a geriatric patient who had dementia and was also a concentration camp survivor. The elderly gentleman had been admitted to control sexually inappropriate and sometimes frighteningly aggressive behavior. Instead of working one-on-one only with a pharmacist who would explain how Zhang might use medication to control the man's behavior, she and the interprofessional student team met with a social worker who kept in contact with the patient's family, gave the students regular updates on the patient's progress, and also obtained consent for procedures, medications, and more. All of this was critical since the patient could neither speak nor advocate for himself.

The occupational therapist and OT assistant worked with the patient and found out that he enjoyed music and singing, which helped to calm him. The nursing student found that he was agitated in the morning when nurses woke him to give his medications. Why was that, the group wondered? Could he be reliving his experiences at the concentration camp, where guards would rip off his blankets at any time of day or night to wake him up? What would happen if nurses used hot towels to warm him when he got up in the morning? Would this ease his anxiety? Or perhaps he could get his medications later in the day when he'd adjusted to being awake. The group discussed these ideas with the nurse, pharmacist, and doctor who were working with the patient. "All of this helped me learn more about the importance of collaborative care and how we all play integral parts in the overall picture of maintaining and/or improving a patient's health and quality of life," Zhang concluded. "Most of all, it has fueled my passion to learn and participate more in interprofessional experiences when I am in practice."

Chapter 8

Threat and Error Management

THREATS, ERRORS, AND HIGH-RELIABILITY ORGANIZATIONS

In their book on high-reliability organizations, *Managing the Unexpected*, Karl E. Weick and Kathleen M. Sutcliffe talk about "mindful management." They are not talking about a bunch of executives sitting around in lotus pose meditating on the contingencies of human existence. They are talking about "high-reliability organizations" (HROs) and how they get that way and stay that way. Weick and Sutcliffe write,

> We attribute the success of HROs in managing the unexpected to their determined efforts to act mindfully. By this we mean that they organize themselves in such a way that they are better able to notice the unexpected in the making and halt its development. If they have difficulty halting the development of the unexpected, they focus on containing it. And if some of the unexpected breaks through the containment, they focus on resilience and swift restoration of system functioning.[1]

Sound familiar? Kind of like the CRM principle that one should prevent, manage, and contain errors. That's because the evolution of CRM into threat and error management is a classic case of moving from an *almost* high-reliability to a truly high-reliability organization. According to Weick and Sutcliffe, high reliability doesn't come just from the kind of communication, teamwork, and workload management that we have described in previous chapters. It comes not just from thinking about how to succeed or congratulating oneself about the mistakes one didn't make. It comes from uncovering, investigating, and discussing mistakes that *were* made.

THREATS AND ERRORS DEFINED

Weick and Sutcliffe spend a lot of time in their book talking about our human tendency to be surprised even by things that, when one looks back on them, shouldn't have been so surprising. We have a tendency, they say, to "overlook accumulating evidence that things are not developing as you thought they would . . . to seek confirmation and shun disconfirmation, . . . to find that your time is off, or that the expected duration of an event proves to be wrong . . . to miscalculate the amplitude of a problem."[2] Organizations that attain high reliability have "a preoccupation with updating." They are constantly aware that "knowledge and ignorance grow together . . . and [they] reexamine discarded information, monitor how categories affect expectations, and remove dated distinctions."[3]

To move toward true high reliability, commercial aviation revisited, reassessed, and refined their list of crew performance indicators. They added the concept of TEM to this new set of tools. To be really safe, researchers realized that once they learned to communicate, work in teams, and manage their workloads, teams needed to expand what they communicated about, what their members focused on, and to be genuinely proactive in managing their workload.

To explore threat and error management, we must first define and understand what is meant by each term. The primary difference between threats and errors is timing.

A *threat* refers to any condition or environmental factor that increases operational complexity and thus has the potential of contributing to an error. In aviation, threats include elements like natural phenomena (e.g., weather), mechanical factors (e.g., structural fatigue in aircraft), or work environment (e.g., crowded and busy airports). Threats can be managed to prevent errors from developing by using tools and techniques such as improved policies and procedures, CRM, and situational awareness. Threats can be overt (obvious) or latent (hidden). Overt threats might include a passing thunderstorm. Latent threats would include improperly written procedures that might unknowingly lead the user to an error. Threat mitigation strategies include the following:

- Maintain situational awareness → recognize.
- Verbalize the threat → communicate.
- Verify the threat → concur.
- Resolve the threat → mitigate.
- Monitor the threat → awareness.

Threats are future events (they haven't happened yet).

An *error*, by contrast, is an action or failure to act that has an unexpected or undesired outcome. Most errors go unnoticed or are harmless. However, errors have the potential of grave and irreversible consequences that commercial aviation has focused on avoiding and eradicating. Errors can be the result of

- misconceptions;
- lack of skill;

- lack of information;
- poor judgment;
- intentional noncompliance.

It is important to grasp that *errors* are past events: they've already occurred, and since we are unable to turn back the clock, our only option is to deal with what we've done. This is a two-step process: the first is to handle the immediate consequences of error as best we can under the circumstances—to mitigate. The second part—and this is the step that now sets commercial aviation apart from other high-reliability organizations—is to learn from our mistakes. This is achieved through the robust reporting and analysis programs that have been developed specifically for that purpose.

Threat and error management is about managing threats to prevent errors and, if an error occurs, capitalizing on that knowledge to develop strategies to keep errors from recurring. TEM provides the tools for reporting, analyzing, and revising policies and procedures to preclude repetition of the same errors at a later time. This is all done in a nonpunitive environment because it has been generally accepted that in spite of our best intentions and efforts to the contrary, errors will occur. TEM concentrates on how to prevent them from being repeated, rather than assigning blame.[4]

THREAT AND ERROR MANAGEMENT VS. CREW RESOURCE MANAGEMENT

TEM is a natural subset of CRM. To understand the distinction between them, it helps to view them as two sides of the same coin. CRM involves the recognition and shared knowledge of the threat or error (problem, challenge, obstacle, etc.) to be prevented, managed, or contained. TEM involves a proactive commitment to manage threats or errors. Consider the following examples.

A passenger notices something that looks like mist coming off the trailing edge of the wing. Never having observed this before, the passenger tells a flight attendant what he's seen. The flight attendant acknowledges the passenger's concern, gathers whatever information she can from the passenger (When noticed? How long? Continuous? Increasing? Decreasing?) and contacts the cockpit to notify the pilots. The pilots gather as much information as possible from the flight attendant and, once they confirm it by using the data provided on cockpit instruments, determine that they have developed a fuel leak in one of the tanks.

The pilots contact company dispatch and maintenance departments to get their input into (1) assessing, resolving, or mitigating the problem and (2) assistance in evaluating alternatives. Maintenance may have a solution that would allow safe completion of the flight to its planned destination, or they may determine that the aircraft is unsafe to continue and may recommend an immediate landing. The dispatcher would assist in finding the best landing alternatives based upon

Air Ontario Flight 1363

A tragic example of dysfunctional communication that often prevailed before CRM occurred in 1989 on Air Ontario Flight 1363, a Fokker F-28, when an observant passenger noticed snow and ice buildup on the wing prior to takeoff and alerted a nearby flight attendant. The passenger "was told (falsely) by the flight attendant that the aircraft had automatic deicing equipment." The flight attendant did not pass on the passenger's concerns to the pilots, and the postaccident investigation revealed that flight attendants were "trained not to question flight crews' judgment regarding safety issues." The aircraft crashed immediately after takeoff, killing twenty-four of sixty-nine souls on board.

weather, ground support, security, and so on.

Up to this point, although threat assessment has been a continuous and integral part of the process, the focus has been on Crew Resource Management. There has been a clear emphasis on gathering and sharing information as well as on the utilization of all available resources to identify and solve the problem, from acknowledging the passenger's concerns and using any information he can provide to the exchange between the pilots and maintenance personnel to determine the best course of action.

Threat management becomes a much bigger part of the picture as all parties begin to weigh the risks of the various alternatives. In this scenario, it is determined that the rate of fuel loss will preclude continuing to the intended destination. Among the numerous possible threats that the crew will now consider are fire, structural failure, difficult approach and landing due to inclement weather at the alternate destination, and language barriers (for international flights). Each of these will be discussed and mitigation strategies planned.

Errors are events that have already occurred. *Error management* thus involves analyzing what happened and developing common strategies—which may include adjusting or changing procedures or policies—to prevent the same error from occurring again. To continue with the example cited above, let's say that the crippled aircraft successfully touched down at the alternate field. All parties involved, however, neglected to consider the effect of reverse thrust (normally used to slow the aircraft after touchdown). The leaking fuel was ingested into one of the engines during the rollout and caused a fire. This oversight would be considered an error. Error management would lead to a process that would ultimately result in changing the written procedure for landing with a wing fuel leak to prohibit the use of reverse thrust in this type of situation.

Error management in commercial aviation has become one of the best-developed and most valuable tools in the safety arsenal. Any psychologist will tell you that the first step in restoring mental health is for the patient to admit that he or she has a problem. This is now true in commercial aviation, where crews are encouraged *and expected* to report when things go wrong. To encourage crews to do this, TEM provides the tools for reporting, analyzing, and revising policies and procedures to preclude repetition of the same errors at a later time. Crews are protected from disciplinary action when they report their own errors, so long as the error was unintentional. *Intentional* noncompliance, however, is not accepted or tolerated.

TEM is used throughout each flight, from flight planning to completion of the "shutdown checklist." As a very simple example, consider a "typical" international passenger flight. Anticipated and potential threats are considered and identified before the flight-planning process has even begun. One threat that always looms over international operations is fatigue. Getting adequate rest is always a challenge for crews who experience constant disruptions in circadian rhythms, unusual foods, novel customs, and unfamiliar rooms and noises. If a crew member has not rested well, he or she is encouraged to speak up, as this is a legitimate threat to safety. The threat might be mitigated in a number of ways (e.g., by providing break times), but there may be no practical way to deal directly with this threat. The fact that the other crew members are *aware* that one of their coworkers may not be fully rested should cause them to be more diligent in monitoring and correcting for mistakes from this individual. Another example of a crew threat might be a lack of either experience (the pilot is new) or "recency" (the pilot has not flown in two months). Another threat would be the distractions that could result from personal problems. As was evidenced in the JetBlue incident in March 2012, pilots are still worried about admitting these problems to other pilots or their chief pilot, even though CRM encourages them to do so. Although there is great resistance to doing so, some will reveal personal problems if they feel these impact safety.

A common operational threat is bad weather. In this case, pilots will consider that thunderstorms are forecast along the route of flight over the ocean. Years ago this was considered nice-to-know information, and the threat would be dealt with if and when it appeared in flight. In the TEM environment, pilots consider the wind direction—which way storm cells are moving—so that if they need to deviate around them, they have anticipated which way to turn to remain upwind of the threat. They consider the track they are on—if the navigation tracks are fifty miles apart, they know to keep situationally aware of just how far they might want to deviate around a storm before conflicting traffic becomes an additional threat. All this is considered and discussed among all crew members. The captain discusses the threat in terms of turbulence with the flight attendants and cockpit crew so that all are aware of the plan should the threat actually materialize. Typically a variety of solutions have been discussed before the aircraft ever leaves the gate.

NONJEOPARDY REPORTING PROGRAMS

"Nonjeopardy" reporting programs are used to collect and collate data on threats and errors. These data are then interpreted to eliminate future threats by revising or changing procedures and are incorporated into future training scenarios. The value of threat and error reporting programs cannot be overstated.

Aviation Safety Action Program

The primary reporting tool used by most commercial carriers is the Aviation Safety Action Program (ASAP), which is a collaborative effort among industry, pilots, and the FAA. All ASAP reports are reviewed by a committee made up of representatives from the companies, the pilot union, and the FAA. The committee *may* contact a crew member who submitted the report for clarification of certain details. Except for *intentional* noncompliance, the committee cannot impose any punitive action on a pilot for an error that he or she has reported using this system. In fact, by the time the report leaves the committee, crews have been "de-identified" as the actual names are irrelevant to the goal of identifying and mitigating trends.

Here's an example of how it works. Let's say that during the flight, the aircraft did encounter the thunderstorms as forecast, including moderate to severe turbulence. Because of a communication problem with air traffic control, the aircraft was unable to contact the appropriate controller to get clearance around the storm. Without clearance, the captain made the decision to deviate around the storm. Before returning on course, the aircraft was forced to take evasive action to avoid a collision with another aircraft in the vicinity.

This is where reporting comes into play. In the past, pilots would have accepted their brush with disaster and moved on. In the TEM culture, they would report the incident via ASAP. In this example, because of the ATC communication malfunction, the deviation resulted in a near disaster, and the subsequent investigation would concentrate on correcting the communication problem going forward rather than allocating blame for what happened in the past.

Flight Operations Quality Assurance

Flight Operations Quality Assurance (FOQA) is a program that has developed as a result of the tremendous advances in technology available to maintainers and operators. FOQA data are available on most late-model aircraft and certain predefined conditions produce recordings that are very similar to those registered on the flight data recorders. FDRs continuously record numerous parameters that are analyzed in the event of an accident or serious incident to piece together the chain of events which led to the occurrence.

FOQA data, by contrast, are recorded when the aircraft or aircraft systems operate outside predefined parameters. In its simplest form, a FOQA event occurs when an aircraft system warning is activated, such as a computer dropping off-line or a takeoff warning alarm being activated.[5] In such cases, a FOQA event would take a snapshot (or series of snapshots) of literally thousands of aircraft parameters.

If, in each of the examples described above, the problem was ultimately resolved and the flight was allowed to continue without incident, the pilots would probably have submitted an ASAP report. There are cases, however, where an error event may occur and be immediately corrected, and because no harm resulted, it would seem fairly insignificant. Such incidents would typically go unreported. (This also happens in health care when errors do not cause actual harm to the patient, and so "nothing really happened." These errors still need reporting because something did indeed happen that points to system problems that could be remedied.)

The pilot personality is, if nothing else, proactive: pilots are hired because of their drive to be mission-oriented—to get the job done without supervision. Therefore, it comes as no surprise that once an immediate problem has been solved, they are inclined to press on rather than be concerned with reports and paperwork. However, there are situations where the system would benefit from knowledge of things that have gone wrong. Although some people may consider these to be isolated occurrences, without a sophisticated reporting system (such as FOQA), we wouldn't know whether they really are. Individual events can help to identify a trend that if left unexplored could eventually lead to an undesirable outcome, even a catastrophe. This is one area where FOQA data are particularly useful.

Consider the takeoff warning system mentioned above, which is required in all commercial airliners. It alerts the pilots that the aircraft has not been properly configured for takeoff. An aircraft must be in the proper configuration—trim and flap settings must be in appropriate positions for the given aircraft weight and balance—or it may simply not fly. This is something you do not want to discover at the departure end of the runway at 160 knots! If the throttle positions are advanced to the takeoff thrust range, but the flaps or trim have not been properly configured, a distinctive warning horn will sound (along with a computer-generated ECAM and voice message in some modern aircraft). Once the crew has been alerted to this critical oversight, it is an easy problem to resolve, and the takeoff can resume in fairly short order.

FOQA would record the takeoff warning as an event. The FOQA data would not necessarily be noticed right away. Typically, maintenance personnel download and place the FOQA recordings in a database for review on a regular basis (every few days). Operators review the data by focusing on certain types of parameters and exceedances. A takeoff warning event would most definitely capture the reviewers' attention.

In the case of the takeoff warning, one incident by itself, although significant, would not necessarily result in further action. If, however, the data began to identify a trend toward several similar events, FOQA analysts would start digging deeper into the causes, including contacting and interviewing the pilots. If it were discovered that this trend was happening with certain regularity on a particular aircraft type (fleet) or a particular airport, FOQA analysts would focus on identifying what set that fleet or location apart and correcting the underlying problem.

The mitigation might involve particular training emphasis or changing procedures to ensure compliance and better performance.

FOQA data, particularly when combined with ASAP reports, present a very valuable and compelling picture as trends develop. This allows timely development of proactive mitigation strategies for error avoidance and results in a significantly safer operating environment.

NASA Aviation Safety Reporting System

The Aviation Safety Reporting System (ASRS) was one of the earliest self-reporting systems developed by NASA. Pilots jokingly referred to it as the "get-out-of-jail-free" card. If a pilot made an unintentional error, he or she was encouraged to report the error to the ASRS. As with ASAP, if the error was reported within the defined time frame, the FAA would not be able to take action against the reporting pilots. ASAP has pretty much replaced ASRS in most commercial airline operations.

Nonjeopardy reporting programs play a vital role in effective threat and error management. Reporting by itself allows effective analysis of trends and issues so that countermeasures and mitigation strategies can be developed and implemented. Being able to report errors without fear of retribution, prosecution, or blame is an essential element of this program, which must be included in any TEM program.

HIGH RELIABILITY IN FLIGHT

Whether it is through training and skill building in communication, teamwork, workload, or threat and error management, the very ground of CRM is the acknowledgment that institutions and industries cannot be safe and highly reliable if the people who work in them—and those who depend on them for their very lives—have no way to deal with the unequal power relationships, cultural biases, and fear of reprisal that are inherent in human society. This effort to make it safe for people to contribute—and to accept and respect the opinions of others—is at the heart of teamwork, no matter what the endeavor or arena in which it is supposed to take place. The skills we have described in the chapters on crew performance indicators have produced skies that, if not necessarily friendlier, are definitely safer. Although CRM training does not lead to perfection, given the obstacles it has had to overcome, the aviation safety movement has been a remarkable success.

In numerous interviews with flight attendants and pilots–whether male or female–almost all explain that CRM has transformed the professional relationships and created real teams. This transformation has endured in spite of another equally dramatic change in relationships between flight attendants and pilots—the isolation of pilots in the flight deck following the terrorist attacks of

September 11, 2001. Before 9/11, pilots circulated more freely in the aircraft, and, time permitting, flight attendants and pilots chatted and socialized during flight. When the meal service was over, the flight attendants would bring the pilots' meals into the cockpit and often stayed for some social banter. That has entirely changed with the current security policies. On-duty pilots stay behind the locked cockpit door at all times except when fairly elaborate security precautions have been initiated to allow them a restroom break. Likewise, because of the tight security arrangements, flight attendants rarely if ever pay social calls to the cockpit. There is no time for chatting in post-9/11 flight.

Scheduling efficiencies have also transformed social interaction. As Patrick recalls, "Flight scheduling was typically done by the month. If I was assigned schedule number 42, I would be flying all month long with a group of flight attendants that were also assigned schedule number 42 for that month. In 1989, when I first got hired, the entire pilot/flight attendant crew would fly together for a month at a time: same captain and same FAs. At the end of a five-day trip, I'd say, 'See you next week,' and indeed we would all be together on the next trip that month. You'd get to know people really well and build a team dynamic in a very natural way."

Michelle Quintas, who worked as a flight attendant for United, echoed those sentiments. "We used to have the time and the ability to build relationships. We knew we'd be working together for that trip, as short as two flights, over a five-day period. You'd fly together from JFK to Hong Kong, to Bangkok, then back to Hong Kong, and home to JFK. Maybe we'd work that trip three times a month. We were able to build more relationships."

Over the past two decades, computers and company financial imperatives changed all that. By the mid-1990s, Patrick says, "We were no longer flying with the same group of flight attendants and pilots throughout the month. Instead, we might be together for a 'trip,' (a 'trip' or 'pattern' covers the time the pilot or FA goes out the door till the time they return. A trip can be two days, or three days or ten days and will include a number of 'legs' or 'segments'—i.e., a discrete flight from point A to point B). So now, instead of the entire crew being paired up for an entire month, we would only be together for just that trip." Then they might never see each other again. In 2011, as we write this book, computers have become so sophisticated that pilots and FAs now may fly only legs together. "This means," says Patrick, "you may only fly one leg with the other crew members and then never see them again! This summer, for example, I made several trips 'solo,' with different cockpit and cabin crew for nearly every single leg for a ten-day trip."

From a teamwork perspective, it is obvious that it is far more effective for crews to fly either on a month-long or at a minimum trip-long basis. But profits trump efficacy, at least in this respect. Because flight attendants and pilots have different work rules, just a fifteen- or thirty-minute difference in the length of their duty periods can have a huge impact on the overall schedule. Different work rules and union negotiations also mean that pilots and flight attendants may not even stay at the same hotels during layovers, which reduces opportunities for informal collegial interaction as well.

Suzanne observed the impact of all these factors firsthand when she herself stayed at a layover hotel owned by a major airline about twenty minutes from the Narita Airport outside Tokyo. For many pilots and FAs, like Patrick, it's a temporary home away from home when they are flying in Asia. To get a taste of aviation culture, Suzanne wandered around the hotel and into the restaurants the crews frequent. It was striking how little socializing crossed occupational barriers. As in the modern hospital—where nurses, doctors, PT, OTs, and many others are now in even more enclosed silos as they hunch over computers entering data or journey through facilities in unidisciplinary pods—pilots seemed to stick with pilots and flight attendants with one another.

Suzanne talked with several flight attendants and asked about CRM. Uniformly they echoed comments like this one: "Since 9/11 we hardly ever socialize with [pilots]. They're locked in their boxes and we don't mingle. But our professional relationships have really improved. When you call them, they listen. They brief us on every flight."

The post-9/11 environment seems to have reminded crews of what Robert Helmreich in 1999 worried they would forget—that CRM is not about making friends but about preventing or reducing the prevalence and consequences of error. From all accounts, as well as the statistics on the reduction in airline accidents, it has done that. Contrary to what is still the norm in hospitals, lack of socialization among disciplines has not negatively impacted professional communication. "Although it's really sad that we are no longer as socially cohesive," says Patrick, "we can really be proud of the fact that we are able to come together as total strangers and make this huge [teamwork] thing happen and do it to relative perfection. Pilots and flight attendants come together from different parts of the country to perform this daily ballet pretty flawlessly without having to know each other." That is a triumph not of wishful thinking but of consistent and effective training—training that, as we will see in the next chapter, was designed, delivered, and reinforced in ways that have assured that it will not, as Patrick once hoped, "go the way of bell-bottom pants" but will be a systematic and enduring part of the airline culture.

Chapter 9

Why CRM Worked

RECOGNIZING HUMAN FALLIBILITY

In his book *Safe Patients, Smart Hospitals: How One Doctor's Checklist Can Help Us Change Health Care from the Inside Out*, the physician Peter Pronovost expresses doubt about the possibility of applying lessons from the aviation safety movement to health care. A Johns Hopkins Hospital intensive care physician and pioneer in the development of patient safety checklists, Pronovost writes that medicine "has not yet acknowledged human fallibility. "In aviation," he argues, the fact that "*this truth had been universally accepted*" made it possible for the industry "to design systems that could prevent or catch inevitable errors before they caused harm, or minimize harm from errors that were not identified."[1]

In fact, the aviation safety movement started out precisely because pilots did *not* accept their human fallibility. Mistaking the end of a very long journey for its beginning, many in medicine do not seem to understand the similarities between attitudes of pilots pre-CRM and those of physicians today. CRM did not succeed because in the 1980s pilots at United and other airlines threw up their hands and said, "We give up." A great many pilots, in fact, dismissed CRM as "charm school" or even a "Communist plot" to erode their authority.

Flight attendants were also initially skeptical. They were being told to challenge pilots, to speak up—that it was no longer just "Honey, why don't you get me the coffee now." They wanted some proof that companies were about to walk the walk, not just talk the talk. Former United flight attendant Nancy Burns, who began her career in 1969 and retired in 2006, explains that her cohort of flight attendants (then called stewardesses) realized that industry was serious because "CRM gave us the language we needed to deal with pilots."

The fact that human fallibility is now universally accepted in aviation is the result of a very long journey that began with a challenge to an ethos that led pilots to believe they had the power of Zeus when, in fact, many only had the hubris of Icarus. So how did Icarus learn to be more humble, and how did the humble learn to be more assertive?

The aviation safety movement has worked not only because of the concrete lessons it teaches but also because of the reconceptualizations and strategic approaches it has utilized. These have been derived from, and refined through, thirty years of hands-on, human-factors research—in other words, evidence-based changes and developments. In this chapter we will briefly outline what we consider the most critical.

REDEFINING HIERARCHY

Bob Francis of the NTSB stated unequivocally that CRM worked because of its approach to what we have called "toxic hierarchy." As Francis said, the captain is still king but one who is far more likely to learn from and with those who share his castle. Pre-CRM it was clear that once the captain entered the cockpit and took command, he claimed de facto ownership of the plane, its crew, and its passengers. The captain was not only permitted to discount, ignore, or silence other people involved in the flight but was actively socialized to do so. As we have also learned, his judgment could easily give way to emotion—such as competitiveness or a sense of invulnerability—and emotion to tragedy. The standard definition of the captain's authority and infallibility had thus created a toxic hierarchy that ultimately led to the loss of many lives and billions of dollars.

What do we mean by this concept? Hierarchy always involves a set of rankings in which someone has an increased level of authority over those below. But authority can be exercised in a variety of ways—including ways that encourage the input of those lower on the graded scale. Rather than bringing people together in the service of realizing a common goal, toxic hierarchies separate people and conceal or devalue their respective knowledge and expertise. In both aviation and health care, toxic hierarchies are characterized by a great deal of action and activity but very little *inter*action and *inter*activity.

Having identified the problem of toxic hierarchy, airline managers had many options at their disposal to try to deal with it. One approach might have been more touchy-feely—the charm school that many pilots mocked. Companies could have used CRM as a kind of finishing school for uncouth aviators—trying to de-macho them and make them more pliant and nicer to their coworkers. One can imagine how this would have sat with a bunch of former solo aviators largely trained in the military.

Another approach would have been to try to make the workplace more egalitarian, with captains being told they had to share authority with their coworkers. This would have encouraged captains to view everybody as an equal player on what would now be the new level playing field of aviation. Again we recall that one of the primary fears that pilots had was that CRM would devalue their expertise and cripple their ability to command. This kind of concern is common wherever there are steep hierarchies and status differentials and where those at the top of the hierarchy generally shoulder the greatest legal liability. Beyond that, those at the top (pilots, physicians) partially define themselves as professionals by the authority and autonomy they have worked to attain and exercise at the cost of greater personal responsibility for outcomes and their consequences, both good and bad.

The safety movement eschewed any head-on assault of the captain-as-king model. Instead, what emerged was a much more subtle and ultimately far more effective challenge to the traditional view of the solo aviator confronting his unique version of wind, sand, and stars. The introduction of the team model, as defined and elaborated in CRM, allowed safety advocates to reconceptualize authority, decision making, and expert judgment and paved the way for a dramatic reworking of the command structure that would detoxify hierarchies while maintaining their effective qualities.

The aviation safety movement dealt with issues of authority—who made the final decision and with whom the buck ultimately stopped—by focusing on *how* authority was exercised, *how* decisions were made, and *how* resources were utilized. Post-CRM, the captain still has the final authority. The fundamental question now is how he or she learns to exercise authority and to interact not only with technology but with human beings in subordinate positions. CRM redefined these subordinates as "resources."

In essence, of course, the traditional definition of the captain's authority was, in fact, being threatened: captains were told that they must not only consider the input of their crew but also were actually expected to solicit it. But the way this paradigm shift was negotiated did not ultimately confirm the fear that CRM was just a scheme that would ultimately erode the captain's authority.

Much to the amazement of CRM skeptics, this approach turned out to actually further empower captains whose decisions were suddenly aided, supported, and enhanced by the knowledge, experience, and insights of fellow crewmembers. In trainings and other settings, captains were taught to see that other airline workers had useful skills, information, insights, and concerns that could be utilized to make everyone safer.

Commenting on the misplaced fear that CRM would result in captains losing authority, a very senior 747 flight instructor, air crew program designee (APD), and CRM consultant, Captain Gary Allen, said, "If anything, captains have increased authority as a result of CRM. Although they still bear the ultimate responsibility for the safe outcome of the flight, they now have the confidence that they have the entire crew watching their backs. That crew is empowered to make suggestions and even decisions. The captain is now at the head of a very effective team."

"INSTRUMENTALIZING" THE CONCEPT OF COMMUNICATION

When pilots dismissed CRM as charm school, many shared the perception that learning to "communicate" better was something other than engaging in a goal-oriented instrumental process that involved mutual learning. Instead, many feared that CRM involved exposure, expressing vulnerability, and being blamed for a variety of perceived faults. Patrick recalls when he first heard about CRM. "My reaction was like [that of] 95 percent of my colleagues—I just rolled my eyes. 'Oh no! Here's another feel-good thing we have to do. Somebody decided that we needed this psychological retrofitting.' Like everybody else, I didn't really care to take the time to do this."

One of the things that Patrick, like many other pilots, disliked was the fact that CRM training involved audience participation. "I think pilots, even more than the general public, dislike anything that involves participatory exercises and role plays." Pilots, Patrick continues, don't perceive that they're doing an exercise *along with* other colleagues. Like the novice ballerina certain that everyone in her class is looking at her–rather than actually looking at themselves in the studio mirror—a lot of pilots don't conceptualize group exercises or role-playing as occasions for learning; rather they are occasions for humiliating self-exposure, judgment, and faultfinding. "It's weird," Patrick muses, "that we are so reluctant to do these kinds of exercises. We are under the microscope all the time, with people monitoring our work in simulators or on checkrides. But this is different. This feels like we're sticking our necks out and being embarrassed in front of our colleagues."

If pilots were wary of doing these group activities with their peers, imagine, Patrick suggests, how worried they were about potential exposure to subordinates. It took a long time, he recounts, for pilots to grasp that group activities and discussion might actually be useful. "I remember we were asked to do an exercise with a group of flight attendants. We all sat around a table and were given a sheet of paper with the description of a hypothetical aircraft problem. It was something like, 'You're at cruise, and a flight attendant has called you two times to let you know that there's a very disruptive passenger in the back. While one flight attendant is bugging the captain about the passenger, another notices the floor is really warm beneath her feet. What do you do?'" The group together discussed what they would have been thinking and doing in these scenarios. In retrospect, Patrick says, it was alarming just how unaware each side of the cockpit door was of what was happening on the other.

> We learned that a lot of the flight attendants would be inclined to say, "I don't want to bug the captain anymore because bugging him about the passenger didn't get us anywhere." The moderator then asked the pilots, "Would you rather the FAs don't say anything?" Of course, we wanted them to alert us, but we quickly realized that we were really unaware of what was on their minds. In the

discussion the flight attendants had the opportunity to say, "Well, even though you personally tell me you want to know, I remember the time I got shut down by another guy who just told me not to bother [him]." We just didn't realize how often flight attendants were shut down by a captain who said, "Don't bother me with that!" These participatory exercises really opened up a dialogue that would never have been opened without them.

At the end of this exercise, the moderator told us that this scenario actually came from a real incident in which there was a fire in the cargo compartment. Because the flight attendants were afraid to call the captain, the fire was much worse than it might have been had the captain encouraged input and been made aware of the situation early on.

This is why the view of CRM as some kind of charm school had to be—and consistently continues to be—challenged. In a retrospective account of the evolution of CRM written in 1999, Robert Helmreich and his coauthors warned against the view that CRM was about making nice or being nice. "Support for this view comes from informal interviews of crews asked 'What is CRM?' A typical response is 'Training to make us work together better.' While this is certainly true, it only represents part of the story. It seems that in the process of teaching people how to work together we may have lost sight of why working together well is important." The authors worried that the "overarching rationale for CRM, reducing the frequency and severity of errors that are crew-based," had been lost.[2]

TRAINING STARTS AT THE TOP AND INCLUDES EVERYONE

About a year ago, a friend of ours was doing some consulting at a hospital where two different units were experiencing serious troubles among the staff. In both instances, although for different reasons, team interaction had become so problematic that basic professional performance was compromised. In one instance the issue was the relationship between nursing staff in the operating room and their nurse manager. In another, a hospital unit that focused on rehabilitation, relationships between nursing staff and occupational and physical therapy had become so tense that the entire unit's functioning was in jeopardy. In both instances, issues had been allowed to fester over months, if not years. Doctors had finally had enough and sought help from administrative higher-ups, who in turn sought help from our friend.

She went into the hospital, did some fact-finding, and discovered that without any team training, groups of individuals who were referred to as teams were teams in name only. They'd never done teamwork well when they were at their best. Now at their worst, relationships were so badly frayed that people were barely on speaking terms. When the consultant suggested team building and team workshops, administrative and physician higher-ups were delighted with the idea, with one proviso: physician leaders adamantly refused to attend any workshops or team-building sessions. The aviation safety movement has succeeded, in large part because, from the very first, this kind of abstention was not tolerated. The "chiefs" were not given a pass.

When United began CRM training for its pilots, the company could have trained each as separate groups—captains, first officers, and flight engineers, as captains would have preferred. "We had to have the power to bully the bullies," Ed Soliday put it bluntly. Not only were captains trained alongside first and second officers from the beginning, but CRM as *Cockpit* Resource Management evolved over the next few years to *Crew* Resource Management to include training of the cabin crew and later, in phase three, of other resources in the system—air traffic controllers, dispatchers, and maintenance workers.[3] Although these different disciplines may not be trained together, they are trained in teamwork skills, and the higher-ups are not only not exempt but also get the most rigorous training of any group.

All flight attendants receive CRM initial training in orientation and annually throughout their careers. FA training usually consists of one day a year. Depending on the airline, FAs sometimes train with pilots, sometimes alone. For logistical reasons, it is often difficult to train pilots and FAs together, as their work scheduling requirements differ, and flight attendants outnumber pilots in any airline. (On domestic flights there are 98,700 flight attendants. There are over 76,800 airline pilots and flight engineers in the US.)[4]

Pilots receive significant CRM/TEM training as part of their curriculum when they learn to fly, either in private or university flight schools or the military. It occurs as part of their initial company orientation and regularly throughout their airline career during "recurrent training." Each airline is allowed a certain amount of discretion regarding recurrent training scheduling, but at a minimum, each pilot will do this training annually. Recurrent training includes academic review of items that are always important (e.g., security, revised performance procedures, items that have been highlighted by recent events, and new knowledge and research such as review of specific aircraft systems and landing on rivers). This training also includes significant time in "the box"—the simulator—where conduct in normal and emergency scenarios is reviewed and perfected. In addition to successful completion of the academic portion, pilots receive a simulator checkride and may even be given an oral exam as well.

CRM/TEM is an essential part of recurrent training, as it is in daily operations. (Some airlines, as part of their predeparture briefing are actually expected to verbalize the most significant threat to the departure phase of the flight.) As part of the Advanced Qualification Program (AQP), CRM is discussed and considered during every aspect of simulator training. It is inconceivable that a captain or first officer would refuse to train in a group with flight attendants or other airline personnel; they would not have that option.

Whether CRM training is part of a recurrent training process or of an initial training program, the cost is borne by the companies themselves. Pilots and flight attendants are paid to attend required trainings as part of their normal work activity.[5] Generally, airlines employ their own staff to develop and administer trainings in accordance with FAA guidelines.[6] As explained in chapter 1, the FAA outlines what a CRM program must contain, but companies are given flexibility to adapt trainings to their individual cultures.

The development and continued evolution of CRM have involved all the players who had critical roles in aviation. Not only were companies, researchers, and government regulators active participants in the creation and implementation of the movement, but so were the labor unions that represented pilots, flight attendants, and other airline workers.

At its inception, when CRM was still conceptualized as Cockpit Resource Management, the Airline Pilots Association—the union that represents most commercial airlines pilots in the United States—took part in planning and implementation of trainings. As soon as CRM evolved into Crew Resource Management, the Association of Flight Attendants was also involved. As Robert Francis describes those early days, ALPA (whose president was then J. Randolph Babbitt) was "pulling, rather than dragging its heels."

Babbitt explained that it became very clear to the union that CRM would create a safer environment by introducing both situational awareness and crew resource management. Part of the union's job, he said, was to help deal with the resistance of senior pilots as opposed to "people at the working level."

> You put people at the working level together and say, "Look, these planes are getting more sophisticated, more complicated. We need to make sure everybody's on the same page." When this began everyone had his own way of doing things. There was no particular standard. Some pilots read the checklist; some pilots didn't. You had to sit on your hands and watch what was gonna happen, try to anticipate what the captain wanted.
>
> You talked to any copilot and they'd been faced with situations where you knew damn well that what the captain was doing was wrong and unsafe. But you just did not challenge him. If the captain said, "We're going to land with the landing gear up," you said, "Yes Sir!"

Today both ALPA and the AFA have active safety departments that teach and reinforce the lessons of CRM.

ADMITTING ERROR AND ASKING FOR HELP

About six years ago Patrick had a serious medical problem that required a three-year hiatus in his career. Before going back to flying, he not only had to be retrained to refresh his skills, but was also quick to let those with whom he was flying know that he'd been off and was just returning to work. "I always told the cockpit crews that I worked with that I'd been away from the flight deck for three years and that if they saw me doing anything that didn't seem quite right, it was probably because *it isn't quite right—so PLEASE, let me know!*"

In fact, it is pretty common practice for pilots to discuss their recent experience during initial introductions. "On the highly technical equipment that we operate these days, just a few weeks off will affect performance," according to Patrick. "It really helps to be familiar with your coworkers' recency of experience. If someone has been off for two months, he or she may be 'current' in the regulatory sense, but is she truly on top of her game? It always helps to know."

Although, as was evidenced in the JetBlue incident in March 2012, pilots are still worried about admitting personal problems to management, at least some do, and there is a greater individual awareness about the impact of personal problems on safety than there was pre-CRM. This change in attitudes was confirmed in a study that compared physicians and airline pilots in their attitudes and behaviors. By 2000, the majority of pilots but a minority of physicians admitted that the effects of fatigue, stress, or personal problems affected professional performance. Pilots agreed that "junior" team members should have input into decisions. (But most medical respondents did not. In particular, attending surgeons were the least likely to tolerate real intrateam discussion around critical issues or disagreements.)[7]

In our view, the focus on problems in the *system* rather than problems with an *individual* was critical in shifting attitudes toward admitting error and asking for help. Traditional attitudes have blamed an individual for whatever problem or accident or harm has arisen. According to this theory, accidents happen because of incompetence, lack of technical proficiency, inattentiveness, or any number of things that can be corrected by identifying the individual responsible and then blaming, disciplining, or even firing that person. If this is the sole explanation of error, then error becomes something shameful, and those who err become, not surprisingly, more concerned with concealing errors (and thereby keeping their jobs and reputations) than learning from them. The first study to systematically challenge this view was done in 1931 by H. Heinrich and his colleagues. This study of industrial accidents and how to prevent them documented that the "occurrence of any injury invariably results from a completed series of factors, the last one being the accident itself."[8] This became one of Heinrich's ten axioms of industrial safety.

Further elaborations on this theory led to James Reason's influential examination and "Swiss cheese model" of how errors happen. Errors don't happen just because of one bad actor or shameful exceptional occurrence. They are in fact inevitable by-products of being human and—particularly in the postindustrial age—of dealing with complex systems.

This approach depersonalizes error. It identifies instead the process through which individuals make errors because systems allow them to. "The basic premise in the system approach," Reason writes, "is that humans are fallible and errors are to be expected, even in the best organizations. Errors are seen as consequences rather than causes, having their origins not so much in the perversity of human nature as in 'upstream,' systemic factors. These include recurrent error traps in the workplace and the organizational processes that give rise to them."[9] Although, as Reason says, "blaming individuals is emotionally more satisfying than targeting institutions," this approach does little to prevent error. A system approach takes something that was hitherto considered shameful—and thus often hidden from sight, discussion, or investigation—into something that actually becomes quite fascinating to review, analyze, and learn from.

According to Reason's Swiss cheese model, error is never due to the holes in one particular slice. It is due to a series of human and system failures—a bunch of slices of cheese, each one of which influences the next, so that when the holes line up perfectly somewhere, error can slide right through. In his model of serious accidents, the chances that the one hole in the many Swiss cheese slices can line up perfectly are minimal.[10] And yet when the conditions are wrong, line up they do.

This combination of focusing on the system as well as helping people to understand that, as humans, we are *all* error-prone has made it possible for aviators and others in the industry to admit to and learn from error. It has also led to an error-reporting system that has become central to safety in aviation. The resulting widespread understanding of human vulnerability to error has produced recognition that no matter where one is in the hierarchy, one should encourage cross-monitoring of activity and input from those considered subordinates.

A HIGHLY INTEGRATED MODEL

CRM training is completely integrated into all aspects of aviation education and socialization. Pilots learn about CRM when they are in flight school as well as when they are oriented in a new airline job. Flight attendants get training in CRM when they come on board as new hires. When pilots are "type-rated" to fly a new aircraft, CRM and TEM are integrated into their training on that aircraft. Type-rating occurs when, say, Patrick goes from flying a 737 to an Airbus 320. One might imagine that the training is purely technical. While technical proficiency is a basic requirement of aviation, error-reduction skills are also threaded throughout the entire training—which can last up to six weeks or more. Trainings are done not only by the airlines but also by the manufacturers of planes.

Suzanne visited the Airbus Training Center in Miami and observed as pilots sat in the simulators and every imaginable emergency or constellation of crises was played out in that virtual reality. For Suzanne what was more impressive than the array of technology was how thoroughly the pilots were schooled in methods of communication. Before takeoff, a captain would brief a first officer. The instructor would intervene because the briefing wasn't brief enough or was too brief. During one event, when it was finally time to fly, an emergency had been programmed into the simulator—say an engine failure just prior to rotation on takeoff. In this scenario the captain was the PF. He correctly made the decision to continue the takeoff (as opposed to a high-speed abort). However, the instructor observed that the PF was also trying to micromanage his copilot (the PM), who was trying to work the emergency checklist. When the event was debriefed, the captain was reminded that his immediate task as the PF was to concentrate on flying and communicating with ATC. The guy in the right seat manages the checklist, the instructor cautioned.

CRM training is integrated and applied far beyond commercial airlines and their pilots and other staff. The value of this concept has not been lost on the military, emergency services, and even NASA. Captain Greg Johnson, a retired navy officer and space shuttle astronaut, stated that one of the first classes he encountered as a new astronaut trainee was Spaceflight Resource Management, or SFRM. "SFRM, or CRM for astronauts," said Captain Johnson, "was not just a tool for us. The difference between an effective shuttle crew and a less effective one came down to our CRM skills and execution. It is that important to us!"

RECURRENT AND CONSTANT TRAINING

In hospitals, too often teamwork and safety training takes place on a one-shot, or reactive-episodic basis. As our consultant colleague described it, "There's trouble on a unit, so it's 'Call in the cavalry! Quick, let's hire a consultant. Do fact-finding. Tell us what's wrong. Do a workshop. Do some follow-up.' And then disappear. If you're successful and actually help them and then suggest that it might be a good idea to continue trainings or work on an annual basis and that new staff should be integrated into the teamwork model now used on the unit, there may be zero interest."

A friend who is a nurse active in patient safety efforts at a prominent West Coast teaching hospital echoes these sentiments.

> We are constantly stymied by the fact that the institution doesn't have an ongoing commitment to patient safety initiatives. We will get a grant for a couple of years to fund some very promising patient safety initiative and things will go really well. And then the grant money runs out and there is no institutional pickup or follow-through. There is simply no institutional commitment to continue the activities, and so very promising progress is consistently stalled because of that.

This failure to continue successful patient safety projects is a constant in health care. In the mid-1990s the U.S. Army funded something called MedTeams, a team training that was developed by Dynamics Research Corporation for use in the emergency room. Eight hospitals piloted MedTeams, and the data on improved outcomes were very promising. Some hospitals did very well, some less so, but in the aggregate improvements were definitely made. Once the government funding disappeared, as one prominent emergency room physician who participated in the grant explained, the trainings themselves faded from view in most nonmilitary hospitals.

> The army adopted MedTeams for use in field hospitals, and the Department of Defense used the training as one of the models used in TeamSTEPPS [a training developed by the DOD and AHRQ, discussed in the next chapter]. Many of us hoped that the College of Emergency Physicians would take it on and adopt it officially, sponsoring it like the Heart Association sponsors Advanced Cardiac Life Support (ACLS). They decided not to do that. The problem was that there was funding for development but no funding for sustained training. Since hospitals are often unwilling to pay for the expense of team training, it doesn't happen. In my institution, you do see some change that has been sustained. Nurses are more assertive and proactive. There is more cross-monitoring and mutual assistance. But many excellent behaviors simply drifted away, and something very positive has had no lasting impact on emergency medicine.

This is not what has happened in aviation. What researchers understood immediately was not only that CRM had to be accepted and endorsed at all levels but also that it had to be continuously repeated if it was to take. People do not simply change behavior because they are exposed to ideas for an eight-hour session—or even for several years of flight school or military training. Old habits and customs take years to break and better new ones, years to acquire. In its most recent document outlining guidelines for CRM trainings, the FAA has this to say:

RECURRENT TRAINING

> CRM training must be included as a regular part of the recurrent training requirement. Recurrent CRM training should include classroom or briefing room refresher training to review and amplify CRM components, followed by practice and feedback exercises, such as LOFT, preferably with taped feedback; or a suitable substitute, such as role-playing in a flight training device and taped feedback. It is recommended that these recurrent CRM exercises take place with a full crew, each member operating in his or her normal crew position. A complete crew should always be scheduled, and every attempt should be made to maintain crew integrity. Recurrent training LOFT, which includes CRM, should be conducted with current line crews, and preferably not with instructors or check airmen as stand-ins. Recurrent training with performance feedback allows participants to practice newly improved CRM skills and to receive feedback on their effectiveness. Feedback has its greatest impact when it comes from self-critique and from

peers, together with guidance from a facilitator with special training in assessment and debriefing techniques.

CONTINUOUS REINFORCEMENT

No matter how effective each curriculum segment is (the classroom, the role-playing exercises, the LOFT, or the feedback), one-time exposures are simply not sufficient. The attitudes and norms that contribute to ineffective crew coordination may have developed over a crewmember's lifetime. It is unrealistic to expect a short training program to reverse years of habits. To be maximally effective, CRM should be embedded in every stage of training, and CRM concepts should be stressed in line operations as well.

CRM should become an inseparable part of the organization's culture.

There is a common tendency to think of CRM as training only for captains. This notion misses the essence of the CRM training mission: the prevention of *crew*-related accidents. CRM training works best in the context of the entire crew. Training exercises are most effective if all crewmembers work together and learn together. In the past, much of the flight crew training has been segmented by crew position. This segmentation has been effective for meeting certain training needs such as seat dependent technical training and upgrade training, but segmentation is not appropriate for most CRM training.[11]

Prestigious orchestras do not stop rehearsing after being hailed for their brilliant performances. Similarly, effective teams must constantly rehearse their performances if they are to reproduce their excellence consistently. As J. Richard Hackman writes in his excellent work *Leading in Teams*,

Some individuals are naturally talented in doing the right thing at the right time and in the right way to help their teams succeed, but others require training to develop their skills in taking action. Much is known about training procedures that can help people develop new skills or hone existing ones, and one of the things that is known is that skills cannot be mastered by reading books, listening to lectures, or doing case analyses. Instead, skill training involves observation of positive models (i.e. people whose behavior illustrates highly competent execution of that which is being taught) coupled with repeated practice and feedback. Training in execution skills is necessarily personalized and for that reason is expensive and time consuming. But it is a critical ingredient in the mix that makes for a great team leader.[12]

And we would add, for great team members as well.

CHANGING THE DYNAMICS OF "COOL"

When Suzanne, Bonnie, and Patrick turned eighteen, each of them decided that the cool thing to do was to start smoking. All of us were raised on images of movie stars and other assorted hotshots with cigarettes dangling from elegantly placed hands or beautifully pursed lips. It was Cool. None of us particularly liked smoking, but we taught ourselves to smoke—and then, with considerable difficulty—to stop. Decades later, Patrick's and Suzanne's daughters wouldn't be caught dead smoking. To them, smoking is the height of un-Cool.

Over the past thirty years, during pretty much the same period when CRM took root, the dynamics of Cool changed radically, and now in the same class, gender, and race cohort, what was amazingly "in" for the parents is totally "out" for the kids. In the case of tobacco, efforts to limit a certain behavior succeeded in great part because that behavior was delegitimized in the eyes of the next generation of potential recruits to smoking—and that took constant repetition of messages about safety and danger, as well as about what constituted desirable and undesirable behaviors.

How one dealt with what we call the "upcoming cohort issue" was critical to changing the behavior of captains who served as role models for those first officers who would become the next generation of team leaders. To change how they would behave when they became captains, it was critical to change the attitudes of first officers, flight attendants, and other crew members whose socialization in deference had been enabling abusive and nonresponsive captains and thus jeopardizing safety. These more deferential crew members also served as role models to anyone entering the workforce at their level in the aviation hierarchy, but they were sending outmoded and no-longer-desirable messages.

In any group, some people will change behavior more easily than others. They are known as early adapters, and they contribute positively to efforts at culture change. Selection standards for entry into professions also must be adapted in order to move an industry-wide change initiative forward. In aviation, companies have increasingly tried to select for people who can work well on teams and are less interested in people who are either deferential or domineering. This new selection process could not, however, alter some of the facts on the ground (or in this case, in the air).

During the initial stages of the change process, a lot of people who had been trained in the old school remained committed to the traditional values and behaviors. Aviation companies could have hinted and hoped—hinting that this behavior was no longer acceptable and hoping it would disappear with the aging and retirement of the pilot workforce. Instead, the industry delegitimated most of the behavior it wanted to eliminate by empowering crew members to speak up and by redefining traditional views of authoritarian behavior. This dynamic was articulated in an interview we had with a pilot who'd flown with a major U.S. airline company for twenty-one years. For fourteen years Steve Johnson occupied the right-hand seat as a first officer. Unlike some pilots who say they were initially skeptical of CRM, Johnson says he was always supportive. Although he believed first officers and flight engineers should be encouraged to speak up, they were at that time socialized to believe that "the captain was god. So if the timid, new first officer sees the captain making a mistake, or something is unfolding that the captain doesn't see, the first officer is afraid to speak up because he doesn't want to make any waves. He doesn't want to get this captain pissed off at him. He's not gonna say anything even though he sees a potential mistake being made."

By redefining this behavior as "insecure authority," the aviation safety movement changed the subordinates' view of the behavior of the superior. If in the initial phases of the implementation of CRM this behavior could not be changed, it could still be delegitimated. What Johnson says he and his younger colleagues learned was that a

> good captain will demand that the first officer say something 'cause he realizes with some humility that everybody makes mistakes and isn't always perfect. The whole idea was for the captain to come on board and give a briefing and say look, if you see anything you don't like, if I'm screwing up, I want you to say something. It's called "secure authority" in our actual training; just demanding participation from the rest of the crew whereas insecure authority is very aristocratic and tries to do everything himself. Which was what a lot of military guys, single-seat fighter pilots had been brainwashed into thinking—"you're the best and that you can do no wrong."

If the captain was an autocrat, pilots like the young Johnson now viewed them as revealing insecurity in their positions of authority. This redefinition of the right stuff reframed behavior that could best be altered by being challenged.

The same dynamic influenced the responses and behaviors of flight attendants. As Michelle Quintas explains,

> Flight attendants tend to be a group of women with a services mentality. Before CRM empowered them a flight attendant could see a wing fire and say, "Oh, I don't know: do you think we should call the cockpit?" Some people might actually have dismissed CRM as "Relating 101," but for many, it was critical. As a group we're not big self-advocators. CRM is all about empowering FAs to feel like they can speak up. While some flight attendants may have a great deal of education, pilots have a lot more when it comes to aviation.
>   . . . CRM training gave us permission to speak up. If you see a fire, it's important to tell the purser and captain. In CLR [United's acronym for CRM], you are a safety professional, you do what you think needs doing.

In a synergistic dynamic, CRM taught captains to listen and flight attendants to speak up—and taught each group *how* to do so as well. To empower the latter and not amend the former, or vice versa, would not have worked. "I think CLR worked so well," Quintas says," because the training went in both directions. What was critical was what went on on the cockpit side of the door. We were told and instructed in how to inquire, advocate, and assert, but more and more of [the captains] reinforced this behavior by telling us we were their eyes and ears in the cabin. 'You can interrupt sterile cockpit if it's an emergency.' They were not so arrogant."

CREATING PSYCHOLOGICAL SAFETY

What both Quintas and Johnson highlight is the fact that companies made it safe for subordinates to challenge superiors by creating an environment of psychological safety—one in which people were no longer rewarded for enabling those with insecure authority and certainly not for emulating their behaviors.

What do we mean by psychological safety? To answer that question we refer to the work of Amy Edmondson, a professor at Harvard Business School, who has elaborated on this concept. Her work builds on that of Edgar H. Schein and Warren B. Bennis, who first described psychological safety in their book *Personal and Organizational Change through Group Methods*. One of the key conditions for learning, Shein and Bennis argue, is "unfreezing" so that people who need to learn new behaviors or ideas develop curiosity about human behavior and about themselves. Essential to unfreezing is the creation of psychological safety within a particular group so that people can *"take chances without fear and with sufficient protection."* Learning new ideas and behaviors requires a sticking-one's-neck-out-without-reprisals attitude, as distinguished from playing it safe. Thus a climate is created that encourages provisional attempts and tolerates failure without retaliation, renunciation, or guilt.[13]

Edmondson argues that psychological safety is essential to the creation of the kind of *institutional learning* that is a nonnegotiable requirement of high-reliability organizations. "Psychological safety describes individuals' perceptions about the consequences of interpersonal risks in their work environment. It consists of taken-for-granted beliefs about how others will respond when one puts oneself on the line, such as by asking questions, seeking feedback, reporting a mistake, or proposing a new idea." In a team, Edmondson continues, "[p]sychological safety describes a climate in which the focus can be on productive discussion that enables early prevention of problems and the accomplishment of shared goals because people are less likely to focus on self-protection."[14]

Elsewhere Edmondson and Josephine P. Mogelof explain, "In psychologically safe environments, people believe that if they make a mistake or ask a naïve question, others will not penalize or think less of them for it."[15] This is the very heart of CRM: making sure that crew members are psychologically safe enough to raise their concerns and that captains are similarly secure enough to listen.

DEALING WITH GENDER ISSUES

Creating this kind of psychological safety inevitably involved dealing with gender issues between cockpit (predominantly male) and cabin (predominantly female), and even inside the cockpit between male and female pilots. Pilots are still overwhelmingly male, with between 6 and 7 percent female.[16] While the number of male flight attendants continues to climb, as of 2007, about 75 percent were female.[17] Flight attendants were not, however, the only ones to force airline companies to deal with sexual harassment and hostile workplaces. Female pilots also fought to change the atmosphere in a cockpit where male pilots used to routinely exhibit pornographic pictures or tell raunchy jokes.

Anne Simpson was one of those women, and her struggle was transformative, at least in her airline. Simpson came from an aviation family and learned to fly when she was twenty-five. She got her first commercial pilot's job with a major airline in 1981. The airline hadn't hired any pilots between 1969 and 1979, and because pilots were needed, male pilots, she says, welcomed her and the other female pilots they hired. (Women represented less than two percent of the pilot group at that time, so we are not talking about large numbers here.)

Although Simpson noticed the soft porn in the cockpit—in the book where pilots keep their checklists or in a cubbyhole where the escape ropes are stowed—she didn't find it too troubling. Then the economy took a nosedive in 1987, and she felt a change in the attitudes of her male colleagues. "The industry had become stagnant in terms of career advancement. The mere existence of female colleagues in the cockpit seemed to suggest to some males that females were preventing them from moving up. This in spite of the fact that no one was advancing! Suddenly, as a first officer, I noticed that the porn was getting more violent and offensive."

What had been slightly irritating before was becoming intolerable. "My attitude was, this is my office. Yes, it's a shared office, but then they shouldn't leave their pornography when they turn their office over to the next crew." Simpson took her concerns to the professional standards department at her union, ALPA. "I said, 'Hey, guys, this is getting out of hand; I shouldn't have to see this when I go to work to do my job.' They agreed and said they would deal with it at the pilot level and work to resolve the inappropriate behavior of some of this group."

That's when her problems really began. Word got out that Simpson was the anti-porn queen. "It became a very miserable experience." For about two and a half years before checking out as a captain in 1991, she would get in an aircraft and see comments in the logbook like, "Simpson doesn't like pornography. Simpson is f—the chief pilot," or something about Simpson and her lesbian lovers. Eventually it got even more personal with messages like "F—you Simpson." Since pilots have no idea in which particular ship number they will be flying, no one was ever sure who would get these messages or if Simpson would ever see them. These written assaults were thus a kind of damning code being broadcast throughout the company.

Simpson was—to say the least—shocked at all this. She thought the problem would be dealt with at the pilot level and that efforts to resolve the problem would not identify her specifically, but she was only to discover that her attempts to seek help from the union had unleashed hostility that was now directed at her personally: "It was quite overwhelming. I always felt that I was a well-liked person. I think I'm considerate, and yet I would be walking through the terminal and see all these other pilots who didn't know me and wonder if they hated me. I was worried when I walked through the company parking lot to my car late at night that someone might physically harm me."

Working through ALPA Professional Standards wasn't effective, so Simpson went to the company's chief pilot, who agreed things were getting out of hand. After more than a year of working with the company to no avail, Simpson sought legal counsel. On the advice of her lawyer, she told the chief pilot that the workplace was increasingly hostile and she would not be coming back to work until things changed. The company management appeared to take the situation seriously by implementing some policy changes, and Simpson returned to work. Unfortunately, these actions did not conclusively resolve the problem: Just three months later she found a tampon in her work mailbox with some very crude and graphic handwritten instructions attached. "Once again I informed the chief pilot that I would be unable to continue working in such a hostile work environment," she said.

After another three months off, Simpson returned to work after the company had reassured her that it had rededicated itself to enforcing their "zero tolerance" policy. Additionally, they established support, resources, and education for current and incoming female pilots. These actions seemed to have finally had a positive outcome, and Simpson eventually rose to become one of the first female 747 captains in the world. "This was a very challenging process, but I feel—and have been told—that I have made a difference for those that came after me."

These kinds of struggles strengthened CRM because they called attention to untenable conditions and their resolution created a respectful environment where everyone—no matter whether male or female, gay or straight, black or white or brown—was now on the team.

THE ROLE OF GOVERNMENT

In his book *Why Hospitals Should Fly*, former military and commercial airline pilot and author John Nance uses a fictionalized scenario to make the case that hospitals should adopt CRM principles. His account centers on a dialogue between two physicians—Dr. Will Jenkins and Dr. Jack Silverman, CEO of St. Michael's Hospital, which has adopted the CRM model with great success. Although his description of the history and virtues of CRM is persuasive, Nance leaves out some crucial facts—particularly the role that the government played in the development and implementation of CRM. Through his characters' conversations, Nance in fact appears to disapprove of government participation. "We know what works and how to make it work," Silverman explains to Jenkins. "We can cajole and teach and lead, but ultimately it's the boards of hospitals across America that will either make hospitals into high-reliability institutions or will thwart improvements to the point that we all end up nationalized and run by some giant bureaucracy in Washington."[18] According to Silverman, FAA regulations on CRM actually stiffened captains' resistance to CRM and hampered its swift uptake. "Fortunately," Silverman says, "we don't have an FAA imposing such a rule and inflaming myopic resistance." Nance's account reflects a strong antiregulatory position that is widely shared in health care, one that ignores the very positive role that government played and continues to play in the creation and evolution of CRM and thus of its successful safety track record.

One of the reasons that CRM succeeded and has evolved so robustly is that it is not optional but mandatory, not only in one airline but in all airlines. In a far more nuanced discussion of CRM's history and staying power, Robert Helmreich explains the government's approach to CRM training. Commercial airlines, he writes, must do some sort of CRM training, but they are free to tailor their CRM programs to local conditions. "The FAA," Helmreich explains, "has an advisory circular on CRM which gives good guidelines for the training. . . . [Circular 120–151] recommends ways of doing it but it is not a government command, 'you will do it this way. This," Helmreich adds, "is a very important lesson for nursing and medicine. There are an awful lot of local factors that influence what happens."

Clay Foushee, who worked with Robert Helmreich and at one point in his career was vice president for flight operations at Northwest Airlines, believes that regulation was critical in the evolution of aviation safety. Suzanne spoke with him several years before he became director of the Office of Audit and Evaluation at the FAA in late 2009. Neither medicine nor hospitals, Foushee notes, operate under a regulatory agency like the FAA. Aviation functions in a "regulatory environment that says that 'you will do this kind of thing and it will be done along policy guidelines.'" These guidelines stipulate that pilots not only must train in CRM/TEM principles and skills but must be tested and retested on their skill in working on teams. Foushee notes,

> I would love, as a patient, to know that my doctor was required to go through an operating room exercise on an annual basis in order to keep his or her board certification valid, and that would involve an exercise where you would go into a simulated operating room with a simulated patient with nurses, anesthesiologists, and had that thing videotaped. I would be reassured knowing that my physician had to sit down with a surgeon who was an instructor and actually review what happened during that procedure with that patient. It seems to me that would be invaluable.

The FAA has not only mandated CRM but facilitated its evolution in a number of critical ways. As we explained in chapter 1, NASA's 1979 meeting was a launching pad for CRM activity. NTSB reports have advanced understanding of why crashes happen and introduced changes, based on their findings, that have made these accidents less likely to reoccur. "NASA was really in the right place at the right time," Foushee explains. "NASA wanted an environment where we could look at crew interaction and performance. The airlines were willing to participate if they saw a problem that the training programs weren't addressing and they were more than happy to have NASA's assistance."

Describing the kinds of synergies that were created between unions, government, airlines, and researchers, Foushee adds, "We put together industry workshops. We created guidelines for flight-oriented trainings. There were proceedings for Crew Resource Management training workshops, and there were a lot of materials that were free for airline training departments to use. We also ran the Aviation Safety Reporting System, which was a large aviation safety data base that was usable in training curriculum, and NTSB databases that were also available."

The FAA also enhances quality control in airlines safety. The agency grants authority to airline company employees who are designated as FAA representatives and who have the power to sign off on pilots' check flights for the federal agency. These personnel—Foushee refers to them as "deputy sheriffs "—are "specifically selected for their skills and have completed rigorous training programs. On a random basis, the FAA also sends out federal inspectors who sit in the flight-deck jump seat during actual flights and check pilots' skills—including safety/teamwork skills." Included in coordinated trainings are flight attendants and other airline personnel.

Most of the prominent researchers who have been involved in the development of aviation safety agree with Helmreich and Foushee. Dave Musson, a physician and pilot and colleague of Robert Helmreich, has worked in both the world of aviation and the world of medicine. When Suzanne spoke to him, he was enthusiastic about the progress in aviation but deeply skeptical about the prospects of similar advances in health care. "There are several generations that have progressed in aviation and it's been because the FAA funds research. Because of the cooperation between the FAA and the airlines, the airlines are happy to provide people like me the opportunity to sit in the cockpit and watch the crews when they fly around. We have meetings with all the aviation trainers where all the different airlines come."

"In aviation," he says, "government has helped to create a culture of collaboration and cooperation," which he has not found in the individualistic, privatized world of medicine and hospital administration:

> In aviation, the safety model evolved because of a need and because of the airlines' desire to make things safer. It didn't evolve as companies selling products to the airline industry. Because of this we have a very open form of discussion. If you're a trainer at JetBlue, you can fly Continental Airlines and speak to the safety manager and he'll happily e-mail you all his training materials. In medicine, the training is done by private companies who are really just interested in selling their product and not [in] making the entire industry safer. The information is

proprietary, and evaluations are done by the companies that are selling the product. It's like keeping a treatment of a disease secret because you want people to come to your office.

Without some regulatory mandate, what happened to MedTeams and other promising initiatives is bound to repeat itself. Today in health care, The Joint Commission—a private, not-for-profit agency that accredits and monitors hospitals—recommends team training and collaborative practice. So do the U.S. Institute for Medicine and accrediting bodies for health care professional education like the Accreditation Council for Graduate Medical Education and the American Association of Colleges of Nursing. None of these organizations can legally mandate—as the FAA has done—that hospitals and professional schools actually implement programs that teach people how to function in teams. Nor have they outlined precisely what interprofessional education or team training must include. Sadly, U.S. hospitals and many U.S. educational institutions seem almost allergic to government regulation or intervention and often choose to ignore the evidence of how team training has positively impacted other high-risk endeavors. Medicine tends to have a very narrow view of what constitutes evidence—preferring the kind of gold-standard randomized, controlled trials that may be useful to evaluate medications and medical procedures but are less effective in bringing about complex behavioral and system change. However, in an era of best practices, it may be useful to consider that government actually has a positive role to play in helping medical personnel keep themselves and others safe.

The government also plays another critical role in establishing the context in which aviation safety is both refined and maintained—that is through workload regulation. In health care, the sky is pretty much the limit when it comes to hours worked and staff-to-patient ratios. With the exception of restrictions on doctor-in-training hours (restrictions that, some safety advocates argue, are still too lax), physicians can work as long as they want during a day and as many days as they want during a week. There are also no work-hour restrictions imposed on nursing or other staff, and in many places nurses may in fact be subject to mandatory overtime on short notice. In aviation, as we have seen, pilots and flight attendants cannot legally work more than a certain number of consecutive hours and are limited as to the total of cumulative hours per seven days, thirty days, and annually as well.

In health care, physicians, nurses, lab techs, and other professionals can be asked to shoulder as large a patient load (or load of X-rays to read, lab tests to check) as the physician or employer deems necessary, or profitable. Except in California (and the state of Victoria in Australia) and under certain union contracts, RN workloads are totally elastic. A nurse can be asked to take care of as many patients as the employer assigns her. Doctors' workloads are similarly flexible. If a doctor decides that his or her income necessitates extra patients or if an employer or physician practice decides that a doctor has to see a certain number of patients and that seven minutes is long enough to establish a good rapport, diagnose and treat, figure out what medications a patient is on, and explain them all—well, seven minutes it is. While there has been a robust debate about staffing ratios in nursing, evidence from California suggests that—in spite of fears of unintended consequences—ratios have increased recruitment and retention of RNs, heightened job satisfaction, and decreased turnover.[19]

In aviation, there are ratios that determine how many pilots must be in the flight deck and how many flight attendants in the cabin. On commercial aircraft, there has to be one flight attendant per 50 seats (if there are 150 seats and only 101 passengers, there still must be three flight attendants on board). In the cockpit, pilots' staffing is regulated under very strict guidelines driven by scheduled flight time and duty times. Likewise, rest periods are similarly regulated and strictly enforced. "There are simply no shortcuts here," says Patrick. "We would never even consider flying short-staffed or without legal rest. The consequences of doing so just once could cost you your job and career (not to mention your life!)."

The combination of company, government, union, and research involvement in aviation has produced a safety program that is evidence-based and constantly evolving. It has become standard operating procedure in the airlines industry and has managed to move past considerable resistance to become not only accepted but routinely regarded as one of the pluses of working in the field.

"Commercial flight," Foushee concludes, echoing a metaphor Patrick used earlier "is like a finely crafted ballet. All of this is so incredibly proceduralized and everybody in the system knows exactly what is going to happen." Ballet is an apt metaphor for what happens both inside and outside the aircraft. To dance in a ballet company demands an extraordinary musculature that has been developed over decades. In aviation, mandated training and retraining, a controlled workload and work hours produce crews who have developed and continually exercise the mental musculature of teamwork.

Chapter 10

The Problems in Medicine

It is now universally acknowledged that failures of teamwork and communication, not simply failures in technical proficiency, are the cause of the majority of medical errors and injuries in hospitals and other health care facilities. Human factors—such as the failure of human beings to relate productively to each other in highly demanding and technological settings—are a major cause of patient harm.

In many of the studies published in the most reputable of scientific journals, CRM is repeatedly mentioned as a model for how to create safer hospitals and health care institutions. It would seem that patient safety advocates recognize that—in spite of their many differences—there are also significant similarities between the aviation industry and the health care system that cannot be ignored and that make the lessons of CRM highly adaptable to health care. Both are hierarchical settings, with one dominant group, which, until recently, was mainly male (and largely remains so in aviation; the number of women physicians has multiplied exponentially in the past fifteen to twenty years). The less dominant but larger group of workers was (and still is) made up of women who have long been tutored in deference. In both, a heroic narrative has encouraged the kind of extreme individual autonomy and lack of oversight for "tops" that has put many people at risk. Finally, there is a huge reliance on advanced technology in both sectors, and there is a historical reluctance to engage in the kind of teamwork that has now been well demonstrated to save lives.

As if recognizing all this, best-selling books promote aviation-inspired checklists and time-outs in ORs and ICUs. We hear about the use of huddles—a series of daily briefings—in labor and delivery. Simulation centers are popping up in medical schools, along with efforts to introduce—and even fund—interprofessional education in university health care training programs and interprofessional care in practice settings. In hospitals, CNOs, CEOs, and medical leaders are finally recognizing the need to create more respectful behavior in their workplaces and are launching civility initiatives. Pilots are continually invited to consult or lecture in hospitals. The Agency for Healthcare Research and Quality's TeamSTEPPS training is now used in many facilities, and The Joint Commission now advises that teamwork and communication training be included in continuing health professional education. The Institute for Healthcare Improvement (IHI) has pioneered many initiatives that have made patient care safer.

Discussions of the lessons of aviation and other high-reliability industries are taking place with greater frequency in health care than ever before.[1] Even the rejection of the CRM model because some believe it cannot be superimposed on health care is a sign that the lessons of aviation are penetrating the medical and administrative awareness of health care institutions. In spite of great resistance, these initiatives are producing positive models that have led to major conceptual shifts and practical improvements and thus offer great promise.

We have already discussed several of those. In this chapter, we look at the limitations in applying CRM to health care. This examination helps us understand why there has been such disappointing progress in actually reducing medical errors and injuries and in reducing tension between health professions or increasing job satisfaction and morale throughout the system. Although the problems we describe exist in many different countries, for the purposes of this discussion we will focus primarily on the U.S. health care system.

If we dissect the reasons for the success of aviation safety as a model for behavioral and cultural change, we find a fairly thorough list of the ingredients needed to create sustainable behavioral and cultural change:

- Challenging the old heroic narrative
- Changing the dynamics of Cool
- Redefining error and changing responses to errors
- Recognizing the existence and value of distributed cognition
- Building team intelligence
- Dealing assertively with toxic hierarchy
- Creating psychological safety
- Introducing training in teamwork and its skills
- Committing to integration of teamwork into organizational work patterns
- Providing for recurrent training
- Managing workloads
- Instituting regulatory incentives and controls

These are the critical elements that make broad systemic behavioral and cultural change efforts work, no matter where they are implemented—whether in aviation, health care, nuclear power plants, or naval vessels. Of course, medicine and aviation are different—and that is why the strategies of CRM have to be *adapted* to the specific health care environments to which they are applied, just as they are adapted for specific aviation settings (commercial, corporate, military, space flight, etc.). We believe that this change in health care will be difficult—very, very difficult. We understand that health care has different complexities than aviation, but we also believe that if aviation and other high-reliability industries can make these changes for the better, then so can health care. As in aviation, the process of change will take years, will meet with resistance, and, on the basis of ongoing research, will be continually refined along the way.

Although we cannot account for every program or initiative that has been developed to improve patient safety in the United States, we have seen a great many. We have seen some very impressive work. Still, change in the whole health care organization or system often does not match the sum of its parts, and there seems to be more talk than action at many sites. Where there is action, it tends to be on a unit-by-unit or service-by-service basis, so even in organizations where there is quite a bit of activity there is still not a whole lot of interaction. This in spite of the fact that health care is positively awash in talk of patient safety, system reform, teams, and teamwork.

THE HEROIC MEDICAL NARRATIVE—THINKING ALONE

In health care, as in aviation pre-CRM, one of the barriers to change is the story that members of the dominant group—the physicians—have inherited and in turn pass on to new cohorts and generations. This heroic medical narrative is part of the folklore of medicine and is encountered in educational and training venues, practice settings, and the popular media. Although this narrative features physicians, its structure and content affect other health care professionals, workers, and of course patients. Rather like the aviators Tom Wolfe described in *The Right Stuff*, in this narrative the lone physician works against all odds, taking great risks and finally triumphing over disease and death. The narrative is inherently antiteam because both the burdens and the victories of patient care are shouldered by or attributed to the doctor alone.

Sadly, this heroic narrative infects not only conventional medicine but even those progressive physicians who seem to be at the forefront of change and patient safety. Consider the work of Jerome Groopman, whose book *How Doctors Think* makes it clear that doctors apparently think only with other doctors. Groopman begins his journey into doctors' thinking by describing the terror that young doctors-in-training experience in their internships. On his own first night in the hospital, Groopman realized that he "would be *alone*, responsible for all of the patients on the floor as well as any new admissions." While he was alone, one of his patients began to crash and he froze. Fortunately, the sudden appearance of a senior physician, whom Groopman characterized without irony as a "deus ex machina," kick-started his paralyzed brain so that he could save his patient.[2]

Reading this, Suzanne and Bonnie, who have spent years in teaching hospitals, could only think, Alone? Where were all the nurses? Many of them, without doubt, had several years' experience in caring for patients (and all of them, with the exception of the very newest hires, would have had more experience than a first-night intern). They were probably available for consultation and assistance at a moment's notice. Indeed, the hospital could not have functioned without its nurses, who are on duty 24/7. The clear, if unstated, message of this narrative is that "alone" for Groopman meant "without other doctors scheduled to be on the premises" and that other doctors were the only ones whose presence in this situation actually counted.

Atul Gawande, a surgeon and staff writer for the *New Yorker*, is another prominent physician champion of patient safety whose fluent writing and publications in the popular press as well as in medical journals have made his ideas integral to current thinking about contemporary health policy and patient safety. Yet, while giving lip service to teamwork, much of his writing is so physician-centric that it is hard to imagine how it could help people effectively lead or function on genuine teams. Gawande's early books, *Complications, Better*, and *Checklist Manifesto*, place him firmly in the tradition of the heroic medical narrative. In one particularly telling passage in the beginning of *Better*, Gawande states,

> We [physicians] also face daunting expectations. In medicine, our task is to cope with illness and to enable every human being to lead a life as long and free of frailty as science will allow. The steps are often uncertain. The knowledge to be mastered is both vast and incomplete. Yet we are expected to act with swiftness and consistency, even when the task requires marshaling hundreds of people— from laboratory technicians to the nurses on each change of shift to the engineers who keep the oxygen supply system working—for the care of a single person.[3]

But physicians do not, in fact, marshal lab techs or nurses or engineers. Nor do these personnel work for physicians; they work for the hospitals that pay them. Most of them do not even remotely conceptualize their efforts as working for physicians but as working for and with patients. The commonly held physician-centric view of the health care enterprise is a serious inhibitor to the kind of teamwork upon which consistently safe patient care depends; it turns hospital care into what Suzanne has called "parallel play among intimate strangers."[4] Gawande's portrayal of health care activity reprises the myth of doctors as armies of one. In actuality, hospital physicians function as players in interdisciplinary settings that include multiple actors, each of whom has an important contribution to make to patient care and to quality and safety improvements. Health care, wherever it is delivered, requires the kind of "distributed cognition" we have mentioned earlier.

In a recent *New Yorker* contribution entitled, "Personal Best: Should Everyone Have a Coach?" Gawande again displays his medicocentric vision.[5] In this well-written piece, "everyone" turns out to mean "physicians." Gawande asks whether physicians should have the kind of personal coaches that are routine in the world of competitive sport. In order to find out if he could improve his game, so to speak, he asks one of the surgeons who served as his mentor during his training to come into the OR and observe him at work. The senior physician—the retired general surgeon Robert Osteen—agrees and watches Gawande in the OR. When the two emerge, they debrief in the lounge and Osteen points to a number of small things that Gawande could have done better. Although neither surgeon mentions the word "teamwork," most of Osteen's points of improvement have to do with interactions with the OR staff of which Gawande had been unaware. To his credit, he owns up to these issues unflinchingly:

> I had positioned and draped the patient perfectly for me, standing on his left side, but not for anyone else. The draping hemmed in the surgical assistant across the table on the patient's right side, restricting his left arm, and hampering his ability to pull the wound upward. At one point in the operation, we found ourselves struggling to see up high enough in the neck on that side. The draping also pushed the medical student off to the surgical assistant's right, where he couldn't help at all. I should have made more room to the left, which would have allowed the student to hold the retractor and freed the surgical assistant's left hand.[6]

He had also been unaware of his patient's blood pressure problems during surgery, which the anesthesiologist had been carefully monitoring. Gawande then muses, "[T]he stranger thing, it occurred to me, was that no senior colleague had come to observe me in the eight years since I'd established my surgical practice. Like most work, medical practice is largely *unseen by anyone who might raise one's sight. I'd had no outside ears and eyes.*"[7] In actual fact, scores of people—entire operating room staffs and innumerable trainees—had to have been observing him quite closely over these eight years. Many of them could have raised his sights and acted as much-needed "outside ears and eyes" and as critical thinking partners had the invitation been extended, or had the culture of the OR encouraged this interaction. Why did it take the presence of a senior surgeon-observer to uncover these teamwork problems? Why didn't anyone else in the OR—medical student, surgical assistant, operating room nurse, anesthesiologist—mention these issues?

The clear lack of team identity and team intelligence among this group of surgical coworkers prevented an entire group of people from enacting simple logistical changes that could have improved working conditions for all of them—and probably patient safety in the OR as well. Gawande concludes that many doctors could benefit from having personal trainers—envisioned as other physicians of equal or greater status. "We could create coaching programs not only for surgeons but for other doctors too—internists aiming to sharpen their diagnostic skills, cardiologists aiming to improve their heart attack outcomes, and all of us who have to figure out ways to use our resources more efficiently."[8] Or, we suggest, perhaps we could create, train for, and enact in daily practice, throughout the hospital, some true teamwork.

These attitudes are not surprising in a system that meticulously teaches doctors that they are *the* responsible parties with respect to patient care and that *they* have the right stuff, which no one else outside their profession shares or can acquire. "You can challenge my orders when you've gone to medical school for four years," is a comment nurses commonly get when they try to cross-monitor physicians. Or they are told that they are "insubordinate" if they openly disagree with a doctor's plan of care. In the see one/do one/teach one apprenticeship model of medical training, some attending physicians will tell medical students and residents—or model by their own conduct—that they should consult with nurses and other health professionals, while others teach students to studiously avoid RNs as representing unwelcome background noise that has more potential to get in the way of than to enhance clinical decision making.

This view of physicians means that very few doctors-in-training learn what exactly nurses or other health care professionals or workers do or why they are employed. One dean of a major nursing school (connected to an equally well-known teaching hospital) recounted, "A chief resident actually came up to me, very earnestly, and asked me, 'Can you tell me what nurses do? I really don't fully understand.'" That someone who had been working in hospitals for years could honestly ask such a question testifies to the lack in health care of the team-focused education and socialization that are now routine in aviation.

The effects of the heroic medical narrative on physician perspectives are also reflected in medicine's categorization of nonphysician health care professions and occupations. Physicians, for example, commonly refer to registered nurses and nurse-practitioners (among others) as "physician extenders." Nurses; physical, occupational, and respiratory therapists; lab technicians; pharmacists and pharmacy technicians; and many others are referred to as "allied health professions"—allied to medicine, that is. Or nurses and other health care professionals are referred to as "midlevel" practitioners (in the midlevel of the status and power hierarchy, for sure). Doctors are taught to view the purpose of nursing and other so-called allied professions as assisting *medicine*—while members of these professions commonly view their purposes as assisting *patients*.

While other health professions may complain of this Adam's rib view of themselves, they often mimic this language and attitudes within their own ranks. Nurses refer to nurses' aides as "nurse extenders." When asked to justify their salaries and work, RNs explain that they are the ones who employ critical thinking skills and are the decision makers when it comes to the care of the patients while licensed practical nurses (LPNs) and nurses' aides apparently have no ability to think critically about their work and neither employ any strategies nor make any important decisions while performing it. In health professions like nursing, as the workforce splinters into ever smaller shards, these kinds of invidious distinctions are made by more and more groups within a profession, as well as between professions. Nurses use the language physicians mobilize to dismiss nursing work to dismiss that of those under them. Plus, a new corps of "advanced practice nurses" (APRNs) uses similar language to explicitly belittle the work of RNs, who are viewed as nonautonomous, not critical thinkers and "just nurses."

As the health care system tries to save money by deconstructing the jobs of various professionals and apportioning aspects of this work to so-called lower-level employees, this self-aggrandizing, other-belittling process is repeated like an endless series of distorted reflections in a fun-house mirror. Physical therapists, pharmacists, and others now have aides and assistants or techs (the name varies but the attitude doesn't) who are seen as extensions of the knowledge and judgment of the professional "superior."[9] Studies in the sociology of work and professions continually document this tendency of (any and all) professions to draw exclusionary boundaries and to assert their own superior status against the necessary—even "natural"—subjugation or diminution of others.

This process can move both ways along the power gradient. In their own professional development, nursing and other so-called midlevel professions turn an equally disdainful gaze on medicine. Nursing education, for example, is often as overtly hostile to medicine as medicine can be to nursing. Nurses are taught that *they* are "the patient advocates," the implicit assumption being that physicians or other health care professionals are somehow not advocating for patients. Many physicians have expressed their frustration with this formulation. One irate surgeon asked Suzanne, "So what does that make me, the patient's enemy?" A physical therapist who'd left the hospital and gone into private practice echoed these sentiments. "Working in the hospital was so frustrating. You'd go into a patient's room and the nurse would be there and she'd make you feel like some kind of interloper, as if she was the only one who cared about the patient and you were there to do the patient harm. I think they teach them that on the first day of nursing school."

As well as being the patients' advocates, nurses consider themselves an antidote to a flawed medical model that provides narrow technical care, while they—the RNs—provide holistic, humanistic care. In listening to RNs talk, as Suzanne has for over twenty-five years, it is clear that medicine and nursing view themselves not as collaborators but as competitors, not as team members but as members of opposing teams. These kinds of tensions are replicated throughout the health care professions. And if professionals treat each other with such wariness, they treat those whom they consider to be doing "mindless work"—such as house-keepers and transport and kitchen workers—even more dismissively.

Patrick has recounted the liberating effect on post-CRM pilots of knowing that they do not have to do everything because there are other human resources available for help and advice. This understanding that one's work involves distributed cognition is largely absent in medicine. If the knowledge of what other health care professionals know and do is invisible, it is easy to understand why little communication may exist between the ranks; why physicians, as "captains," feel so responsible and so vulnerable; why patients may suffer from this significant misunderstanding; and why there is so little evidence of genuine teamwork and team intelligence on health care teams.

THE TEAM—REALLY?

Everywhere you look in health care there are discussions of patient care as a team activity and mention of the team that is responsible for this or that patient or outcome. When you probe further, it becomes clear that the same people who talk about teams lack even the most basic agreement on what a team is, who is on it, and what it should do. In most health care settings, "team" refers to that group of individuals who just happen to be assigned to the same patient or group of patients ("the care team"), work on the same unit ("the ICU team") or are in the same discipline ("the respiratory therapy team").

Another common tacit definition of "team" in health care is of an *intra*disciplinary group of people who are in charge of the patient—for example, the medical team. Ask a nurse to identify the team and she may well point to the group of physicians doing their rounds on the floor. She may not consider herself a member of the team, nor will these doctors necessarily view her as a teammate. But then when nurses, PTs, or other professionals talk team, they similarly refer to people in their own clinical discipline.

Another, unwritten definition of a team goes something like this: a stable group of people who have worked together in one setting over time and have thus earned one another's trust by demonstrating their competence and credibility in that setting. Suzanne has often heard nurses recount their excellent relations with a particular doctor, in a particular unit, whose trust they say they have earned over many years. This type of trusting and effective working relationship does actually make up a true team of a kind, but it typically includes only a specific group of individuals who have forged very good working relationships in a circumscribed environment.

In health care the kind of psychological safety that leads to institutional learning is often replaced by disrespect, historical antipathies, and even outright abuse.

In a recent study on disrespect in the workplace, Lucien Leape and his colleagues noted that

> a substantial barrier to progress in patient safety is a dysfunctional culture rooted in widespread disrespect. . . . At one end of the spectrum, a single disruptive physician can poison the atmosphere of an entire unit. More common are everyday humiliations of nurses and physicians in training, as well as passive resistance to collaboration and change. Even more common are lesser degrees of disrespectful conduct toward patients that are taken for granted and not recognized by health workers as disrespectful.
>
> Disrespect is a threat to patient safety because it inhibits collegiality and cooperation essential to teamwork, cuts off communication, undermines morale, and inhibits compliance with and implementation of new practices. Nurses and students are particularly at risk, but disrespectful treatment is also devastating for patients.[10]

This kind of disrespect is a gift that keeps on giving in healthcare. Sometimes, when nurses mention good teamwork with physicians, they claim that it is a result of the fact that they taught a resident what's what by paging him over and over again in the middle of the night. One nurse told us that when a resident was tardy filling a pain order for one of her patients, she paged the attending to complain. She then boasted that "the attending must have reamed him a new one because he came down right away." These passive-aggressive strategies may work to bring "recalcitrants" to heel or to badger initiates into specific behavior patterns, but playing "gotcha" does *not* create a team (and in fact seriously undermines trust, a fundamental aspect of team building).

So-called teamwork created through punitive means applies to health care in both the inter- and intradisciplinary context. One of the mantras in nursing is that "nurses eat their young." This phenomenon generally refers to more experienced nurses who do not support, listen to, or accord respect and civility to the new kid on the block, who may be a newly minted nurse or simply a new recruit to their work unit. Residents similarly complain about attendings who blow them off or are rude or condescending. One young woman entering an internal medicine residency at a prominent Harvard teaching hospital in 2011 told us that during her orientation the physician in charge of her clerkship blithely informed the group of incoming interns that things might be tough on them but that they would "just have to learn to play in the sandbox" because that's the way things were and nothing was going to change. Given this opening message, she said she felt she had nowhere to turn when faced with what she considered problematic and unprofessional behavior on the part of attendings or more senior residents.

Even when people are trying to rectify these problems in their institution—say, through a civility initiative—they often believe that problematic behavior on the part of physicians, nurses, or other staff members is a question of personalities—

personalities that can't really be changed—rather than a *system issue*. The old adage "leopards can't change their spots" is frequently invoked. In actuality behaviors can be taught, learned, and changed, irrespective of individual personalities, as CRM has demonstrated. And institutions, if they are serious about professional behavior, can readily communicate that message by placing noncompliers on leave, ordering remediation, or delivering an official reprimand. Actions speak louder than words.

When teams are established in the unquestioned sandbox, the process tends to make it difficult, if not impossible, to reframe what is Cool because the system is constantly reproducing undesirable behaviors. In medicine, these are behaviors that jeopardize patient safety as well as staff and trainee morale. In aviation, the bad captain's behavior is now the example of what *not* to emulate—an embarrassment to the profession. In most medical settings, this kind of behavior may still be criticized in personal venting sessions (or in trainings like TeamSTEPPS), but it is not yet typically the subject of widespread delegitimation that can change the dynamics of Cool in a workplace culture.

In the see one/do one/teach one model, the new recruit may feel he or she is entering a boot camp, rather than a learning/teaching/healing institution. Interns are often deeply disheartened—and many experience true crises of conscience as they live through what the hospital culture *actually* metes out to them and makes available to patients. When teams are created on the foundation of this kind of hazing—even bullying—team members may become so stressed that they are unable to perform up to par.[11] This in turn places patients at further safety risk and contributes to downward-spiraling morale among personnel.

Pity the poor patient who is dependent on a resident who not only has been up for twenty hours but has just gotten scolded by an attending during morning rounds because he or she has made a mistake (of the kind that are essential to the trainees' learning process). Or the poor patient who is cared for by Dr. X and a nurse she's worked with for only a few days or even weeks. Or the new nurse whose RN colleagues are showing him who's boss on the unit. (Or the doctor or nurse who has not only been up for hours but also has not eaten a thing. As Daniel Kahneman has documented in his book *Thinking, Fast and Slow*, the human brain actually needs fuel to function. Without it, people are irritable and disinclined to consult with or listen to colleagues.)[12]

If true teamwork were actually a matter of years spent earning the trust of a higher-status professional, patients would not be safe under the common conditions of health care, where people continually rotate to work with people they have never worked with before. Fortunately, CRM has demonstrated clearly—and over at least two decades—that *with the right training, strangers meeting for the first time can rapidly create high-functioning teams.*

In discussions of the problems of the health care system, safety advocates and quality improvement experts constantly point to the problem of what are called health care "silos." Disciplines like nursing, medicine, physical therapy, and pharmacy each work in their own universes of upward reporting lines, as do different hospital units. Since hospital reengineering began in the 1990s, corporate models encourage hospital administrators and medical leaders to view different hospital services—cardiology, oncology, and transplant, for example—as competing "product lines." Competitors are usually not in the habit of sharing information with one another. Thus the preexisting condition of failure of physicians and others to share information in an era when information sharing is critical becomes even more exacerbated.

As we have observed this process, we have become convinced that health care disciplines and divisions seem to resemble fortresses more than silos, each strongly defended and in pursuit of its own political and fiscal well-being in the larger system. We will see how this plays out when we consider how the components of genuine teamwork are taken from theory to practice in health care.

TEAM BUILDING AND COMMUNICATION

A team is a trained aggregate of persons with specific individual and interactive roles, a distributed set of skills, and shared and explicit language, purposes, and goals. The basic components of teamwork are

- introductions;
- shared language and mental models;
- shared information, plans, and protocols;
- cross-monitoring; and
- feedback/correction mechanisms through the use of briefings and debriefings.

Introductions

As we saw in chapter 3, the very first thing people in aviation learn is the non-negotiable building block of teamwork: people who work together need to know one another's names. This would seem to be such a simple activity—the very basis of everyday manners and civility—that one would think it went without saying. In health care, however, people of many professions and occupations often work together without ever exchanging names outside their own professions. Here's a common scenario. Doctor walks into patient's room. Nurse, PT, or respiratory therapist is at the bedside. Doctor (irrespective of gender) begins to talk to the patient and present family members, ignoring the other professional, who does not offer name or ask name of doctor. Doctor talks to patient and family, then walks out of the room. End of story.

Suzanne recalls standing in a patient room in a major teaching hospital that had just received recognition for the excellent quality of its nursing care, i.e., Magnet hospital status. She was following a nurse on a vascular floor. The patient was seriously ill and also had a hospital-acquired infection. Anyone entering the room had to don protective gloves and a disposable gown over his or her clothes. Naturally these gowns also covered any hospital ID badges.

The patient was receiving a blood transfusion, and the nurse, fully gowned and gloved, was standing at the bedside administering and monitoring the transfusion. As she was talking to the patient, a young man and woman—also suitably covered and without visible ID—entered the room and breezed past the nurse, approached the patient, and blithely announced, "Hi, we're Hem-Onc" (translation: Hi, we're hematology-oncology, or in English, blood diseases and cancer). Suzanne was thinking, Well, hi, Hem-Onc, I'm Journalism, she's Nursing, and he's Illness. Hem-Onc began to talk with the patient, giving him some very bad news. The patient began to cry, and Hem-Onc made their exit.

These doctors never gave their names or asked for that of the nurse, the patient, or the visitor in the room (Journalism). The nurse did not ask their names or offer her own. Before approaching the patient, they did not request a status report (briefing) from the nurse, nor did she suggest that she brief them. When they left, she didn't talk with them, and they made no attempt to talk with her.

This was not an isolated event.

The issue of naming practices and introductions is so peculiarly construed in the medical system that Patrick, when addressing a group of surgeons, was surprised to receive the following question: "Do you have protocols for introductions when you first enter the plane and meet another crew member for the first time?" Patrick said, "Well, yes, I usually get on the plane, see someone else in uniform that looks like they belong there, put out my hand and say, 'Hi, I'm Patrick.'"

In aviation, introductions reflect efforts to create a flatter hierarchy and psychological safety so that members of the crew can exercise their obligations as team members to inquire, advocate, and assert. Airplane captains routinely use their first names when introducing themselves to first officers, gate agents, ground personnel, or flight attendants. This is quite deliberate. It levels the playing field and makes it a lot easier for other staffers to raise concerns or safety issues. "It's a whole lot easier to tell Tom he might be making a mistake than [to tell] Captain Smith," one pilot explained.

In spite of concerns about patient safety, the opposite goal—asserting and reinforcing status hierarchies   seems to be the primary intention of introductions and other uses of language in health care. In years past, title plus last name was the standard form of address in most hierarchical work settings. Today, as much of society has moved to a first-name culture, medicine has not. Physicians are commonly addressed, and introduce themselves to others, by title and surname, and nurses, PTs, OTs, social workers, and other workers by first name only. If a nurse calls a physician by his or her first name outside the patient room, he or she will almost always revert to referring to the physician as "Dr." while they are with the patient together; the physician, on the other hand, will still use only the nurse's first name. Nurses (and other health care workers) often complain that while they are expected to call doctors by last name and title, doctors may not even bother to register that they have a name and will simply call out "nurse" when they want to get someone's attention.

No Shared Language

Throughout our discussions of CRM and in the case studies on the Osher Clinical Center and interprofessional education in Toronto, we have seen the importance of shared language to safety and the impact having no shared language has on team communication. In health care, different professionals use language in entirely different ways. What is even worse, the two largest professions in the system—medicine and nursing—are obliged to speak different languages.

In the health care workplace, the professional lexicon of medicine is the talk form, whose use is recognized by physicians to signal possession of authoritative knowledge and professional expertise. For well over a century now, nurses have been firmly instructed—both in their professional educations and in the policies and norms of their workplaces—to refrain from using such "medical language." This proprietary language has been reserved for physicians because its use, in some circumstances, constitutes diagnosis ("the patient has pneumonia"), a function and privilege assigned by law as well as by long and carefully enforced custom to physicians only. On the basis of this legal privilege, nursing has been classified and categorized as subordinate to medicine, and its activities have been rendered largely invisible through what Geoffrey C. Bowker and Susan Leigh Star, authors of *Sorting Things Out: Classification and Its Consequences,* describe as the valorization of one point of view, which often renders another entirely invisible.[13]

Under penalty of disciplinary action, nurses have been enjoined, for instance, from saying or noting in a patient's chart that the patient "has developed a respiratory infection" or a "urinary tract infection," or is "hallucinating." This medical-speak. Rather, nurses must report in descriptive terms the indicators that lead them to their suspicions. Thus a nurse would say, "The patient is experiencing frequency of urination and burning," or "The patient is seeing little white elephants." They are taught to leave the doctor to reach the diagnosis and apply the correct medical label. Both physicians and nursing managers may reinforce these lessons by reprimanding or disciplining nurses who violate these linguistic norms. Nurses can even lose their licensure if found to be "practicing medicine without a [medical] license" (which includes making medical diagnoses). This penalty for "practicing medicine" (vs. practicing nursing) is explicit in states' nursing practice acts.

Since doctors and nurses have historically used different languages to describe their patients' problems and events, each has developed its own professional lexicon and forms of discourse. For nurses, this discourse began to be formalized and codified in the early 1970s under the name "Nursing Diagnosis." Formulated and overseen by an officially authorized peer review organization, taught in schools of nursing, and now in international use in multiple languages, Nursing Diagnosis allows nurses to discuss and document significant patient findings and care plans without trespassing on medical turf. In most U.S. hospitals, Nursing Diagnosis is the language in which nurses chart their professional activities in the official written record as well. Like medical language, it follows stepwise formulas for presenting relevant information leading from assessment data to care plans and desired or expected outcomes.

Ironically, the methods and lexicon of Nursing Diagnosis have been specifically formulated to indicate scientific grounding for nursing assessment and practice, but its enforced use of substantially laicized terminology—just a few syllables per word more complex than common speech—instantly distinguishes it from medically recognized expressions of expertise. This separate and unequal language permits nurses to express to each other their structured observations and conclusions about a patient's status and to annotate their particular concerns regarding the patient's condition and care. It also virtually ensures that physicians either will not understand what nurses are talking about or will be prompted by obvious linguistic cues to dismiss its clinical relevance and informational value (Data don't sound like this . . .).

Use of Nursing Diagnosis is thus an inherently conflicted process: both not medicine in its restricted terminology and range of specific concerns and emulating medicine in title (diagnosis) and in form (analysis of patient data and observation to arrive at a diagnostic conclusion). Nurses are obliged by hospital and interprofessional circumstances to be bilingual—fluent both in the language of Nursing Diagnosis *and* in the terminology of medicine, in which physician orders are received, documented, and interpreted for implementation. Physicians, as the higher-status group in hospital culture, have neither the mandate nor the need to become conversant in the language of nursing. The *flow* of communication remains essentially unidirectional since the *language* of valid expert communication belongs to only one of the two professions. Juxtaposed to the rarefied argot of medicine, the language of Nursing Diagnosis seems unsophisticated, even unlearned; it is barred from access to medical shorthand, and its compensatory circumlocutions sound irritating to get-to-the-point physicians.

While physicians *do* routinely ask nurses to tell them about observations the physicians select as relevant, they do not generally read nursing notes in the patient record, which one junior faculty physician in an Ivy League academic medical center told Bonnie were "noncontributory" to essential patient care. Residents in one New England hospital characterized nursing notes in their patients' charts as "not worth the time it takes to read them" because they are "way too wordy" and "never say anything useful." In another New England teaching hospital where we have worked, nursing notes are in fact kept in an entirely separate chart from the one used by physicians to record medical actions and patient progress. (In a perhaps unconscious symbolic statement, the physicians' charts are in gray-blue notebooks, while the nursing charts' binders are a subdued rose color.)

Neither the residents nor the faculty physicians in this hospital, participating in a 2007 discussion of strategies for improving interprofessional communication, had any inkling that nurses were actually *not permitted* to use the language they as physicians would have preferred, respected, and found authoritative; nor could they use the same shorthand forms (such as SOAP notes) for communicating their clinical impressions and recommendations.[14] As this hospital made its transition in 2010 to electronic medical records, two *separate* electronic systems were put in place for physician and nursing patient records, thus further ensuring the separation of the two professions' assessments, plans, and activity records, and reinforcing for physicians—by making them now physically invisible—the sense of the nursing notes' irrelevance to patient care. The two systems are not linked electronically, and for the first six weeks or so of their deployment physicians could not gain entry into the nursing note system if they wanted to because they had not been issued password access.

The lack of a common language and communication medium—or at least of mutual professional intelligibility—both creates and sustains friction between nurses and physicians, and the cumulative irritation runs in both directions. Nurses resent having their knowledge, expertise, and competence shrugged off by physicians, while doctors resent having to wade through written chart notes that do not come succinctly to the point with respect to patient data and the treatment directions they may indicate. Medicine continues subtly and not so subtly to attempt to laicize nursing knowledge and expertise, as nursing continues to create and implement structures to professionalize its knowledge and fully incorporate it into the inpatient health care environment.[15] Given this lack of a shared language, it is difficult to imagine the members of any so-called multidisciplinary team creating a shared purpose and a shared mental model. This failure can have serious consequences. According to the 2012 report by the inspector general of the U.S. Department of Health and Human Services, Medicare estimates that 86 percent of adverse events in hospitals in the United States go unreported. Why? Not because staff are afraid to admit mistakes but because they actually *do not share common understandings of what an adverse event is,* who should report it, and what should be done about it.[16]

Briefings

Recall that in aviation briefings are conducted at the beginning of, during, and sometimes after every flight. If we consider each patient's daily care plan as analogous to an airplane flight, we do not see the same frequency of communication or team building in hospitals. The preflight briefing would be analogous to morning rounds. In many hospitals, nurses do not routinely accompany physicians when they make their morning visits to patients to discuss their status, progress, and plan for the day. Nurses who have vital information about patients whom they have cared for during their overnight shifts are not necessarily approached before doctors make their rounds. Morning rounds are usually conducted on physicians' schedules. Because of differences in work hours and shift definitions, they often take place at a time when nurses are not available for the discussions: they have just reported to work and are busy giving their morning medications and getting their patient briefings from the nursing shift that is ending. Doctors may come to see a patient at other times to report on the results of a test or procedure or to update the patient and family on the plan of care. The particular patient's nurse is often not available at these times either because of other patient care activities. Even if he or she is, doctors do not routinely brief that nurse either before or after this discussion. The idea that nurses should be briefed—or that they should ask for a briefing, as team members do in aviation—is almost entirely foreign in health care.

Here is a fairly routine example a nurse recounted to Suzanne. A patient had been admitted to the hospital for liver problems. The nurse explained that the team (in her frame of reference med students, residents, and the attending physician; she did not include herself as a member) had ordered an MRI. While she was in the room taking care of the patient, the attending walked in and without asking the RN to briefly talk with him outside told the patient the results of the MRI. The team, he said, had gone over the MRI and seen a suspicious mass and thought he had cancer. The attending chatted with the patient and then—again without requesting a discussion with the nurse—left the room. The nurse did not follow him or request a debriefing, even though she later said she felt sideswiped by the fact that the attending "laid this information on the patient without talking to me first." (When Suzanne told this story to a friend who is an internist, she responded, "What's wrong with telling the nurse and the patient at the same time?")

In some areas, like labor and delivery and the operating room, briefings have become slightly more common. At Franklin Square Hospital in Baltimore, Maryland, the labor and delivery unit typically does a "huddle" three or four times a day. Nurses and doctors group at the nurses' station to update one another on patient conditions. According to the chief of service, Dr. James Chisholm, "The huddle creates an atmosphere where everyone feels that all patients are the team's responsibility." He points out that before the huddle, "if a doctor looked into a patient's room and saw that the patient was in trouble, they might say, 'thank god, that's not my patient,' and walk away. Now we all feel comfortable going to someone and saying, 'You know, this doesn't look right.'"

These huddles are paralleled by surgical briefings where doctors, nurses, and others in the operating room are supposed to meet, clarify roles, and outline procedures and, most important, conduct a time-out where everyone makes certain that the right patient—and body part—is about to be operated on. While many operating rooms and lead surgeons perform briefings and time-outs, these are not *always* conducted. Surgical nurses routinely complain that surgeons do not like the interruption and may resist conducting the briefings and time-outs irrespective of the dictates of hospital policy. Moreover, even when briefings or huddles are conducted in hospitals, they are used in isolated units or settings—the operating room, critical care, labor and delivery—that are considered high-risk.

And herein lies a problem. It has been estimated that there is at least one medication error per hospital patient per day.[17] If communication and teamwork are keys to reducing these injuries—as the research evidence irrefutably reveals—then why aren't huddles, briefings, time-outs, and other such innovative practices required on every hospital unit? Why isn't this a part of practicing evidence-based medicine?

In aviation, CRM/TEM isn't just activated on "important" flights—say, long international flights that cross several time zones and exceed three thousand miles. It is required on every flight, irrespective of distance or duration. In health care, the use of innovations like briefings or checklists is still limited to specific units or settings. Example: A surgeon makes introductions, completes a time-out or briefing in the OR, but does not stop to introduce himself or talk to the nurse on the floors when he is visiting his postop patient, who is now in a bed on a hospital ward.

In the most terrible patient safety disasters—for example, the case of the kidney patient that Peter Pronovost describes in his book *Safe Patients, Smart Hospitals* (discussed below) or the case of Lewis Blackman (a fifteen-year-old boy who underwent what was supposed to be uncomplicated elective surgery and died a few days later), the main communication problems did not occur *in* the operating room but once the patient had left it.[18] Patients will never be safe if communication training is restricted to the highest-risk environments and if hospitals do not begin to expand auspicious beginnings across the institution. Imagine what would have happened if CRM had maintained such artificial limits on teamwork and communication. On a flight leaving New York for Tokyo with a stopover in San Francisco, CRM would be practiced only as the plane crossed the ocean, but all teamwork bets would be off as it flew across the continental United States. Fortunately, that is not the way it works in aviation; unfortunately, that is still the way it works in health care.

Why? Largely because even to those with the will to change the status quo the project seems too monumental. The resistance to change is so strong among physicians and others across health care institutions that just getting a surgeon to consistently complete a checklist or time-out seems a daunting task. To extend teamwork and communication techniques throughout the hospital seems to be— as one insurance company executive, whose company is encouraging some hospital services to use TeamSTEPPS, puts it—overwhelming.

A companion problem is that excellent initiatives like TeamSTEPPS are too often considered by health care administrators to be end points rather than points of departure. These models are conceptualized as appropriate tools for specific applications but seldom viewed as valuable institution-wide initiatives. More important, they are often examples of a cafeteria approach to teamwork training: some hospitals will use checklists, others will use huddles, others time-outs, others TeamSTEPPS or Crucial Conversations for specific units. Very few have implemented the kind of complete and integrated package that made aviation safety a reality and not just a good intention. For this reason, researchers like Lorelei Lingard have pointed out that specific innovations like checklists, when detached from the more intricate weave of the whole cloth of teamwork training and culture change, can actually *interfere* with teamwork rather than reinforce it.[19]

TEAM TRAINING—ONCE AND THEN AGAIN AND AGAIN

As we have seen in aviation, CRM is a process, not an event; a tightly interconnected series of heavily reinforced lessons, not a discrete innovation like a time-out or checklist. Pilots, flight attendants, air traffic controllers, and other airline personnel are socialized with multiple exposures to CRM principles. They get them in their initial training and education. CRM training is repeated when they are hired at an airline, when they are type-rated for new aircraft, and throughout their careers. Because they have the most important job, pilots have the most rigorous training. Their skills—in terms of both technical equipment and communication/teamwork—are constantly monitored.

Although there are attempts to bring similar changes to health care, there is no teamwork or communication training in the basic education of physicians, nurses, or other health professionals. Some hospital systems have hired training corporations to present voluntary-attendance CRM workshops such as Indelta Learning Systems' "Lessons from the Flight Deck."[20] While these are clearly useful introductions to the key concepts, they are one-off events, and there is little effort to integrate CRM-like practices on hospital floors or in other health care institutions. Nor is there any required or recurrent training in these concepts.

Some hospitals have signed on to seminars about conflict management—like those promoted by the for-profit company Vital Smarts, whose Crucial Conversations workshops are aggressively marketed to hospitals. While these workshops are also useful, they focus only on conflict situations and do not deal with team building.

As we write, the latest fad is seminars that promote emotional intelligence. One of the prime agents in the EI movement is Daniel Goleman. Emotional intelligence is a useful concept, with several theoretical variations, but one that is generally limited to self-perception, assessment, and control of one's own emotions in order to manage emotion in individual and group settings—largely for the avoidance or resolution of conflict. It is not a teamwork training model.

These efforts are limited not only in scope but also in their ability to make sustained change because they tend to be one-shot offerings and their curriculum is not consistently revisited. As we discussed early on, behavioral and cultural change does not come about after one workshop or afternoon seminar or after reading the "facts" in a journal article. Changing deep-seated cultural and behavioral customs requires frequent repetition and recurrent training, as well as systems-level supports (incentives, recognition, mandates, rewards, etc.). Even if every medical, nursing and other health professional school in the world offered interprofessional education and systematic teamwork training in its curriculum, if these subjects are not regularly revisited through an individual's professional career, their lessons will not keep—any more than other clinical or technical skills will remain current without refresher courses and continual use. If faculty and staff are not trained interprofessionally, as they are in Toronto, then they may unwittingly contradict messages that students learn in school assuring that the hidden curriculum will reassert itself. Teamwork, like any essential clinical skill set, requires rehearsal and renewal at regular intervals.

AUTHORITY AS EXEMPTION VS. EXPECTATION

In aviation, as we have seen in the prior section, the captain of the ship is expected to set the tone when it comes to team building and communication. In health care, communication patterns seem more to reflect efforts to reassert authority and status than to encourage teamwork, cross-monitoring, the maintenance of situational awareness, or creating a sense of psychological safety. Indeed, when one examines many potentially positive initiatives, doctors seem to define their authority as the thing that makes them de facto team leaders and that exempts them from requirements to communicate or function as team members. Several years ago Suzanne was visiting a large hospital that was the site of a Robert Wood Johnson/ Institute for Healthcare Improvement initiative entitled Transforming Care at the Bedside (TCAB). These TCAB units were devoted to improving safety and efficiency. On this particular unit, Xeroxed signs—a version of the triangular traffic sign that announces a no-passing zone—had been taped to the door of each patient room. When she asked the nurse accompanying her what these signs were for, she proudly announced that this was a TCAB innovation to make patients safer. All hospital staff members, she said, were told that they should look into a patient's room while walking by to make sure nothing unsafe was occurring. "For example" she continued, "if you see a frail ninety-eight-year-old woman trying to crawl over her bedrails, you shouldn't say to yourself, 'that's not my job,' you should do something to stop it."

When Suzanne asked her if this expectation extended to physicians, she immediately exclaimed, "Oh no, just to hospital staff. Doctors are not under our control." In other words, the captain of the ship, the putative leader of the team, was explicitly exempt from this particular safety practice. Suzanne wondered what kind of message this was sending to nursing and medical students who were training on the floor, not to mention so-called lower-level staff. What was even more ironic was that this was the same hospital that was promoting huddles on its labor and delivery service. A good example of the proverbial right hand not knowing—or caring—what the left is doing.

When Suzanne used this example at a university conference on patient safety, an irate vascular surgeon approached her after she'd spoken. How dare she suggest that doctors should stop at patients' rooms as they were walking by to make sure they were safe! "Don't you know how busy we are," he demanded?

This kind of flouting of protocol or expectation of exemption from many safety practices is intrinsic to the definition of authority, autonomy, and leadership prevalent in medicine. In their article on disrespectful physicians, Leape and his colleagues argued that

> Disrespectful behavior may actually affirm status by rewarding the person behaving disrespectfully, who is typically highly sensitive to the hierarchy and keenly aware of the consequences of disrespect directed up the status gradient. In a hierarchical environment, the ability to disrespect others with impunity is a measure of status. The department chair or world-class cardiac surgeon can often "get away with" conduct that is not tolerated among those lower down the ladder.[21]

A case in point occurred in 2010, at the Rhode Island Hospital, the major teaching hospital for Brown University's medical school and the most important hospital facility in the state, which was cited by the state Department of Health and the Centers for Medicare and Medicaid Services because of a repeated history of wrong-site surgeries and retained foreign objects (RFOs) during surgery, along with other so-called never events. The incidents described in the Department of Health report to RIH management (a public record document) illustrate the kinds of patterns that continue in many institutions despite growing concern about medical errors and injuries:

The hospital policy for surgical counts appears to be appropriate and the rate of RFOs after surgery does not appear to be greater than the national average. The significant problem we identified, once again, was the failure of RIH staff to follow hospital policy. During this most recent "never event," the staff and surgeon were aware in the operating room that the drill bit had broken. They could not locate the broken piece. The surgeon said he thought it might be in the surgical flap. The operating room nurse asked for guidance from her manager who reportedly told her to put the drill bit pieces in a bag. No discussion occurred about obtaining an X-ray to make sure the drill bit was not in the patient despite the fact that your hospital policy (which is consistent with the national standard of care) clearly articulates that an X-ray should be obtained prior to the patient leaving the operating room with a suspected RFO. In addition the surgical count was reported as normal. These actions resulted in the patient being placed at significant risk of harm when she had a "routine" MRI the next day while having a metallic piece of a drill bit in her surgical wound. The continued failure of the hospital to ensure that operating room staff (including physicians) follow existing policies remains very troubling.[22]

In this institution nurses were not empowered to enforce time-outs and briefings or compliance with proper surgical count procedures. Although "staff reported that the surgical count process for sponges and medical equipment was often incorrect" Health Department investigators "did not find any evidence that appropriate action was taken by hospital management to address this significant problem."[23] The report noted that one surgeon ordered operating room staff to "stop the count" because he was "in a hurry," and they complied.[24]

In another incident, an anesthesiologist who had repeatedly been told after previous violations to put his surgical mask on when he entered a sterile operating room once again entered without putting on his mask. When he was told to put on his mask, he "made like he held his breath and walked through the operating room, again being told not to do so. The anesthesiologist at that time 'made a joke about it and continued on.'"[25] According to the report, these repeated infractions "were never addressed by [the] medical leadership."[26]

Doctors were routinely allowed to flout standard protocols, and no one intervened to discipline physicians. It is interesting that this is a hospital that has routinely offered seminars in which airline pilots have partnered with physicians to conduct day-long CRM-style trainings.

TEAMWORK AND LEADERSHIP

Over the course of writing this book, Bonnie and Suzanne have related a number of health care stories to Patrick. In many of them, the people who are supposed to captain the health care ship have ignored policy and dangerous incidents, while hospital administrators have been nowhere to be found. In each case, Patrick's immediate response was, "Where is management? Who is in charge here?" That is indeed the question.

Not surprisingly, in hospitals and other health care institutions the leadership problem starts at the very top and is exacerbated by the fractured employment structures that are the norm in American health care. In many instances, hospital and health care executives have abdicated responsibility to exercise leadership authority over physicians whom their CEOs consider substantial revenue generators. Numerous CEOs have told us that doctors are perceived to be the geese that lay the golden eggs. If anyone ruffles their feathers, they will take those eggs and play elsewhere.

This problem is exacerbated by the fact that many physicians—called "voluntary" or "community physicians"—are not employed by the hospital or health care institution. Instead they have what are known as "admitting privileges," which means that they can admit their private-practice patients to a hospital and treat and visit them in that hospital. To get admitting privileges, physicians need to be thoroughly vetted to make sure that they are properly credentialed, are board-certified in their specialties, have no disciplinary records, and so forth. The Board of Trustees has ultimate responsibility for these physicians, and the physicians are governed by the Medical Executive Committee (MEC). Doctors as a profession, however, are notoriously poor at self-policing. As one hospital CEO notes, it is very difficult to revoke or suspend a voluntary physician's admitting privileges even if he or she does something egregious. For issues that are considered more touchy-feely—yelling at a nurse, throwing things in the OR, not communicating well—it is almost unheard of.

"Voluntary" physicians may have admitting privileges at a number of different local or regional hospitals. The hospital does not pay them anything and they are not hospital employees. The institution's MEC is charged with monitoring these physicians and could revoke or suspend their privileges. In actual practice, "physicians on the MEC are loath to police their colleagues because those colleagues are a source of referrals. To revoke their privileges would mean that they lose revenue," another hospital CEO explains. The lengthy due process afforded physicians also complicates matters. Unlike other hospital employees who, in a nonunion hospital, can be fired summarily, physicians get special treatment. Sometimes the lengthy due process exists because without it competitive forces would trump quality or patient safety. "If you're in a small town, and doctors in one practice admit to Hospital A, they may not want doctors from another practice to get admitting privileges because they want a competitive advantage. Or they might argue for revoking someone's privileges for the wrong reasons," says this CEO. "It's also hard to get voluntary physicians on the program of teamwork if they are admitting to a variety of hospitals, some of which emphasize teamwork and some of which don't," he continues. "If a surgeon admits to five different hospitals, and our hospital is the only one that insists on OR checklists, he can easily say, 'I'm not going to do checklists; it takes too much time; I don't want to,' and all he has to do is leave our hospital and work at the four others."

All of this makes disciplining physicians who refuse to practice teamwork very difficult. Hospital executives don't want to do it because they know it will involve lawyers and potential litigation, and medical executive committees don't want to do it because it can hurt their pocketbooks or cause enormous, long-drawn-out hassles. One hospital board member recently told us that with great reluctance and after anguished discussion, the community hospital that she helps to oversee suspended the admitting privileges of a doctor who had been rude—if not outright abusive—to nurses, pharmacists, technicians, and other staff members for years. Finally she began abusing patients, and that was the last straw. When Suzanne asked the board member why the board had not acted earlier, she said, "Well, she was such a good *clinician*." When Suzanne and Bonnie discussed the incident, their response was quite the opposite. This doctor might have been a good technician, but since clinicians work in clinics (hospitals) and clinics deal with people—including staff and patients—this doctor could not, by definition, be a good clinician, particularly if her behavior negatively affected patients or prevented other people from doing their best work.

The same tolerance is not accorded to lower-level staff members, who often report that management does not support them, particularly when there is a conflict with a physician. Many nurses at the ground level feel that neither their nursing managers nor top nurse executives will support them if they raise safety concerns about physicians but will instead support the physician. In one study, a team of researchers led by Linda Flynn surveyed 9,854 direct-care RNs working primarily in hospitals. "Forty percent of the RNs reported that their frontline nurse manager was not supportive of their nursing staff, 42 percent reported that their nurse manager would not back them up in a conflict with a physician, even when the manager knew they were right, and 43 percent of the nurses concluded that their nurse manager did not have the skills to be a competent manager."[27] People lower on the hierarchy (not only nurses but medical students, interns, and residents) are aware of the unspoken mandate not to anger an attending physician, whether by overt disagreement with a treatment plan or by making significant patient findings that the senior physician might have missed.

Given the persistence of these attitudes, it is not surprising that even prominent physicians have trouble saving their patients. In his book *Safe Patients, Smart Hospitals,* Peter Pronovost describes a horrific incident that happened at the Johns Hopkins Hospital on his watch. An otherwise healthy twenty-nine-year-old woman had been admitted for laparoscopic removal of a kidney. She quickly developed complications, and the surgical resident called Pronovost, who was at the time on call at home as an ICU attending. He told Pronovost that the surgeon in charge had requested that the patient be admitted to an intermediate care unit for extra nursing monitoring in spite of the fact that the surgeon insisted the surgery had gone well and the patient would be fine. Four hours later, at 2:00 a.m., the same resident called Pronovost to request the patient's admission to the ICU with life-threatening problems.[28]

Pronovost understood that the patient's problems could only be a result of a surgical complication and that she needed to return to the OR or she could die. The surgeon, the resident insisted, did not agree and refused to take the patient to the OR. Because the surgeon was in charge of the patient, neither Pronovost nor the resident could get the patient to the OR immediately. Pronovost called the surgeon, who continued to insist that his surgery had gone without a hitch. Holding his temper, Pronovost argued his case, and the surgeon finally retorted, "I am not going to the OR. I have to leave town. From now on talk to the surgeon on call."

After additional delays, the woman was taken to the OR, and another surgeon discovered that during the first surgery the trocar, a harpoon-like rod used during laparoscopic surgery, had accidently punctured her intestine and pancreas. "Accidents like this happen: surgery is not a perfect science. However, if this had been discovered quickly the patient might have suffered less harm."[29] Because the surgeon did not tolerate cross-monitoring and was allowed even by a world-renowned colleague to refuse it, the patient who weighed 110 pounds on her arrival at the hospital ended up weighing 80. Instead of spending three days in the hospital, she spent six months and an additional year in a rehab facility. In addition, she lost both kidneys, was on dialysis, and needed a kidney transplant.

This incident did not happen at some remote or tiny hospital but at Johns Hopkins Hospital, several years after the Josie King incident when Hopkins had become a leading example of an institution devoted to patient safety.[30] Josie King was a toddler who had suffered serious burns and was admitted to the hospital and died because of dehydration—something that could have been prevented by better teamwork and communication among staff and between the family and staff. The problem here is not a single medical institution but, as Pronovost himself explains, the "toxicity" of the medical system itself. In this kind of hierarchy, there is no two-challenge rule so that someone else can take charge of the patient when the captain of the ship is on a deadly course. Nurses who are concerned about patient safety in an urgent situation have to go up a cumbersome chain of command—charge nurse to nurse manager to clinical director and then–which rarely happens—to chief nursing officer, which could take more time than the patient has. She cannot call in another physician to oversee the case. In fact, even famous physicians like Pronovost cannot wrest a patient in danger from a surgeon or other physician's control.

WORKLOAD MANAGEMENT

Work Hours

High-reliability industries like aviation are very concerned about the now well-recognized effects of worker fatigue on safety. Regulation of work hours is an integral part of organized efforts to prevent, manage, and contain hazardous errors instigated or exacerbated by fatigue. To cite only a few examples, in the U.S. military, air force pilots are limited to flying 12 hours in a 24-hour period and 75 hours in a thirty-day period. This is also true in combat, where all flight and non-flight personnel are limited to a 10-hour workday, six days a week, for a total of 240 hours a month during continuous operations. Crews manning intercontinental ballistic missile silos must have at least 6 consecutive hours for sleep during their duty period. In the nuclear power industry, workers may not put in more than fourteen consecutive days at work without having two days off, more than 72 hours in any seven-day period, or more than 12 hours straight, and they must have a minimum of 12 hours off between work shifts. The Federal Aviation Administration restricts air traffic controllers to 10 consecutive hours of work in a 24-hour period and a maximum of six days' work in each seven-day interval. And as we have seen, the FAA has a complex set of regulations that strictly limit pilot duty hours. Long-haul truckers cannot exceed 10 hours' driving out of every 18-hour period, with a weekly limit of 60 hours in seven consecutive days or 70 hours in eight consecutive days.[31]

As a high-risk industry, health care is an outlier in ignoring and avoiding work-hour regulation. With the exception of the much-resisted imposition by the ACGME in 2003 of the 80-hour workweek duty-hour restrictions on physician trainees in residency and fellowship, which were increased in 2010 and 2011, there is no organization of health professionals that defines limitations on consecutive work time. Nor is there a federal or state law that limits the hours of physicians who are not in training or of nurses, laboratory technicians, pharmacists, or other health care professionals.

In spite of a considerable body of research documenting the adverse effects of fatigue on doctors' and nurses' judgment, error rates and severity, patient safety, work relationships, and worker health and safety, there has been almost no serious discussion of regulating the hours of attending physicians. Virtually no hospital in the country has implemented its own significant work-hour restrictions for either profession; none has policies regulating work hours of senior physicians. Yet surgeons, to take one particular example, have both very long work hours *and* a type of work that carries a high level of inherent risk for patients. At least two fields have reported increases in senior physician work hours in academic medical centers as a result of resident duty-hour restrictions, but they continue to resist the notion of caps on senior physician hours.[32] Suzanne recently talked to a primary care physician at a major West Coast teaching hospital who was about to quit because her work days began at 7:00 a.m. and ended at 10:00 p.m.. Some primary care physicians in the hospital, she reported, where actually sleeping in their offices.

Nursing hours are also unregulated and escalating. Researchers Alison Trinkoff at the University of Maryland School of Nursing and Ann E. Rogers at the University of Pennsylvania School of Nursing have documented that the once-standard eight-hour nursing shift is practically a quaint antique.[33] On paper (i.e., as scheduled), most U.S. nurses now work three twelve-hour shifts per week. In actual fact, these shifts routinely creep up to thirteen and fourteen hours' duration as nurses linger to catch up on patient care and documentation duties or to complete their detailed handoffs to the incoming shift. The implications for patient safety are ominous. The research of Rogers as well as Trinkoff and Geiger-Brown has suggested that error rates go up after ten consecutive hours at work and increase even more after twelve.[34] Although nurses and their unions staunchly oppose what is known as hospital-mandated, or mandatory, overtime, they are equally opposed to restrictions that will limit their ability to choose longer hours or additional shifts when they want them. This seems particularly ironic given the claim of many nurses that they are patient advocates.

Many physicians also oppose work-hour limitations and reject the notion that fatigue impacts their performance.[35] Their resistance to work-hour limitations is also ironic in light of the growing popularity among physicians of evidence-based medicine, a movement whose strong form contends that *all* patient care decisions should be made on the basis of reliable research evidence and not on long-standing traditions of practice or received wisdom. Apparently this rule applies only to evidence whose implications are popular with physicians or that do not affect their own freedom to design their workdays and workforces as they see fit.

Workload

In its 128 instructional scenarios, presented as examples of both productive and counterproductive interactions in the TeamSTEPPS training manual, many of the scenarios that go wrong show that the problem they illustrate can be attributed to excessive workloads. A patient's blood draw is delayed because the lab is too busy.[36] An X ray interpretation error is made because of the pressures of very high volume in the ER.[37] Unable to access appropriate protocols in an understaffed medical-surgical unit, a nurse hangs blood for the wrong patient.[38] A new staff nurse on a neonatal intensive care unit (NICU) is criticized for not doing things quickly enough and in her subsequent haste and distress fails to adequately attend to a problem in an infant patient's arm. When the next nurse comes on at change of shift, she's too busy to monitor the situation closely, and as a result of this chain of events, the infant's right hand has to be amputated.[39]

The problem of overwork, thus identified, is serious and real. In their discussion of disrespectful behavior, Leape and his colleagues brilliantly identified how hospitals disrespect the people who work in them by forcing them to work "unduly long hours," burden them with "unreasonably heavy work loads," and force them to "experience multiple conflicting demands on their time and psyche."[40] Hospitals, the authors write, also fail to protect them from things like needlestick or back injuries. How can nurses maintain situational awareness for each patient if their normal workload requires them to run between seven and ten patients' rooms all day? How does a new NICU nurse get the mentoring and oversight she needs when even the seasoned nurses have so many patients to manage that they can't intervene appropriately in a preventable gangrene? How do people watch each other's backs—cross-monitor—in their teamwork if they can't even carry out their own work safely? How do nurse managers manage when, as is now the case, they may routinely supervise as many as 120 RNs, LPNs, aides, and others? Appropriate workloads at baseline, plus protocols for peaks, are necessary conditions for success; individual adjustments will not remedy system-wide problems.

Workload and work intensification are seldom openly recognized as patient safety issues. At a 2006 meeting of a Massachusetts patient safety coalition, for example, an ambitious program was outlined to eliminate medical errors and injuries. In the discussion period following the presentation, a health care administrator and conference participant pointed out that the success of this proposed initiative would stand or fall on nurses' ability to implement its numerous component parts. He observed that the nursing shortage, which began in the 1990s with extensive hospital restructuring and continues unabated in the present day, would—unless addressed in all of its complexity—make the proposed ambitious agenda entirely futile. *No one* in the room took up the issue or responded to his concerns; no discussion of nursing overwork or of the realistic prospects for nurses to implement such a proposal in the current work environment took place. With the exception of California, no state in the United States has mandated safe staffing ratios, and hospital associations and hospital leaders have opposed the implementation of such ratios in every state in which they have been proposed.

Not only is workload management important in the two main professions in health care, but it is also critical in every other. Lab technicians running too many tests, X-ray techs with too many X-rays to read, outsourced cleaners who have too many rooms to clean—whatever the profession or occupation, in health care the pressure is on for workers to constantly do more with less and to work more hours for less compensation. What is little recognized is that long hours and intensified workloads not only harm patients but also lead to greater rates of injuries and stress-related illnesses for health care staff. In a great but unrecognized irony, it seems that conditions in health care, certainly in the United States but also in other countries, are turning the people who care for patients into patients themselves—thus increasing costs for health care systems that say they are trying to contain costs and making an already risky job even (and unnecessarily) riskier.

THREAT AND ERROR MANAGEMENT

In order to manage threats and errors successfully, the issues considered in this chapter—along with many others identified in the substantial literature on patient safety—will have to be addressed systematically, and soon. The study on non-reporting of medical errors conducted by the Department of Health and Human Services (mentioned above) was particularly disturbing because it suggested that, even when errors are reported, the conditions that led to them are rarely addressed and remedied. In many cases, as Tucker and Edmondson point out, healthcare facilities encourage and reward the kind of work-arounds and first-order thinking that do not solve system problems and in fact often exacerbate or conceal them.[41] Short-term fixes are relatively inexpensive but may not save money—or patients' lives—in the longer run, and they often add to the fiscal costs of proper and comprehensive resolutions. System-wide, comprehensive assessment and improvements are needed—and they are inescapably expensive, labor-intensive, and tremendously complex. Many organizations are already striving to implement systemic responses to these daunting challenges, sometimes against great odds. We suggest that an understanding of how aviation successfully addressed similar issues can provide a workable, adaptable model for health care, and we encourage its application in health care change implementation. In our final chapter, we offer some ideas about how these efforts can be strengthened.

Conclusion

NOT A PERFECT WORLD . . .

Throughout this book, we have argued that aviation has produced a safety model that has worked for a complex, multidisciplinary, safety-critical, often-unpredictable work environment. Because both aviation and health care share so much as *types* of systems, we believe the model is adaptable to health care in its principles and many of its practices. We do not claim that the concrete content of CRM can or should be mapped directly onto the health care environment; indeed, CRM has had to be *adapted* even for different settings involving aircraft and flight (commercial, military—including service-specific adaptations—corporate, etc.). It is no longer arguable that the safety training programs in aviation have made commercial flying safer. These facts notwithstanding, we do not want to idealize CRM/TEM. As in any human endeavor, maintaining high reliability and team intelligence, as Thomas Jefferson said about safeguarding freedom, requires constant vigilance. No matter how much or how often staffs are trained in teamwork and conflict resolution, there will always be people who aren't with the program, who are uncooperative, become angry with those with whom they work, or who don't navigate conflicts well. This is as true in aviation as it is anywhere else. In spite of CRM, there are pilots who are brusque in their briefing style, make contact only with the purser and not the entire crew, or even neglect to brief altogether, among other problems.

Patrick recently spoke with an airline flight attendant about her thoughts on CRM. Although an avid proponent, she said, "There isn't much you can do about what goes on on the other side of the [cockpit] door." She had recently worked with one captain who said "all the right stuff" in his briefing but performed much differently during a crisis. On climb-out, the aircraft experienced what this flight attendant much later learned were "compressor stalls" in one of the two engines.

It was a nighttime departure and about halfway through the climb, there was a series of loud "pops" accompanied by bright flashes of flames that were visible throughout the aircraft. It was the left side and flames shot out the front and back of the engine! The aircraft shook violently and yawed from side to side.

I tried to call up to the cockpit on the interphone to tell the pilots what we were seeing. The first officer answered and said they were "on it" and hung up. We never heard another word until we were on the ground . . . right back where we started twenty minutes before. This was a legitimate emergency; many of the passengers were terrified; the cabin crew did not have a clue about what was happening. Yet the pilots didn't take ten or fifteen seconds to call the Lead [flight attendant] or even make a public announcement to the passengers until we were finally on the ground again. This was a definite failure in communication and ultimately a threat to safety!

Patrick tells a story of working with a captain who appeared to be a CRM skeptic and who later explicitly confirmed that suspicion:

A couple of years ago, I had a six-day trip with a particularly grumpy captain that I can accurately describe as "old school." Personally, he was a nice enough guy, but in the cockpit, he was gruff, brusque, demeaning and made it very clear that he was very much in charge and in control of every aspect of the operation. To his credit, he pulled it off and was a technically very talented aviator, but from a CRM perspective, I believed that he was about a heartbeat away from screwing up, simply because he was such a one-man show.

On the subject of briefings, this captain actually stated, "I think that you shouldn't have to go into any great detail on an approach briefing. If you don't know how to do this by now, you are in the wrong business."[1]

The night before our last leg home, I was having dinner in the hotel restaurant by myself, reading a book that we have referred to many times throughout this tome, *Cockpit Resource Management*.[2] The captain unexpectedly walked in and I discreetly put the book down in the seat next to me. He sat down across from me and asked, "What are you reading?" I sheepishly picked up the book and showed it to him.

The captain just grinned and said, "You know what I think of that? A bunch of bullshit!" Well, I guess we cleared the air on that. I replied, "I could have guessed."

Thankfully for all of us, this captain is now retired.

Just as global events have transformed the passenger's experience of flying, pilots, flight attendants and other airline personnel report that these events may also have a negative impact on airline safety. Today they worry that concern for the bottom line is negatively impacting safety. Commercial airlines are in the business of making money. Like many other large corporations in the early twenty-first century, in their pursuit of profits they seem to be on a collision course with quality and safety. This is another thing that aviation and health care have in common. Work intensification—the attempt to get more out of personnel with reduced resources—is a major trend that threatens both quality and safety in our competitive global economy. Regardless of their place in the hierarchy, people are pushed to attain an increasing variety of productivity measures (e.g., on-time departure in aviation, hospital throughput in health care). Their work is subject to more and more distracting interruptions, and they are given less time for rest and respite.

Similarly, most major industries are trying to save money by cutting back on what they now regard as "nonessentials." To cite just one example, all commercial airliner cockpits are equipped with what is called a *Quick Reference Handbook* (*QRH*), which contains over one hundred checklists (depending upon the aircraft) for pilots to use to navigate emergencies. As Chesley Sullenberger explains in his book, prior to his famous Hudson River ditching, US Airways had QRHs with numbered tabs for each aircraft system, making it easy to go quickly to the right system in an emergency:

> That made it easier to find the exact page we needed. You could hold it in your left hand and use it like an address book, grazing over the numbered tabs with your right hand before turning to the tab for, say, procedure number 27. In recent years, however, in a cost-cutting move, US Airways had begun printing these booklets without the numbered tabs on the edge of the pages. Instead, the number of each procedure was printed on the page itself, requiring pilots to open the pages and thumb through them to get to the right page.[3]

Captain Sullenberger and First Officer Jeffrey Skiles had three minutes and twenty-eight seconds to maneuver their aircraft to safety after hitting a flock of Canada geese. The airline's cost-cutting measure cost Skiles valuable seconds; without tabs to guide him to the relevant section he had to frantically flip through the book to find the right checklists.

This is only one indication of many problems that pilots, flight attendants and other personnel are experiencing as airlines contend with higher fuel prices, terrorism, and a host of other difficulties. In all his discussions with the media after his historic landing, Sullenberger highlighted problems arising from this dynamic. He was able to navigate this near disaster so successfully because he is a highly experienced pilot with decades of experience in both military and commercial aviation. Yet he has warned that airline companies are now outsourcing the jobs of experienced pilots to regional carriers with less-experienced pilots. In July 2011 a major airline's pilots' union took out a full-page ad in *USA Today* warning the public about what it believed were unsafe practices at the airline. The first paragraph of the ad read as follows:

> Unfortunately, our employer does not share our passion for safety. While [this airline's] management touts their safety record and certain programs they have in place, they have nonetheless created a culture of intimidation and pressure, where a Captain's authority takes a backseat to economic considerations and on-time performance. We know that being on-time is important to our passengers, but

[this airline] is pressuring its labor groups beyond reasonable limits and to the detriment of safety. We cannot support their desires for profits over safety, and we will not put the lives of our passengers at risk to satisfy the on-time performance goals that produce lucrative executive bonuses.

The rest of the ad cataloged a series of incidents in which the pilots' union claimed the airline had attempted to intimidate pilots who tried to maintain a safety culture. Though we have not been able to observe cases like these directly, we have talked with a number of pilots and flight attendants who report that the industry is now pushing personnel to work harder and longer, and sometimes to ignore safety concerns, because of competitive pressures to maintain on-time departures.

The current trend toward airline consolidation is creating enormous instability as different individual safety cultures combine. The two most recent mergers (Delta with Northwest and United with Continental)—which are also the largest in history—have resulted in cultural migraines that probably far exceeded what anyone could have anticipated. The Delta-Northwest consolidation was afflicted by confusion, turmoil, and angst, common byproducts of such an undertaking. Each airline has, over decades, developed its own FAA-approved procedures for just about every action, from when to extend the flaps for takeoff to when certain fixes get circled on the flight plan.[4] To an outsider, these differences may seem subtle and relatively insignificant, yet to a pilot—for whom habit, consistency, routine, predictability, and discipline are conditions that allow complex successions of tasks to be accomplished day in and day out with a high degree of reliability—they matter a great deal. "At Northwest," one pilot said,

we were trained to utilize checklists word for word. If a pilot replied, "SET," when the proper expected checklist response was "ON," it would literally stop the checklist reading until the proper switch setting was verified and the correct response was stated. Seems like a small thing, but if a response didn't match the challenger's expectation, it caused you to dig deeper into why.

Now, imagine how disruptive a whole series of changes could be when trying to blend the "best practices" of both organizations. The first challenge was that each company believed strongly that their way was the best practice. Otherwise, we wouldn't have been doing it that way, right? So there were the politics of figuring out which procedure for each item would prevail. Then there was the challenge of implementing the new common procedures so that both groups were doing the same thing the same way.[5] Pilots had to be trained and checked to make certain that they had it right, and it was an understandably painful process.

The process, although difficult, was unavoidable and I must say that even though we are a long ways from working out all of the kinks, the fact that we went through this without bending one aircraft is a testament to the benefit of operating in a CRM culture. I seriously doubt if things would have gone this smoothly had this merger occurred thirty years ago.

At this writing, the United-Continental consolidation is going through similar growing pains. An article published online describes the concerns of United Airlines pilots who have had to absorb a large volume of changes all at once, including some procedures that make them "uncomfortable." To minimize costs, the airlines do not want to spend any more time in training than is absolutely necessary. Therefore, pilots are burdened with numerous changes that must be implemented and absorbed all at once. In addition, the article states that pilots received no classroom instruction on the new procedures. Instead, they received a fifty-four-minute computer-based slide show; some pilots have been designated to answer questions, and that's it. Wendy Morse, the head of the pilots' union at United said, "No single change would be difficult but there's a whole plethora of changes in a row, and one on top of another, and that is what's creating the angst. Our guys are not comfortable because of a whole list of those kinds of things."[6]

Several United flight attendants have told us that they feel that safety at the airlines is not what it used to be and that CRM efforts have been less rigorous since the airline's merger with Continental. One flight attendant with forty years of experience explained, "We used to always have our [CRM] sessions during our emergency training with at least some pilots there. But that seems to have gone by the board during this current merger."

We raise these issues to point out that no magic bullet can ever guarantee long-lasting safety and high reliability. No matter how much improvement an innovative program like CRM produces, it will always require constant maintenance, updating, and attention, as was clear in the recent JetBlue incident and many others. In spite of many threats to the integrity of the aviation safety movement, CRM/TEM still remains a model from which health care has much to learn. This is why we conclude this book by exploring what it would take for health care to utilize the intelligence of its teams in every setting in which human beings depend on safe and effective services.

IMAGINE

In CRM training, concepts like cross-monitoring; mature leadership; assertive followership; briefings and debriefings; situational awareness; being aware of the danger of assumptions, task saturation, and fatigue; and distributed cognition—to name only the highlights—are now integrated into the consciousness of those who fly planes and who make it possible for planes to actually get off the ground and then land safely. What would it look like if these concepts, adapted for health care, were integrated into the workaday consciousness of those in that field?

In the introductory chapter we recounted the experiences of a patient in a prestigious American hospital—one that has tried to implement serious patient safety initiatives—and the many errors that beset her treatment for a bowel obstruction and caused her tremendous additional harm. We'd like to ask you to go back and reread that case study. Then take a moment to imagine what would have happened if something like CRM/TEM training had been routinely offered in that hospital. What would all the characters in the drama have done if they had had team intelligence? How would the outcome have changed if just one character had acted differently? Two? Three? What would a debriefing of the case look like? What elements of CRM might be involved?

How much pain, suffering, and money would have been saved had the patient's physician listened to the concerns of the home care nurse? If CRM (maybe we could call it team intelligence in action, or TIIA) were routinely taught in health care settings, the physician would not only have listened to but actually *solicited* the input of the home care nurse. Alternatively, when the physician had blown off the home care nurse, she would have challenged him. Because of training in MedTeams, some participating emergency room staff still utilize today the techniques they learned in the mid-1990s. One ER physician told us, "If we don't listen to them in our ER, nurses will challenge us and actually say, 'We're two-challenging you,'" referring to the two-challenge rule MedTeams borrowed from aviation." If health care institutions embraced the concept of cross-monitoring, such challenges would not be considered acts of insubordination, but would be welcome acts of mutual support—along the lines of, "Hey you're about to forget something, and I am saving your bacon."

What would have happened to the patient with the bowel obstruction if hospitalists and other staff members had actually communicated with one another face-to-face? If they had been trained in team intelligence, they would have been doing routine briefings and debriefings that included all staff with relevant information. What if they had paid attention to the nutritionist's note? This would have obviated the problem that nearly proved fatal—the failure to consider the nutritionist's recommendation that the patient receive tube feeding. Since physicians and nurses would have met with the nutritionist in a face-to-face briefing, she would have been able to convey her concerns and explain the nutritional issues, which would have been taken seriously by the medical and nursing staff.

If airline captains now willingly recruit other pilots who aren't part of the cockpit crew to add their insights and expertise to managing an emergency, why is it that some physicians fail to enlist the expertise of another physician, like the patient's friend and advocate? What would have happened in this instance if the captains of the ship had been trained to listen to, and consider as resources, not only other hospital staff but also the patient's oncologist and physician friend? When team intelligence is put into action, members of the more formal institutional team learn how to be flexible enough to expand their thinking to include the input of other people who have valuable information that can be used to improve decision making. These voices would have been welcomed instead of being viewed as intrusive or as constituting a critique. So would the voices of the patient's family.

Multiple other concepts adapted from CRM—like avoidance of dangerous assumptions, fatigue, and continuation bias—would also have been useful in caring for this patient. We know that her nurses were working twelve-plus-hour shifts, that residents taking care of her were working eighty hours a week, and that even her attending physicians were working long, exhausting hours and carrying heavy patient loads. Task saturation is inevitable in such circumstances, as is the kind of fatigue that makes people less apt to consider why poor outcomes—multiple readmissions, a patient who is failing rather than thriving—are occurring. Considering the *real* reasons for the patient's declining health status would also have been aided by recognizing the dangers of the staff's assumptions that, because she had had five previous cancers she was expected to decline. Recognition of the continuation bias that leads to persisting in a course of action that is not producing results would also have proved immensely helpful.

In today's health care universe, the kinds of cognitive problems outlined above and the training that would remedy them are often considered "soft" or "touchy-feely," not as important as the "hard" skills of diagnosis and treatment. Just as many pilots considered CRM to be "charm school," many physicians do not recognize the validity of the kinds of insights that the social sciences and more ethnographic approaches have to offer. Yet, as we are learning from studies of how the brain actually works, most of us are not the completely rational choice makers we like to think we are. Failure to attend to the more "touchy-feely" aspects of behavior *does* in fact have a direct effect on accuracy of diagnosis, on appropriateness of treatment plan, on costs of care, on patient suffering, and ultimately on health care outcomes.[7]

What aviation teaches us is that so-called "soft" and "hard" skills and abilities go hand in hand, which is why the study of error in high-tech enterprises is known as Human Factors Research. What aviation also teaches us is that mastering the soft skills may be as difficult as, or even more difficult than, mastering the "hard" ones. And, it shows us that none of these difficult things will be done voluntarily, which is why we believe government regulation is needed to deal with many patient safety issues and why Captain Chesley Sullenberger, who has spent a great deal of time since 2009 consulting on patient safety, recently joined Dennis Quaid and others to call for the equivalent of an NTSB for in healthcare.[8]

JETTISONING THE HEROIC MEDICAL MODEL

Creating a high-reliability safety culture will require taking a number of steps, and one of these will be replacing the heroic medical narrative with one that validates the importance of teamwork. To do this, the health care discourse will have to include a very different story about health care innovation, success, and even failure. Geraint Lewis and colleagues, in an article in the health policy journal *Milbank Quarterly*, outline fifteen "error countermeasures" that are incorporated into present-day commercial aviation but not typically followed in health care.[9] These are classified into three broad types, of which the first two are "counterheroism," ("safety concepts that seek to downplay the role of heroic individuals and instead emphasize the importance of teams and whole organizations") and "common knowledge" ("concepts that seek to increase and apply *group knowledge* of safety information and values").[10] Citing an ethnographic study of operating rooms, they note that:

> when items of surgical equipment were missing, surgeons modified, reshaped, or adjusted equipment designed for other uses. The surgeons described these actions as "adventurous," "daring," and necessary for "getting the job done." In contrast, other members of the operating room team said they felt anxious about these "heroic" modifications of established practice. However, the frequency of system failures had bred a culture in which complaining about system failures was regarded as a criticism of the surgeons' ability to innovate rather than as a condemnation of the system failure itself.[11]

Lewis and his coauthors conclude that the ways in which physicians respond to safety threats and errors is inextricably tied to the "culture of heroism" in medicine and in fact that "system failures and a culture of heroism may be self-reinforcing. [. . .] Fostering [an aviation-style culture of safety] in health care therefore requires curbing individual heroism, which may be achieved through increased codification and other measures [such as increasing a common knowledge/team approach] that downplay the role of individuals in ensuring safety."[12] This article contains excellent suggestions for how CRM/TEM principles and practices could be adapted to health care.

Doing this would go a long way to address the toxic hierarchies that are now so prevalent in medicine. This new narrative would reconceptualize those who work in healthcare as team resources rather than as competitors or as invisible, relatively mindless, backstage actors who play only a minor role in a drama that centers on physician leaders. This in turn will require an understanding of the function of each profession and occupation in health care and a respect for their work and insights—much as the Osher Center (chapter 5) has modeled. (In our dream world everyone in a health care leadership position would be required to read Mike Rose's excellent book *The Mind at Work*).[13] With even a modicum of understanding of the scope of work and the importance of others in health care, a resident asking a dean of nursing what nurses do should be beyond belief. (Imagine a quarterback asking the coach to explain the function of a linebacker or defensive end because he really had no idea what it was.) A hospital's demanding that all personnel except doctors work to prevent a frail ninety-eight-year-old from crawling over her bedrails would be equally incredible.

Any new health care narrative has to be centered on another intellectual leap. This involves the explicit acknowledgment that in a complex endeavor, which is heavily dependent on technology, cognition is *distributed*. In the village it takes to care for the sick and vulnerable, no one player or discipline can possibly have all the information, data, or knowledge needed to make complex decisions in dynamic situations. Health care team leaders and team members need a concept of competence that mirrors this reality—a concept of safety and quality that is grounded on what Lorelei Lingard calls "collective competence."[14]

SHARED LANGUAGE

This recognition would begin to create another cornerstone of team resource management: creating a shared language. If medical language is off-limits to a whole host of health care workers because talking is conflated with acting (e.g., when "naming" is considered to be "diagnosing"), then how can people ever hope to effectively create teams or put team intelligence into action? Imagine if mathematicians were to tell physicians they could no longer use numbers and equations because that is "mathematical language" and physicians after all are not mathematicians. Or if chemists insisted that doctors had to find new words for the elements because the language of the periodic table was off-limits to non-chemists. Constructing a common lexicon, as those at the Osher Center did, is not just a nicety or an interesting intellectual endeavor; it is a nonnegotiable necessity for safe and effective patient care and thorough information transfer. People involved in the care of the sick simply can no longer do without mutually intelligible terminology, available to all who need to use it in the care of patients.

RESEARCH

While the development of programs like TeamSTEPPS has been informed by serious research, we believe that not enough has yet been done in health care. We simply don't know enough about how, precisely, the hidden curriculum and socialization of health professionals and those in other health care occupations negatively or positively affect teamwork, team intelligence, and safety. Bonnie and Suzanne have both observed amazing examples of performance in what would, were they formalized, be team performance indicators. We have also seen some truly shocking behavior. Between these two poles, we've observed routine behavior that is often anti-TRM:

- A nurse decides she doesn't need to tell an intern why she doesn't have the time to change the dressing on a patient at change of shift because "why does he need to know?"
- An attending advises a resident that he has to "remember you're the boss" when a nurse suggests he use a different medication than the one he wants to prescribe.
- A nurse-manager has no skill in intervening when an RN and an aide get into a dispute because the latter keeps hoarding the blood pressure cuffs.
- One orthopedic surgeon routinely rounds with nurses, pharmacists, and PTs when seeing his patients on an orthopedic unit in a major teaching hospital. The other twelve who admit to the unit think rounding with other members of the health care team is a waste of time. No one has the authority to insist that rounding with the team should be standard operating procedure.

None of these examples involves patient harm—yet. What they all do involve is delivery of subtle messages that reinforce traditional toxic hierarchies and jeopardize the effort to create new paradigms for workplace relationships. We need to know more about these subtle messages and how the anti-team hidden curriculum works in different health care settings. Who are high effectiveness (Hi E) team leaders? What do they say and do? Who are Low E physicians, administrators, managers, nurses, etc.? How does the kind of language (including body language) used in the health care professions hamper teamwork? What about health care education? What do people learn about one another in the classroom or on the ward? Dedicated faculty can construct successful common learning activities in a well-thought-out interprofessional education curriculum, but if students return to the classroom where theories and practices declare one group superior to another, their primary educational experience won't be one of distributed cognition but one of cognitive dissonance.

This is why research has to move beyond broad surveys like the one conducted by the American Association of Critical Care Nurses, entitled *Silence Kills*,[15] to the kind of detailed, direct, *in vivo* qualitative observations that were done in aviation and other high-reliability industries. Unfortunately, most sociological and cognitive studies in health care focus not on the collective but either on the individual profession or the provider-patient dyad. The majority of this research focuses on physicians, with some on nurses. Whatever the discipline, most researchers home in on dyadic relationships—doctor-patient, nurse-patient, PT-patient. Few studies target the team, and fewer still address interprofessional communication in teams or assess and evaluate interprofessional education and practice programs. This kind of research is, however, critical, as Scott Reeves, founding director of the Center of Innovation for Interprofessional Education at the University of California at San Francisco, points out:

Just because someone tells you they have an interprofessional education program or practice teamwork doesn't mean they are actually working interprofessionally or on teams. We know that people will often give the socially desirable response when questioned. That's why we really need to peel off the surface layer to see what is really going on beneath. Implementing rigorous research that can provide evidence for what's really going on is crucial if we are going to make progress in this area.

Conducting and heeding the lessons of such research will require an expansion of the limited view that the only research that counts is the quantitative variety, which often is not suited to capturing the kinds of behavioral nuances and organizational problems that impact patient safety and effective workplace organization. If we don't know—in great detail—what the problems are and how traditional socialization creates and reinforces them on a daily basis, we will never be able to solve them. If we don't know what really works, how can we export it outside the unit or institutional frame in which it has been developed and nurtured?

TEAM TRAINING AND TEAMSTEPPS

Armed with this kind of research, health care professionals can design and implement essential training in skill building. One example of this is the TeamSTEPPS program, developed by the Patient Safety Program of the Department of Defense and the Agency for Healthcare Quality and Research after the 1999 release of the Institute of Medicine report *To Err Is Human*. TeamSTEPPS is an excellent beginning, and we believe it should be one of the models that, like United's CRM training, is widely adopted and *adapted* throughout hospitals and other health care institutions. After three years of research funded by the DoD and AHRQ, in January of 2003 the two government agencies gathered a panel of thirty experts in human-factors, human-error, and medical-team training. "At this meeting . . . experts discussed the needs, requirements, and strategies for effective teamwork in health care. Topics included competency requirements for medical teams, appropriate training strategies for teams, how to reliably measure teamwork, and what health care could learn from aviation and other disciplines. The result was a roadmap that helped guide the research that followed."[16]

Much influenced by the aviation model (whose application to health care has been studied by one of those experts, Eduardo Salas), TeamSTEPPS focuses on four major core competencies that are similar to CRM CPIs. These are: leadership, situation monitoring, mutual support, and communications.

The training was initially carried out by the Department of Defense in sixty-eight facilities. This effort produced 1,500 trainer-coaches who have trained more than 5,000 staff members. In November of 2006, AHRQ publicly released the TeamSTEPPS resources and began its effort to promote the use of the training program in all health care institutions throughout the United States via its National Implementation Project. To disseminate the program across the United States, TeamSTEPPS has set up five team resource centers: Duke Medical Center, Durham, North Carolina; Carilion Clinic, Roanoke, Virginia; University of Minnesota Fairview Medical Center, Minneapolis, Minnesota; Creighton University Medical Center, Omaha, Nebraska; and University of Washington Medicine, Seattle, Washington. These centers train "master trainers," who then go out and run the training at various health care facilities. This national network also produces Webinars and a toll-free telephone line. Because it is a government program, training in TeamSTEPPS is free, as are materials. Institutions who send staff to be trained in the program have to pay for their time and daily expenses but not for the training itself.

TeamSTEPPS is perhaps the only standardized teamwork training model in health care, at least in the US. While the training curriculum may seem overly complicated to some and may not include—in our view—enough about workload management, it is an important template that can be utilized in and adapted by many different health care institutions. Whatever the training program, hospitals and health care facilities need to begin to team-train staff at every rung of the health care ladder—and ideally, to train them *together*. Separate discipline-specific trainings are better than nothing but run a poor second to collective training, which by its very nature and inclusiveness begins to break down some barriers of professional exclusivity. Adding the direct *experience* of others' skills, knowledge, mandates, and challenges becomes itself a part of the formation of team intelligence and identity. To be even more effective, hospital-based efforts should accompany efforts to train health care students interprofessionally, as has been done at the University of Toronto as well as other universities in Canada and is now being launched in the United States. Wherever it is done, interprofessional education has to be envisioned not as an occasion for students to learn together about some external subject matter (say the importance of introducing HIV testing into primary care settings) but rather, as Scott Reeves and Ivy Oandasan point out, as an "occasion when two or more professions learn *from and about each other* to improve collaboration and the quality of care."[17]

Efforts to teach and model interprofessional education and practice are great beginnings, "beginnings" being the operative word. If they are to be truly successful, they have to move beyond the world of university health care education to a wide variety of different educational settings—to the community colleges and other schools or institutions that train many of the health care workers who nowadays have the most contact with patients and thus the most critical information to share. This training and education also must be done in the workplace where it includes non-professional staff. Moreover, having a workshop or IPE placement in medical or nursing school does not accomplish the goal of fostering teamwork for a lifetime. The lessons needed to create and cultivate team intelligence must be consistently revisited in the continuing education of both professional and supporting staff. No health professional gets certified in CPR for life; these skills and the advancing knowledge that informs them require regular refreshment. Patients are commonly advised nowadays to question surgeons about how many times they've performed a given operation because we know that once—or even a few times—is not enough. Recurrent training is equally important for teamwork and for all of the team performance indicators we've discussed. (Whether they have been trained in teamwork should also be something patients ask when consulting a physician about an elective procedure or considering which primary care provider to sign up with.)

WORKLOAD MANAGEMENT

In aviation, workload management is a separate but equal crew performance indicator. Fatigue, work intensification, continuation bias, and more are addressed in crew trainings and in the regulatory context. How long someone works, how much sleep he gets, whether she feels she is negatively impacted by stress, should not be left to the judgment of the individual professional or health care worker. Sadly, studies have documented that, like the residents of Lake Woebegone, most health care personnel think they are above average: that they can work effectively when they are in fact falling into microsleep; that they can effectively multitask under almost any circumstances (even though brain scientists are now teaching us that multitasking is a myth). People who try to handle too many tasks at a time—for all practical purposes a fundamental demand in today's health care system—experience more stress, fail to learn as effectively, and may use up energy figuring out how to task-switch that could be more profitably expended on sticking to one task at a time. Safety is similarly compromised when doctors are restricted or restrict themselves to ten to fifteen minutes when seeing complex patients or when they see thirty or thirty-five patients a day, are sleeping in their offices, or perform too many surgeries in a day. Since we know that fatigue has a significant impact on interpersonal interactions and that people who are exhausted tend to be irritable and thus unlikely to work effectively on a team, one wonders how anyone can talk about effective teamwork in health care without dealing with the kinds of workloads and schedules that keep people from getting enough sleep.

Another thing we should be worried about is the fact that so many doctors, nurses, and other health care staff are so busy at work that they do not have time to take breaks to eat. Amazingly, the health care system, which is supposed to be evidenced based, has forgotten the incontrovertible evidence that the human machine requires fuel—known as food—to function. Excessive workloads may, however, preclude taking time to refuel in many health care workplaces. Many nurses working twelve-plus-hour shifts tell us they eat breakfast at 5:30 am, arrive at work at 6:45 am, and do not eat again until 1:30 or two in the afternoon. Physicians are similarly working without stopping to refuel.

Not eating, particularly when combined with chronic fatigue, can have a negative impact on people's ability to be attentive and empathic as Daniel Kahneman points out in his book about how the brain works, *Thinking, Fast and Slow*. In it, he cites a study conducted on the decision making of Israeli parole judges. A group of researchers studied judges who were determining whether prisoners deserved parole. The judges were assigned random cases, and their default position was to deny parole. "The authors of the study plotted the proportion of approved requests [for parole] against the time of the last food break. The proportion spikes after each meal, when about 65 percent of requests are granted. During the two hours or so until the judges' next feeding, the approval rate drops steadily, to about zero just before the meal. As you might expect, this is an unwelcome result, and the authors carefully checked many alternative explanations. The best possible account of the data provides bad news: tired, hungry judges tend to fall back on the easier default position of denying requests for parole. Both fatigue and hunger probably play a role."[18] When we read this we couldn't help thinking about the fate of patients who rely on both the judgments and kindness of strangers, many of whom, on a daily basis, function when hungry and tired, in the contemporary health care system. Indeed, part of the heroism that CRM-like programs could counter is the notion that heroic physicians and nurses (who have their own heroic narrative), can somehow rise above bodily needs and functions.

It is exceptionally difficult to temper, through effort or will, the impact of stress and fatigue, and yes, hunger, on behavior. Everyone in health care claims to be on the side of the patient and uses the benefit to the patient to justify his or her practices or prejudices. Yet how many decision makers consider the fact that *anything* that interferes with the high-level functioning of the human machine puts patients and teamwork in jeopardy. Martyn Diaper, a British general practitioner and a member of the Primary Care Team, Safer Care, at the British National Health Service Institute for Innovation and Improvement, explains,

> I went into this profession because I care. Like a lot of doctors, I respect all my colleagues and patients. I also understand that working as a team to get the best for patients means that we have to communicate effectively and show each other respect and support. I also know that my behavior and communication falls below the standards I aspire to when I am stressed or tired. The communication I espouse and the communication I use can be two very different things. I can be crabby and gruff at times. That is not because my belief in good communication wavers but because my energy and stress level does, and with it my ability to communicate well.

This is why fatigue and workload need to be carefully attended to at every possible opportunity.

Hospitals and health care institutions have to take action to deal with work organization, workload, and fatigue. We are not as allergic to regulation—as many physicians and health care administrators seem to be. We feel that there needs to be more wise regulation of the health care workload and of patient safety hazards like sleep deprivation. The United States and Canada have much to learn from other countries like those in the European Union, Australia, and New Zealand when it comes to limitations of both physicians' and nurses' work hours. It is a part of the definition of a "profession" that it is able to be self-regulating. Yet heretofore health care professions and organizations have not done well at this task. If institutions or the health professions themselves refuse to establish regulatory policies and practices that protect patients and staff from technological and human-factors hazards, then the government will have to do it. What is the alternative?

LEADERSHIP AND LEVERAGE

We believe leaders must *lead*. As Lucien Leape, one of the medical leaders in the patient safety movement, has consistently argued, they must be at the front of the pack in patient safety and building cultures of respect and teamwork in their institutions. In two articles on respect in health care Leape and his colleagues argue that hospital CEOs and physician leaders must create the kind of codes of respect and teamwork initiatives that have been described in the case study of Maimonides hospital.[19]

In doing so they are implicitly, if not explicitly, recognizing that cognition and competence are not only evaluated and monitored at the individual level but also *distributed* within a team and that these distributed competencies must be accessed and used by that team. If hospitals implement codes of conduct or civility initiatives, these should be founded in the recognition that disrespect is not only an individual problem but also a *system issue*. Up until now many health care institutions have not merely tolerated but actually enabled, and even rewarded, bad behavior. The attitude has been that just as boys will be boys, nothing can be done to temper the behavior of hot shots who produce revenue for the institution. Hospital and health care administrators have to take the attitude that was expressed by Maimonides CEO Pam Brier, who explained that no physician (or any other skilled technician)—no matter how much revenue he or she generates—is worth his or her salt if that person cannot function on a team. Such a person is particularly not worth it if his or her actions are having a negative impact on staff ability to maintain situational awareness. Under the best of circumstances, caring for the sick and vulnerable is difficult work. Does it need to be made even more so because the people doing the work don't have the skills necessary to deal with either the sick or each other?

Patients cannot afford to rely on institutions that continue to coddle geese just because they lay the golden eggs. Those who do not attend to the details of teamwork and the best practices for patient care actually put the hospital and their patients at risk. What, precisely, is so golden about surgeons who refuse to complete a checklist or time-out because they are in a hurry or are personally annoyed by the protocol? Why reward the medical and nursing staff on units where there is no genuine communication about a patient's status or about staff safety concerns? Why does a hospital continue to employ a nurse manager who's great at making OR schedules but can't deal effectively with her staff? A good technician is not necessarily a good clinician, and a good clinician is not necessarily a good manager. Top institutional leaders have leverage, and they need to use it—not to punish and blame but to coach, train, and maintain. If some people can be neither coached nor retrained, then perhaps they need to find another occupation that better fits their skills.

Institution-wide or unit-based implementation and standardization of teamwork training—and, yes, even regulation—may be the only ways to assure that health care professionals change their behavior and that health care institutions change their cultures. Recall the CEO who lamented that physicians may refuse to abide by voluntary standards at one hospital if another hospital down the road doesn't have the same strict standards. Many hospital leaders comment that physicians threaten to leave and take their patients with them if they do not like a particular hospital's policies and practices. But if every hospital—like every airline—had to abide by similar policies and practices, there would be nowhere more attractive to run.

CEOs of hospitals have a positive role to play. So do health care insurers. As we discussed in the previous chapter, physicians cannot just waltz into a hospital and begin to order drugs and procedures and wield scalpels in an OR. They have to be either employed by the hospital or credentialed in order to practice there. Hospital administrators—like airlines—can preferentially hire or extend privileges to those who have a team mentality or have explicit teamwork training in their backgrounds. At some point, if they are dealing with bullies, they have to be willing to "bully the bullies" in order to change the culture.

Insurers also have a role to play in the unfolding of this medical drama. Just as one of the drivers of change in the airline industry was the threat of litigation from families of passengers who died or from passengers themselves who had been injured, so too the threat of malpractice litigation and the cost of medical errors and injuries for providers, health care institutions, and the system as a whole is a powerful lever for change. Malpractice insurers thus have a significant role to play in encouraging physicians and other clinicians or hospitals to walk the walk of patient safety through communications and teamwork training. Some are already doing that and are extending their traditional role of claims management to also include risk management. If you check out the website of the malpractice insurer CRICO, you will find a list of communication/teamwork training and support materials, along with reference to a Harvard study showing that "negative team factors in the operating room contributed to delays in 40 percent of all cases studied and 30 percent of adverse events."[20] An executive at an East Coast malpractice insurer explained that his company is now encouraging the hospitals and physicians it insures to carry out team trainings like TeamSTEPPS. "Four hospitals in our group have decided to send thirty people from the OB to do the TeamSTEPPS training. These people will return to their institution and train more staff. Then they may move on to training people in other hospitals we insure." This kind of dissemination of the team model holds great promise and should be widely pursued.

One surgeon in a community hospital, whom Suzanne met at a safety meeting, expressed great interest in team training and interprofessional continuing education. He was stymied by the traditional hierarchy in his institution. Where could he find a forum to bring doctors and nurses together? "We can't do it at the medical staff meeting. Nurses don't come to that. We can't do it at a medical retreat. They don't come to that either." When Suzanne suggested physicians might consider inviting nurses to a medical staff meeting (it's hard to imagine they would refuse such an invitation), he seemed both stunned and then pleasantly surprised. "What a good idea!" he exclaimed.

THE ISSUE OF TIME

One of the primary rationalizations for hewing to the status quo in health care is time pressure. "We don't have time" to add anything more to the educational curriculum, faculty of health professional schools insist. We don't have time to do a team training for staff in our institution. We are "resource strapped," one patient safety officer told us. We can't possibly get an hour for nurses and physicians to get together to learn about teamwork. Can't they watch something on their own, listen to something as they are driving to and from work? Apparently, there is simply no time, no forum available for this kind of discussion. It would cost too much money, another insists.

Time and money *are* big obstacles. But adaptability to new circumstances is a critical factor for business success in strapped economies; one can't afford *not* to make the necessary changes. Quite apart from the medical and ethical issues, what is the cost in time and money spent on *just one case* of patient harm? Might preventing that save both (not to mention a patient's life or functional capabilities)? As one obstetrician said of his institution's recent innovation of including nurses in rounds, "You can't imagine how much time it saves physicians, because nurses now know what's going on and don't page us as often."

We are convinced that health care professionals and other health care workers owe it to their patients to engage—really engage—in this act of mastery. We also believe they owe it to each other and to themselves. We cannot imagine a more eloquent statement on this subject than a comment Mark Sand, a cardiac surgeon and chief of staff at Orlando Health, made at a patient safety forum: "When we wound one another, the wounds heal very slowly. When we invest in one another, the rewards may come back for a lifetime. Someday, sometime, perhaps when we least expect it, we will all be patients. If for no other reason, we must unite with one another at the bedside."

Appendix

MAIMONIDES MEDICAL CENTER
CODE OF MUTUAL RESPECT

Maimonides Medical Center recognizes the importance of professional behavior and desires to expand upon the principles outlined in the Maimonides Medical Center By-Laws and Corporate Compliance Program Code of Conduct and consistent with professional society codes of ethics. Following the endorsement of a Medical Staff Code of Mutual Respect in 2004 (which is incorporated into this document), the Medical Center now expects all members of the MMC Community to comply with the following code ("Code"):

I. PREAMBLE

The Medical Center recognizes the considerable interdependence amongst health care providers in the rapidly changing health care environment. It acknowledges that the ability to deliver high-quality health care and success in competing in the marketplace depend in large part upon the ability of all health care providers to communicate well, collaborate effectively, and work as a team to optimize and monitor outcomes.

The Medical Center further acknowledges that there are many participants in the process of effective health care, including patients, their families, physicians, nurses, allied health professionals, hospital staff, students, vendors and consultants, volunteers, and others, collectively herein referred to as the "MMC Community." Further the Medical Center understands that working harmoniously is a necessary aspect of modern health care. The Medical Center affirms that everyone, both recipients and providers of care, must be treated in a dignified, respectful manner at all times in order for their mutual goal of high-quality health care to be accomplished. "MMC Community" includes the employees, vendors, and consultants of MMC Holding of Brooklyn, Inc. and its subsidiary corporations ("MMC Holding"). "Medical Center" shall be deemed to include MMC Holding wherever appropriate.

The Medical Center affirms that it is the MMC Community's mutual responsibility to work together in an ongoing, positive, dynamic process that requires frequent, continual communication and feedback. The Medical Center agrees to devote the necessary time and resources toward achieving these goals and maintaining a positive, collaborative relationship amongst its members and with other providers and recipients of care.

II. PRINCIPLES

In order to accomplish these goals, the MMC Community agrees to the following principles and guidelines and to work collaboratively to promote them in the organization and in the community.

1. Professionalism

The MMC Community recognizes its commitment to the highest levels of professionalism with regards to the delivery of care. Therefore, the MMC Community encourages cooperation and communication amongst all health care providers and recipients of care, and displaying regard for each other's dignity. The MMC Community recognizes that acting professionally entails treating others with courtesy and respect, and refraining from the use of abusive language, threats of violence, retribution, or litigation, and actions that are reasonably felt by others to represent intimidation. The MMC Community also recognizes that it is unproductive to make inappropriate remarks concerning the quality of care being provided in public or in front of others not involved in the patient's care and agrees to address concerns about clinical judgments with associates directly in an appropriate setting and to avoid inappropriate entries in medical records. Additionally, favoritism and sidestepping of rules should be avoided.

2. Respectful Treatment

All members of the MMC Community including but not limited to health care provider team shall be treated in a respectful, dignified manner at all times. Language, nonverbal behavior and gestures, attitudes, etc. shall reflect this respect and dignity of the individual and affirm his/her value to the process of effective, efficient health care.

3. Language

All members of the MMC Community are expected not to use language that is profane, vulgar, sexually suggestive or explicit, intimidating, degrading, or racially/ethnically/religiously slurring in any professional setting related to the hospital and the care of its patients.

4. Behavior

The MMC Community is expected to refrain from any behavior that is deemed to be intimidating including but not limited to using foul language or shouting, physical throwing of objects, or making inappropriate comments regarding physicians, hospital staff, other providers, other employees, patients, or families.

5. Confidentiality

The MMC Community is expected to maintain complete confidentiality of patient care information at all times, in a manner consistent with HIPAA and generally accepted principles of medical confidentiality. The MMC Community further recognizes that physicians, students, hospital staff and employees have the right to have certain personal and performance problems and concerns about competence dealt with in a confidential manner in a private setting. The MMC Community agrees to maintain this confidentiality and to seek proper, professional, objective arenas in which to deal with these issues.

6. Feedback

The MMC Community is expected to give all parties prompt, direct, constructive feedback when concerns or disagreements arise. The MMC Community recognizes the necessity of describing such behavior in objective, behavioral terms and that such feedback should be given directly to the person(s) involved through appropriate channels, in a confidential, private setting.

7. Communication

The MMC Community encourages frequent, respectful, and clear communication amongst all its members, especially those involved with the direct care of patients. Specifically, the Medical Center Professional and Ancillary Staffs expect their members to respond to pages in a timely and suitable manner, and to respond to patient and staff requests appropriately. Patients and their families are encouraged to speak to professional and ancillary staff members so that they feel engaged in their or their family members' care.

III. MECHANISMS FOR PREVENTING DEVIATIONS FROM THE CODE OF MUTUAL RESPECT

The MMC Community recognizes that frustration in a high-tension environment can predispose to deviations from the "Code." The MMC Community therefore urges all departments and areas of the hospital to develop mechanisms (e.g. staff meetings, glitch book) that allow MMC Community members to have such frustrations addressed in an appropriate and timely fashion.

The MMC Community encourages all of its members to work together in a collaborative fashion such that unfavorable interactions can be either avoided, or addressed by the parties involved in a professional, productive manner.

It is the intent of these guidelines to help focus reasonable efforts to fix the systems issues that lead to frustration. However a few points must be understood by involved parties:

A. Problem system issues do not excuse bad behavior; just help understand it.
B. There must be acknowledgement that certain circumstances/conditions may not be under hospital control, but where they are, a process will be in place to keep the issue visible and those responsible for correcting it responsive.
C. Systems issues may be handled differently due to the specifics of a particular incident.
D. In all cases, attempts will be made to look at the root cause and contributing circumstances to help understand to what extent involved parties have a role to play.

General expectations:

A. An alleged system failure will only be investigated if it has been formally reported to the appropriate Administrator.
B. Once a system issue has been established and formally reported, the appropriate manager will investigate it.
C. Repeat occurrences that have not been effectively addressed (i.e. become a predominant cause for frustration) will have follow-up by senior level staff including the appropriate Vice-President and/or the Chief Operating Officer.

IV. MECHANISMS FOR ADDRESSING DEVIATIONS FROM THE CODE OF MUTUAL RESPECT

The Code is only intended to provide mechanisms to deal with disrespectful behavior as outlined generally in Section II. Measures to address other forms of inappropriate behavior including but not limited to sexual harassment, racial discrimination, and workplace violence are already described in the Medical Center's Human Resources Policies, Corporate Compliance Code of Conduct, Medical Staff By-Laws and other relevant policies. It is understood that the mechanisms set forth below may not be the exclusive remedy for certain behaviors.

Behavior inconsistent with the Code should be reported via the Respect Hotline (718-283-6677) or via e-mail to respect@maimonidesmed.org to ensure consistency of response. All reporters of disrespectful behavior are protected from retaliation. (For Medical Center staff this is specified in COMP-10—Protection Against Retaliation). When a report is made, an investigation will be initiated according to the following protocol:

A. Physicians

The Medical Staff Subcommittee on Respect (SOR) will monitor physician compliance with this Code. Three Directors preside over the SOR. One Director is a physician appointed by the President of the Medical Staff. Another Director is a full time physician appointed by the President of the Medical Center. The first two Directors jointly appoint the third Director. Both the President of the Medical Staff and President of the Medical Center have the authority to remove their respective Director appointees. Together the three Directors, in consultation with the VP for Professional Affairs and his/her staff, appoint up to 25 members of the SOR. The composition of the SOR is representative of the Clinical Departments and both the full time and voluntary staff.

When a report is made, one of the SOR Directors assigns a member of the SOR to investigate the report. This assignment should be made within two business days of the receipt of the report. The results of the initial investigation are discussed with the Directors and if the complaint is validated, action will be taken according to the following scheme:

1. First time occurrence

   a. A collegial discussion takes place between a SOR Director and/or the investigating SOR member and the physician to explore the situation and discuss ways to prevent further disrespectful behavior.

2. Second occurrence

   b. A meeting is held with the physician, his/her Chairman or designee, and at least one of the SOR Directors.
   c. The discussion emphasizes that if such behavior continues, more formal action will be taken to stop it.
   d. A follow-up letter to the physician is placed in the physician's departmental file which states the problem and that the physician is required to behave professionally and cooperatively.
   e. The involved physician may submit a rebuttal to the letter also maintained in his/her departmental file.

3. Third occurrence

   f. A meeting is held with the physician, his/her Chairman, Medical Staff President, Medical Director, and at least one of the SOR Directors.

g. This meeting is not a discussion but rather constitutes the physician's final warning.

h. A follow-up letter reiterates the warning and is placed in the physician's departmental file.

i. The involved physician may submit a rebuttal to the letter also maintained in his/her departmental file.

4. Fourth occurrence

a. A meeting is held with the physician, his/her Chairman, Medical Staff President, Medical Director, and at least one of the SOR Directors. The group confers and may recommend a suspension of up to but not exceeding 4 weeks to be considered by the Credentials Committee, EMC and Board of Trustees. The physician would thereafter be entitled to the hearing and appeal processes under Articles IV and V of the Medical Staff Bylaws should there be a recommendation made for an adverse action against the physician's privileges.

5. Fifth occurrence

a. A meeting is held with the physician, his/her Chairman, Medical Staff President, Medical Director, and at least one of the SOR Directors. The group confers and may recommend termination of privileges to be considered by the Credentials Committee, EMC and Board of Trustees. The physician would thereafter be entitled to the hearing and appeal processes identified under Articles IV and V of the Medical Staff Bylaws should there be a recommendation made for an adverse action against the physician's privileges.

6. General guidelines for dealing with disrespectful behavior

a. Once disrespectful behavior has been confirmed, all meetings with physicians should include the following:

   i. Goal of the meeting e.g., to make sure the physician understands what he/she did and the consequences.
   ii. Definition of the problem e.g., the nurse said you yelled.
   iii. Getting the physician to acknowledge the problem e.g., at a minimum, "I understand my behavior was seen by others as disrespectful."
   iv. Next steps e.g., Consequences if behavior continues, apology.

b. Mediated conversations should be used as needed to help all parties understand their potential roles in any given situation. This is particularly important for first time occurrences.

c. Throughout the process resources (i.e. counseling) are offered to assist the physician to help him/her deal with his/her disrespectful behavior.

d. In cases where a physician's behavior is particularly egregious, some of the steps outlined above can be bypassed at the discretion of the Medical Staff President in concert with the Department Chairman.

e. In all cases feedback is given to the person who reported the incident so that he/she knows that the report has been addressed and of the Medical Staff's commitment to address the disrespectful behavior.

f. Reporters are encouraged to report disrespectful behavior as soon as possible.

g. If the physician reported for alleged deviations from the Code of Mutual Respect is a resident in a Maimonides or Maimonides affiliated residency program, the residency program director would be included in any actions taken under the Code. This includes investigation regardless of outcome.

B. Employees

The reported incident will be given to the Director overseeing the department where the employee who allegedly violated the Code works. An investigation will be performed which ideally will include all involved parties in the alleged incident. In all cases, the investigation will attempt to determine whether or not the employee violated the Code and whether any other member of the MMC Community did so. In addition, any systems issues that may have been a catalyst for disrespectful behavior should also be identified and reported to the appropriate department. (see III). The results of the investigation will be discussed with the employee's Director and if the complaint is validated, action will be taken according to the protocol outlined in the progressive discipline policy found in HR12—Disciplinary Action (or Disciplinary Action #06–10 for MMC Holding). The employee may grieve any action taken as a result of this investigation as outlined in HR11—Grievance Procedure (or Dispute Resolution (Grievance) #06–09 for MMC Holding). In the case of unionized employees, any disciplinary action and grievance process will be according to the applicable Collective Bargaining Agreement.

C. Volunteers

The reported incident will be given to the Vice-President in charge of patient relations. An investigation will be performed to include all involved parties in the alleged incident. In all cases, the investigation will attempt to determine whether or not the volunteer violated the Code and whether any other member of the MMC Community did so. In addition, any systems issues that may have been a catalyst for disrespectful behavior should also be identified and reported to the appropriate department. (see III). The results of the investigation will be discussed with the volunteer's supervisor and the Director of Volunteer Services and if the complaint is validated, the volunteer will be informed that his/her services are no longer needed.

D. Students

The reported incident will be given to the Maimonides supervisor overseeing the student who allegedly violated the Code. An investigation will be performed to include all involved parties in the alleged incident. In all cases, the investigation will attempt to determine whether or not the student violated the Code and whether any other member of the MMC Community did so. In addition, any systems issues that may have been a catalyst for disrespectful behavior should also be identified and reported to the appropriate department. (see III). The results of the investigation will be discussed with the student's supervisor and if the complaint is validated, action will be taken consistent with the terms of the Affiliation Agreement with the school and discussions with the school representatives, which action may include but not be limited to removal of the student from Maimonides' premises.

E. Vendors, Consultants, and Others

The reported incident will be given to the Medical Center supervisor who has arranged for the vendor/consultant to work at the Medical Center. An investigation will be performed to include all involved parties in the alleged incident. In all cases, the investigation will attempt to determine whether or not the vendor/consultant violated the Code and whether any other member of the MMC Community did so. In addition, any systems issues that may have been a catalyst for disrespectful behavior should also be identified and reported to the appropriate department. (see III). The results of the investigation will be discussed with the Medical Center supervisor and if the complaint is validated, the vendor/consultant and/or his/her employer will be notified that he/she is no longer welcome at Maimonides Medical Center. The Legal Department will be advised so any contract issues can be addressed.

V. INSTITUTIONAL COMMITMENT TO RESPECT

1. The commitment to respect will be supported through the following mechanisms

   a. Skills training–All members of the MMC Community will have access to training in interpersonal communication skills and problem solving on a continuing basis.

b. Mediated conversations—In the course of investigation of alleged Code violations, mediated conversations between the involved parties are encouraged to help them better understand how the unfavorable interaction occurred and how it might be prevented in the future.

c. Measurement—Periodic surveys of members of the MMC Community will be conducted to continuously evaluate the effectiveness of and compliance with this Code.

2. Expectations for performance

a. Physician credentialing and re-credentialing will encompass compliance with this Code under the core competency of Professionalism.

b. Medical Center employees, as part of their yearly performance appraisal will be evaluated for compliance with this Code.

c. Volunteers, as part of their yearly performance appraisal will be evaluated for compliance with this Code.

d. Student evaluations will include comments concerning their compliance with this Code.

Endorsed by the Executive Medical Council (EMC)—September 25, 2008
Adopted by the Board of Trustees—November 10, 2008
Revised EMC—July 23, 2009

Glossary

Accreditation Council for Graduate Medical Education (ACGME). The organization responsible for the evaluation and accreditation of postgraduate (after medical school) medical training programs in the United States.

Agency for Healthcare Research and Quality (AHRQ). Part of the U.S. Department of Health and Human Services; supports research to improve the outcomes and quality of health care, reduce health care costs, address patient safety and medical errors, and broaden access to effective services. It also acts as the regulator for patient safety organizations that are certified under the Patient Safety and Quality Improvement Act.

air crew program designee (APD). An FAA-designated representative within a particular aircraft, organization, fleet, or program. An APD is appointed in accordance with FAA regulations, meets the stringent qualification requirements, and is authorized to certify qualified individuals for aircraft operation and give type ratings.

air traffic control (ATC). A service provided by ground-based controllers who direct aircraft on the ground and in the air. The primary purpose of ATC systems worldwide is to *separate* aircraft to prevent collisions and to organize and expedite the flow of traffic.

Aviation Safety Action Program (ASAP). The goal of this program is to enhance aviation safety through the prevention of accidents and incidents. Its focus is to encourage voluntary reporting of safety issues and events that come to the attention of employees of certain certificate holders. To encourage an employee to voluntarily report safety issues even though they may involve an alleged violation of Title 14 of the Code of Federal Regulations (14 CFR), enforcement-related incentives have been designed into the program. An ASAP is based on a safety partnership that will include the Federal Aviation Administration (FAA) and the certificate holder and may include any third party such as the employee's labor organization.

black box. A term that refers to either the cockpit voice recorder or the flight data recorder or both.

captain (CA). Pilot in command of the aircraft.

center of gravity (CG). A point along the aircraft's longitudinal axis at which weight is distributed equally fore and aft—CG is critical to aircraft stability and performance.

check airman. A person who is qualified, and permitted, to conduct flight checks or instruction in an airplane, in a flight simulator, or in a flight training device for a particular type of airplane.

checkride. That portion of an FAA examination used to demonstrate competency to qualify for pilot certification, recertification, or additional flight privileges.

cockpit voice recorder (CVR). An instrument that records the audio environment in the cockpit of an aircraft for the purpose of investigation of accidents and incidents. Typically only the last thirty minutes of data is available.

crew performance indicator (CPI). A critical factor that ensures safe, efficient, and effective completion of a team task, such as flying an aircraft.

Crew Resource Management (CRM). According to the FAA, "a system of management that makes optimum use of all available resources to the Flight Crew to ensure safe and efficient flight operations."

decision speed: V1. The maximum speed at which an aircraft pilot may abort a takeoff without causing a runway overrun.

Department of Defense (DoD). In addition to its other missions, a major funder of medical research in the United States.

electronic centralized aircraft monitor (ECAM). A computer system that monitors aircraft functions and relays them to the pilots. It also produces messages detailing failures and in certain cases lists procedures to undertake to correct the problem.

Federal Aviation Administration (FAA). The national aviation authority of the United States. An agency of the Department of Transportation, it has authority to regulate and oversee all aspects of civil aviation.

first officer (FO), or copilot. The officer second in command of the aircraft after the captain, who is the legal commander. In the event of the captain's incapacitation, the first officer will assume command.

flight attendant (FA). A member of an air crew employed by an airline primarily to ensure the safety and comfort of passengers aboard commercial flights, on select business jet aircraft, and on some military aircraft.

flight data recorder (FDR). An electronic device that records multiple aircraft environmental parameters such as airspeed, altitude, attitude, and accelerations. It also records instructions sent to electronic systems on an aircraft. It is one of the black boxes that provides critical information for accident investigations.

flight engineer (FE). The person primarily concerned with the operation and monitoring of all aircraft systems, who is required to diagnose and where possible rectify or eliminate any faults that may arise. The FE position has been eliminated in most modern transport aircraft as his or her duties have been replaced by computer technology. The flight engineer is also known as the second officer.

Flight Operations Quality Assurance (FOQA). A method of capturing, analyzing, and visualizing the data generated by an aircraft and applying the information learned from this analysis to find new ways to improve flight safety and increase overall operational efficiency.

flyby. A low, close-in pass in which an aircraft is flown close to a ground observer either for the purpose of flight demonstration or to allow the observer to verify a certain aircraft condition or status. Also known as a low pass.

hint and hope. The tendency to avoid confrontation by hinting rather than clearly stating a problem or issue, then hoping that the other person will understand and respond appropriately.

indicated airspeed (IAS). The airspeed read directly from the airspeed indicator on an aircraft, driven by the pitot-static system. It is not the same as true airspeed.

Institute for Healthcare Improvement (IHI). An independent nonprofit organization helping to lead the improvement of health care throughout the world. Its primary agenda is to eliminate needless deaths, needless pain or suffering, unwanted waiting, waste, exclusion of anyone, and feelings of helplessness on the part of both those served and those serving.

instrument flight rules (IFR). Rules governing flight operations in which aircraft navigation is done exclusively with reference to flight instruments; these are in contrast to visual flight rules (VFR) covering the use of visual reference.

interprofessional education (IPE). A recent and rapidly growing movement in health care, whose goal is to provide interprofessional education as a part of basic and undergraduate or graduate health care professions training, so that key disciplines in health care learn with and about each other and improve care and collaboration. Some interprofessional education programs also take place in hospitals and other health care settings and may include other health care workers who are not generally viewed as "professionals."

Joint Commission, The (TJC). Formerly called the Joint Commission on Accreditation of Healthcare Organizations, this is a private, not-for-profit organization that monitors and accredits hospitals and other healthcare organizations, according to their degree of compliance with a consensual and published set of standards. In 2007, formally changed its name to The Joint Commission.

knots (KTS). Nautical miles per hour (one knot equals about 1.15 mph).

Line Oriented Flight Training (LOFT). Training in a full flight simulator with a complete crew using representative flight segments that contain normal, abnormal, and emergency procedures that may be expected in day-to-day line operations.

low pass. See **flyby**.

National Atmospheric and Space Administration (NASA). An agency of the United States government that is responsible for the nation's civilian space program and for aeronautics and aerospace research.

National Transportation Safety Board (NTSB). The federal agency that investigates airline accidents and makes recommendations about how to prevent them

part 91 regulations. These FAA regulations apply to general aviation, private, and owner-operated aircraft.

part 121 regulations. These FAA regulations apply to scheduled air carriers (commercial airlines).

part 135 regulations. These FAA regulations apply to commuter and on-demand (charter) operators.

pilot flying (PF). The pilot physically in control of the aircraft (not necessarily the captain).

pilot in command (PIC). The pilot ultimately responsible for the aircraft and well-being of passengers and crew, usually the captain.

pilot monitoring (PM). Generally, the pilot not in physical control of the aircraft, who may or may not be the captain; duties include backup or monitoring the PF's performance.

primary care provider (PCP). A health care professional who provides first-line, walk-into-the-office health care. A PCP in the United States today may be an MD or DO, a chiropractor (DC), a nurse-practitioner (NP), a naturopath (ND), or a physician's assistant (PA), depending on the state in which he or she practices. The PCP is typically the first person a patient sees when entering the medical system.

purser. The flight attendant crew manager, also known as the lead flight attendant.

risk. The potential that a chosen action or activity (including the choice of inaction) will lead to a loss (an undesirable outcome).

ROMEO and ROZO. The names of particular navigational fix points.

second in command (SIC). The next person in the line of succession for command of the aircraft, generally the first officer.

second officer (SO). See **flight engineer**.

SOAP Notes. SOAP (subjective, objective, assessment, plan) notes are a method used by health care providers to document assessment and treatment plans for patients in the medical record. Subjective indicates the patient's own description of his or medical condition, subject to his or her personal, cultural, and emotional biases. Objective is the physician's description, presumed to be free from emotional, cultural, or experiential bias. Assessment is evaluation of the patient's medical, physical, emotional, and social situation. Plan indicates the proposed plan of treatment.

standard operating procedures (SOPs). A written document or instruction detailing all steps and activities of a process or procedure for the purpose of standardization.

team intelligence (TI). The ability of a group of individuals to manage complex and non-routine situations together. Intelligent teams can outperform their most knowledgeable members.

TeamSTEPPS. A health care teamwork training system developed jointly by the Department of Defense (DoD) and the Agency for Healthcare Research and Quality (AHRQ).

true air speed (TAS). The speed of the aircraft relative to the air mass in which it is flying. In "still air" (no wind), it is the same as ground speed.

type rating. Qualification to fly a certain aircraft type that requires additional training beyond the scope of initial license and aircraft class training. Any person acting as pilot in command of an aircraft operated under part 121 rules (commercial airlines) must be type rated for that particular aircraft.

Notes

Introduction

1. Captain Chesley "Sully" Sullenberger with Jeffrey Zaslow, *Highest Duty: My Search for What Really Matters* (New York: William Morrow, 2009), 209.

2. Institute of Medicine, *To Err Is Human: Building a Safer Health System* (Washington, D.C.: National Academies Press, 1999).

3. National Academies, press release, "Medication Errors Injure 1.5 Million People and Cost Billions of Dollars Annually; Report Offers Comprehensive Strategies for Reducing Drug-Related Mistakes, July 20, 2006." http://www8.nationalacademies.org/onpinews/newsitem.aspx?RecordID=11623, accessed April 20, 2012

4. Archie Clements et al., "Overcrowding and Understaffing in Modern Healthcare Systems: Key Determinants in Understanding Methicillin-Resistant *Staphylococcus aureus* Transmission," *Lancet Infectious Diseases* 8 (2008): 427–34.

5. Kathleen McPhaul, University of Maryland School of Nursing, personal communication, June 20, 2011.

6. Rebecca Voelker, "Updated Guidelines Target Reductions in Catheter-Related Bloodstream Infections," *JAMA* 305 (17) 2011: 1753–54; P. J. Pronovost et al., "Sustaining Reductions in Catheter Related Bloodstream Infections in Michigan Intensive Care Units: Observational Study," *BMJ* 340 (February 4, 2010): c309, doi: 10.1136/bmj.c309; P. J. Pronovost et al., "A Research Framework for Reducing Preventable Patient Harm," *Clinical Infectious Diseases* 52 (4): 507–13; A. Lipitz-Snyderman et al., "Impact of a Statewide Intensive Care Unit Quality Improvement Initiative on Hospital Mortality and Length of Stay: Retrospective Comparative Analysis," *BMJ* 342 (January 28, 2011): d219, doi:10.1136/bmj.d219; M. Romig, C. Goeschel, P. Pronovost, and S. M. Berenholtz, "Integrating CUSP and TRIP to Improve Patient Safety," *Hospital Practice* (Minneapolis) 38 (4) 2010: 114–21.

7. Sharona Hoffman and Andy Podgurski, "E-Health Hazards: Provider Liability and Electronic Health Record Systems," *Berkeley Technology Law Journal* 24 (4) (2009): 1524.

8. Michael Harrison and Ross Koppel, "Interactive Sociotechnical Analysis: Identifying and Coping with Unintended Consequences of IT Implementation," in *Handbook of Research on Advances in Health Informatics and Electronic Healthcare Applications: Global Adoption and Impact of Information Communication Technologies*, ed. Khalil Khoumbati (Gandhinagar, India: Institute of Information and Communication Technology, 2008), 33–51; Ross Koppel et al., "Role of Computerized Physician Order Entry Systems in Facilitating Medication Errors," *JAMA* 293 (10) (2005): 1197–1203; Ross Koppel, "Defending Computerized Physician Order Entry from Its Supporters," *Journal of Managed Care* 12 (7) (2006): 369–70, cited in Ross Koppel and Suzanne Gordon, eds., *First, Do*

Less Harm: Confronting the Inconvenient Problems of Patient Safety (Ithaca: Cornell University Press, 2012), 74.

9. Department of Health and Human Services Office of the Inspector General, "Hospital Incident Reporting Systems Do Not Capture Most Patient Harm," January 2012, OEI-0609–00091, 12. http://oig.hhs.gov/oei/reports/oei-06-09-00091.asp, accessed March 25, 2012.

10. Interprofessional Education Collaborative, *Core Competencies for Interprofessional and Collaborative Practice* (Washington, D.C.: AAMC, 2011); Interprofessional Education Collaborative, *Team-based Competencies: Building a Shared Foundation for Education and Clinical Practice* (2011 conference proceedings).

11. J.C. Morey, et al., "Reducing Errors in Emergency Medicine through Team Performance: The MedTeams Project," in *Proceedings of the Second Annenberg Conference on Enhancing Patient Safety and Reducing Errors in Health Care* (Rancho Mirage, CA: National Patient Safety Foundation, 1998), 142–46.

12. Geraint H. Lewis et al., "Counterheroism, Common Knowledge, and Ergonomics: Concepts from Aviation That Could Improve Patient Safety," *Milbank Quarterly* 89 (1) (March 2011): 4–38.

13. Our ideas about teams have been influenced by our own observations, readings, and books such as Scott Reeves et al., *Interprofessional Teamwork for Health and Social Care* (Oxford: Wiley-Blackwell, 2010), 4.

14. Edwin Hutchins, *Cognition in the Wild* (Cambridge, MA: MIT Press, 1996), 176.

1. History of Crew Resource Management

1. National Transportation Safety Board, Aircraft Accident Report, United Airlines, Inc., McDonnell-Douglas DC-8–61, Portland, Oregon, NTSB-ARR-79-7, December 28, 1978. http://libraryonline.erau.edu/online-full-text/ntsb/aircraft-accident-reports/AAR79-07.pdf, accessed March 9, 2009.

2. Ibid., 2.

3. Ibid., 26, 27.

4. Ibid., 8

5. Ibid., 26.

6. When the ECAM senses a malfunction, it not only alerts the crew to the abnormality but provides initial steps toward dealing with the problem, to be followed up with the use of a more expansive checklist.

7. One knot equals about 1.15 miles per hour.

8. At the time, all commercial transport jet aircraft in service required three cockpit crew members: captain, first officer, and engineer. Later model airliners have been designed to eliminate the need for the engineer position and now require only two crew members for operation.

9. National Weather Service Lighting Safety, http://www.weather.gov/om/lightning/medical.htm.

10. "Chances of a Plane Crash,"City-Data.com, http://www.city-data.com/forum/travel/1277998-chances-plane-crash.html.

11. The first three-crew cockpits actually had two pilots and one flight engineer; the flight engineer was not necessarily trained or qualified as a pilot. Eventually almost all three-crew cockpits required the FE to be a qualified pilot as well.

12. *Wikipedia*, s.v. "Jacob Veldhuyzen van Zanten," accessed December 21, 2009, http://en.wikipedia.org/wiki/Jacob_Veldhuyzen_van_Zanten.

13. A pilot's initial checkout in a new aircraft type actually involves several stages of "checkrides" during which he or she must demonstrate proficiency in various circumstances. The pilot is tested on his or her ability to handle emergency situations in the simulator, and the final stage of the process is in the actual aircraft under the tutelage of a very senior and experienced instructor pilot, or "check airman," such as Captain van Zanten.

14. Shari Stamford Krause, *Aircraft Safety: Accident Investigations, Analyses and Applications,* 2nd ed. (New York: McGraw-Hill, 2003), 210 (emphasis added).

15. The flight crew is defined pretty broadly: it could be only the pilot in a single-piloted aircraft, the three-man crew of a 747-200 or the cockpit crew, as well as the flight attendants.

16. "History of Aviation," Global Aviation, accessed March 15, 2010, http://www.globalaircraft.org/history_of_aviation.htm.
17. Robert L. Helmreich and H. Clayton Foushee, "Why Crew Resource Management? Empirical and Theoretical Bases of Human Factors Training in Aviation," in *Crew Resource Management*, ed. Earl L. Wiener, Barbara G. Kanki, and Robert L. Helmreich (San Diego: Academic Press, 1993), 5 (emphases added).
18. *Wikipedia*, s.v. "Aviation History," accessed September 5, 2010, http://en.wikipedia.org/wiki/Aviation_history.
19. Tom Wolfe, *The Right Stuff* (New York: Picador, 1979), 25.
20. Ibid., 24.
21. The black boxes are anything but black: they are in fact brightly colored for easy visual identification after a crash. When introduced, FDRs were pretty basic; today they record hundreds and sometimes thousands of data parameters. In addition to relying on the FDR, which is a sealed, "crashproof" piece of hardware, modern aircraft continuously monitor thousands of parameters and transmit anomalies to ground stations in real time, transparent to the flight crew. The CVR typically records the last thirty minutes of conversation on a continuous loop.
22. John K. Lauber, foreword to Wiener, Kanki, and Helmreich, *Crew Resource Management*, xvi.
23. Ibid. xvii. In commercial airlines first officers, or copilots, always sit in the right seat and captains always in the left.
24. Hugh P. Ruffell Smith, "A Simulator Study of the Interaction of Pilot Workload with Errors, Vigilance, and Decisions" (Moffett Field, CA: NASA-Ames Research Center, NASA Technical Memorandum 78482, 1979).
25. Thomas R. Chidester in Wiener, Kanki, and Helmreich, *Crew Resource Management*, 315–16. Many large transport aircraft, such as the 747, carry so much fuel for long flights that their takeoff weights are far higher than the weight at which a safe landing can be made. If there is an emergency on takeoff, for example, the crew may need to jettison as much as a hundred thousand pounds of fuel in order to get the aircraft down to a "safe" landing weight.
26. Helmreich and Foushee, "Why Crew Resource Management?," in Wiener, Kanki, and Helmreich, 7.
27. R. L. Helmreich, A. C. Merritt, and J. A. Wilhelm, "The Evolution of Crew Resource Management Training in Commercial Aviation," *International Journal of Aviation Psychology* 9 (10) (1999): 19.
28. Robert R. Blake and Jane S Mouton, *The New Managerial Grid* (Houston: Gulf Publishing, 1964).
29. http://en.wikipedia.org/wiki/United_Airlines_Flight_811
30. The landing gear would have free-fallen into place if lowered at this point, but the loss of the two hydraulic systems on the right side of the aircraft would have made it impossible to raise it again if needed.
31. With the loss of two of the engines and unknown structural damage, the copilot noted that the aircraft might not be able to maintain altitude to make it back to land, particularly with the substantial additional drag of the extended landing gear.
32. Not noted in the Soliday interview: Normal procedure called for the FO to pull the fire handles for the two damaged engines. In addition to shutting off fuel and ignition to the damaged engines, this procedure would have completely disabled the two hydraulic systems associated with engines three and four. The FO wisely suggested—and the crew concurred—that they deviate from procedure and manually shut off fuel and ignition *only*, leaving available any remaining hydraulic pressure being produced by the windmilling engines.
33. Robert L. Helmreich and H. Clayton Foushee, "Why Crew Resource Management," in Wiener, Kanki, and Helmreich, 20.
34. Robert L. Helmreich, Ashleigh C. Merritt, and John A. Wilhelm, "The Evolution of Crew Resource Management Training in Commercial Aviation," *International Journal of Aviation Psychology* 9 (1) (1999): 19–32.
35. Judith M. Orasanu, "Decision-making in the cockpit," in Wiener, Kanki, and Helmreich, 155.
36. Ibid., 159.
37. Ibid., 161.
38. This became quite evident at Northwest Airlines in the early 1990s. Clay Foushee was hired in 1992 as vice president of flight operations, where his influence as a leading human-factors

scientist led Northwest to embrace CRM as a way of life. Dr. Foushee has researched and written extensively on CRM issues and in his position as vice president has had a direct and lasting impact on hiring practices. Fighter-pilot types were at times (depending upon the bias of the individual in charge at the time) given preference because in the military culture they tended to be at or near the top of their classes, meaning that they had been "prescreened" for their flying skills.

39. Pilots and flight attendants are required to undergo annual recurrent training that reviews and reinforces subjects such as security, emergency procedures, technical proficiency, policies, and now CRM.

40. IS-BAO certification is required for business aircraft operations in many countries. IS-BAO included CRM training in its audit requirements in 2007.

41. Federal Aviation Administration Advisory Circular 120–51e: Crew Resource Management Training, 8–10.

42. In aviation, standard operating procedures are written, published, and tested procedures that are expected to be universally and consistently applied within an organization. "Aviation Glossary, Standard Operating Procedures," accessed October 9, 2011, http://aviationglossary.com/federal-aviation-administration-faa-definition/sop-standard-operating-procedures.

43. Ibid., 5.

44. Depending upon the analysis, there may be more than four CPIs, but the ones articulated here appear to be the most consistent and relevant.

2. Communication

1. Anderson: "[W]e had a two-inch plastic tube attached to the UHF-VHF [radio] switch to make it easier to locate without looking; thus the noodle, and if you forgot to switch over at the appropriate time, i.e. on the flight line performing a maneuver (Boss and Lead solo in diamond/solo maneuvers) or all in Delta formations/maneuvers, you had committed a noodle, which was a safety debrief item normally brought up by the offending party."

2. Earl L. Wiener, Barbara G. Kanki, and Robert L. Helmreich, eds., *Cockpit Resource Management* (San Diego: Academic Press, 1993), 112.

3. "Thick Description: Toward an Interpretive Theory of Culture," Clifford Geertz, SocioSite, accessed December 9, 2010, http://www.sociosite.net/topics/texts/Geertz_Thick_Description.php.

4. Wiener, Kanki, and Helmreich, *Cockpit Resource Management*, 29.

5. Ibid., 115.

6. Ibid., 119–20.

7. Daniel E. Maurino, "Crew Resource Management: A Time for Reflection," in Daniel J. Garland, John A. Wise, and V. David Hopkin, *Handbook of Aviation Human Factors* (Mahwah, New Jersey: Lawrence Erlbaum Associates, 1999), 216.

8. J. Bryan Sexton, Eric J. Thomas, and Robert L. Helmreich, "Error, Stress, and Teamwork in Medicine and Aviation: Cross-Sectional Surveys," *BMJ* 320 (2000): 745–46.

9. For an excellent discussion of this see Robert M. Sapolsky, *Why Zebras Don't Get Ulcers* (New York: Holt, 2004).

10. Captain Chesley "Sully" Sullenberger with Jeffrey Zaslow, *Highest Duty: My Search for What Really Matters* (New York: William Morrow, 2009), 25.

11. David M. Musson and Robert L. Helmreich, "Team Training and Resource Management in Health Care: Current Issues and Future Directions," *Harvard Health Policy Review* 5, no. 1 (Spring 2004): 26–27.

12. "Currency" refers to when a pilot last flew a particular type of aircraft. In today's highly technical aircraft, proficiency drops off perceptibly after a few weeks off the job. Pilots typically share currency status during their initial introductions as just another tool in their threat assessment process.

13. V1, known as "decision speed" or "abort speed," is a speed that is computed on the basis of numerous variables (such as weight, runway length, environmental conditions) beyond which a safe abort cannot be achieved should an engine fail; above V1, the aircraft is committed to fly if an engine fails; conversely, an abort is *required* if an engine fails below V1.

14. The abort is a critical maneuver, and more than one pilot has turned a minor malfunction into an emergency by choosing to execute a high-speed abort for a relatively minor problem.

15. The aftermath of this accident revealed that there were cultural dynamics going on within the aircraft cockpit that contributed to the fatal miscommunications. Eight crew members and sixty-five passengers lost their lives. *Wikipedia,* s.v. "Flight 52," http://en.wikipedia.org/wiki/Avianca_Flight_52.

16. The purser is the lead flight attendant, the flight attendant crew manager.

17. "SBAR Technique for Communication: A Situation Briefing Model," Institute for Healthcare Improvement, accessed July 8, 2011, http://www.ihi.org/knowledge/Pages/Tools/SBARTech niqueforCommunicationASituationalBriefingModel.aspx.

18. Glide slope is an angular vertical reference to the runway point of landing. Cockpit instrumentation will indicate to the pilots whether they are above or below this imaginary plane in space. Deviations are referred to as "dots" on the glide slope indicator.

19. Barbara G. Kanki, Robert L. Helmreich, and Jose M. Anca, *Crew Resource Management* (Amsterdam: Academic Press, 2010), 311–12.

3. Case Study: Maimonides Medical Center

1. Psychological safety is a concept developed by Edgar H. Schein and Warren B. Bennis and elaborated by Harvard Business School professor Amy Edmondson. It describes a workplace environment in which employees are not afraid to speak up about mistakes and workplace problems and who do not feel they will be belittled, humiliated, or put down when they try to express their views or concerns.

2. Jeffrey H. Silber et al., "Hospital and Patient Characteristics Associated with Death after Surgery: A Study of Adverse Occurrence and Failure to Rescue," *Medical Care* 30 (1992): 6165–629.

3. S. P. Clarke, "Failure to Rescue: Lessons from Missed Opportunities in Care," *Nursing Inquiry* 11 (2) (2004): 67–71; Sean Clarke and Linda Aiken, "Failure to Rescue: Needless Deaths Are Prime Examples of the Need for More Nurses at the Bedside," *American Journal of Nursing* 101 (1) (2003): 42–47.

4. Kathryn Kaplan, Pamela Mestel, and David L. Feldman, "Creating a Culture of Mutual Respect," *AORN* 91 (4) (April 2010): 498.

5. David Maxfield et al., *Silence Kills: The Seven Crucial Conversations for Healthcare* (AACN, VitalSmarts, and Crucial Conversations, 2005).

4. Team Building

1. Amy C. Edmondson, "Managing the Risk of Learning: Psychological Safety in Work Teams," in *International Handbook of Organizational Teamwork and Cooperative Learning*, ed. M. A. West, D. Tjosvold, and K. G. Smith (New York: Wiley, 2003), 258.

2. Suzanne Gordon, *Nursing against the Odds: How Health Care Cost-Cutting, Media Stereotypes and Medical Hubris Undermine Nurses and Patient Care* (Ithaca: Cornell University Press, 2006).

3. Robert C. Ginnett, "Crews as Groups: Their Formation and Their Leadership," in *Cockpit Resource Management*, ed. Earl L. Wiener, Barbara G. Kanki, and Robert L. Helmreich (San Diego: Academic Press, 1993), 73.

4. Ibid., 77.

5. "Leading Teams," J. Richard Hackman, Harvard Business School, http://hbswk.hbs.edu/archive/2996.html.

6. Scott Reeves, Simon Lewin, Sherry Espin, and Merrick Zwarenstein, *Interprofessional Teamwork for Health and Social Care* (Oxford: Wiley-Blackwell, 2010), 4.

7. J. Richard Hackman, ed., *Groups That Work (and Those That Don't): Creating Conditions for Effective Teamwork* (San Francisco: Jossey-Bass, 1990), 6–7.

8. J. Richard Hackman, "Teams, Leaders, and Organizations: New Directions for Crew-oriented Flight Training," in *Cockpit Resource Management*, ed. Earl L. Wiener, Barbara G. Kanki, and Robert L. Helmreich (San Diego: Academic Press, 1993), 47–69.

9. Edwin Hutchins, *Cognition in the Wild* (Cambridge, MA: MIT Press, 1995), 176.

10. Drew Whitelegg, *Working the Skies: The Fast-Paced, Disorienting World of the Flight Attendant* (New York: New York University Press, 2007), 7.
11. Ibid.
12. Kathleen M. Barry, *Femininity in Flight: A History of Flight Attendants* (Durham, NC: Duke University Press, 2007), 178.
13. A. Pawlowski, "Why Aren't More Women Airline Pilots?" CNN Travel, http://articles.cnn.com/2011-03-18/travel/female.airline.pilots_1_women-airline-pilots-american-airlines-captain-helen-richey?_s=PM:TRAVEL, accessed April 16, 2012.
14. *Merriam-Webster's Twentieth Century Dictionary*, s.v. "authority."
15. Title 14, Code of Federal Regulations, U.S. Federal Aviation Regulation part 91.3(a).
16. Ibid.
17. *Dictionary.com*, s.v. "authoritarian," http://dictionary.reference.com/browse/authoritarian?s=ts, accessed May 25, 2011.
18. *Dictionary.com*, s.v. "autocratic," http://dictionary.reference.com/browse/authoritarian?s=ts, accessed May 25, 2011.
19. Webster's New World Dictionary of the American Language, 2nd College Edition (Cleveland, Ohio: The World Publishing Company, 1980.), s.v. "command."
20. Robert C. Ginnett, "Crews as Groups: Their Formation and Their Leadership," in *Cockpit Resource Management*, ed. Earl L. Wiener, Barbara G. Kanki, and Robert L. Helmreich (San Diego: Academic Press, 1993), 84.
21. Ibid.
22. Joseph P. Dunlop and Susan J. Mangold, *Leadership/Followership Recurrent Training Instructor Manual* (Washington, DC: Office of the Chief Scientific and Technical Advisor for Human Factors to the Federal Aviation Administration [AAR-100], 1998), www.crm-devel.org/ftp/instman.pdf, 44, accessed April 12, 2012.
23. Robert C. Ginnett, "Crews as Groups: Their Formation and Their Leadership," in *Cockpit Resource Management*, ed. Earl L. Wiener, Barbara G. Kanki, and Robert L. Helmreich (San Diego: Academic Press, 1993), 89.
24. Ibid., 90.
25. Ibid.
26. Ibid., 90–91.
27. PowerPoint on Crew Resource Management Teambuilding by CRMLLC, Seattle, WA, 2006.
28. Deferred, or "placarded," maintenance items: Regulators give airlines a certain amount of latitude to defer specific "nonessential" maintenance items. The airline is allowed to operate with the item missing or broken under certain conditions and for a defined time or cycle limit, which is published and strictly adhered to. For instance, an aircraft may fly without an operating radar but only under daytime visual conditions and only for three days.
29. Joseph P. Dunlop and Susan J. Mangold, *Leadership/Followership Recurrent Training Instructor Manual* (Washington, DC: Office of the Chief Scientific and Technical Advisor for Human Factors to the Federal Aviation Administration [AAR-100], 1998), www.crm-devel.org/ftp/instman.pdf, 14–15, accessed April 12, 2012.
30. Fortunately, the army has since abandoned that marketing strategy!
31. *Online Etymology Dictionary*, s.v. "advocate," http://www.etymonline.com/index.php?term=advocate, accessed April 25, 2011.
32. Dunlop and Mangold, *Leadership/Followership*, 18.
33. Jad Mouawad, "Fracas Aloft Shows Gap in Screening," *New York Times*, March 28, 2012, http://www.nytimes.com/2012/03/29/business/jetblue-incident-raises-questions-about-screening-pilots.html?pagewanted=all, accessed March 29, 2012.

5. Case Study: Osher Clinical Center for Complementary and Integrative Medical Therapies

1. This chapter was jointly authored by Bonnie B. O'Connor, Donald B. Levy, and David M. Eisenberg, all of whom were involved in the events described.

2. National Center for Complementary and Alternative Medicine (NCCAM), National Institutes of Health (NIH), "Model of Integrative Care in an Academic Health Center," Grant #AT00905, 2001–2005, principal investigator, David M. Eisenberg, MD.

3. Funded by the NCCAM grant and a philanthropic gift from the Bernard Osher Foundation.

4. Definition provided by Wanda Buczynski, organizational development consultant to the CPC and training program facilitator.

5. This is an *extremely* simplistic definition of *qi*, a topic to which whole chapters and books have been devoted. The Japanese variant of the word is Anglicized as *ki* (pronounced "key").

6. This is also an *extremely* simplistic definition of a concept to which, like *qi*, thousands of pages of definition, theory, varied interpretations, and elaboration have been devoted.

7. Exercise supplied and facilitated by organizational development consultant Wanda Buczynski.

8. A burr hole is a hole drilled into the skull; it is unlikely anyone would want to try this simply to "experience" this therapeutic option available to neurologists!

9. For example, a pair of studies now under way funded by NCCAM), National Institutes of Health (NIH), Use and Effectiveness of a Model Integrative Care Clinic in an Academic Hospital. Grant #1R01 AT005065-01A1, 2011–2015, principal investigators, Julie E. Buring, PhD, and Peter J. Wayne, PhD. These studies test cost and cost-effectiveness of the OCC team approach and explore clinician team decision-making processes.

10. We wish to acknowledge the following groups: *Curriculum Planning Committee (CPC)*: Sally Andrews, MBA; Wanda Buczynski; Mark Cunningham; David M. Eisenberg, MD; Arthur Madore, LMT; Bonnie O'Connor, PhD; Randall Paulsen, MD; Robb Scholten; Megan Tabor, DC; *Curriculum Implementation/Steering Group*: Wanda Buczynski; Mark Cunningham; Bonnie O'Connor, PhD; Randall Paulsen, MD; *Current OCC Clinician Team* (*indicates members who joined after the team training program had been completed): Meredith Beaton Starr, MS, OTR/L; Xiao Ming Cheng, LAc; Brendan Carney, LAc*; Lynda Danzig, LMT, LAc, MAc; Jie Fan-Roche, PT, NCMT; Thomas Jacobson, LMT; Caitlin Hosmer Kirby, MS, RD; Matthew H. Kowalski, DC; Donald B. Levy, MD; Arthur Madore, LMT; Thomas Mecke, DC*; Randall Paulsen, MD; Megan Tabor, DC. For more information about the OCC visit http://www.brighamandwomens.org/Depart ments_and_Services/medicine/Services/oshercenter/default.aspx.

6. Workload Management

1. National Transportation Safety Board, Aircraft Accident Report: United Airlines 232 of July 19, 1989, NTSB/AAR, November 1, 1990.

2. Captain Al Haynes, "The Crash of United 232 by Captain Al Haynes," http://clear-prop.org/aviation/haynes.html, accessed March 10, 2011.

3. Captain Chesley "Sully" Sullenberger with Jeffrey Zaslow, *Highest Duty: My Search for What Really Matters* (New York: William Morrow, 2009).

4. Aviation Fatigue Management Symposium: Patrnerships for Solutions, P3, http://www.faa.gov/about/office_org/headquarters_offices/avs/offices/afs/afs200/media/aviation_fatigue_symposium/8-19_Sumwalt.pdf, accessed May 15, 2011.

5. For more on the impact of sleep on safety, particularly patient safety, see Christopher Landrigan, "Physicians, Sleep Deprivation, and Safety," and Allison Trinkoff, and Jeanne Geiger-Brown, "Sleep-deprived Nurses: Sleep and Schedule Challenges in Nursing." in *First, Do Less Harm: Confronting the Inconvenient Problems in Patient Safety*, ed. Ross Koppel and Suzanne Gordon, 150–79 (Ithaca: Cornell University Press, 2012).

6. Drew Dawson and Kathryn Reid, "Fatigue, Alcohol, and Performance Impairment," *Nature* 388 (July–August 1997); The Buck Stops Here (blog), "Losing Sleep Makes You Drunk," http://stuartbuck.blogspot.jp/2009/01/losing-sleep-makes-you-drunk.html, accessed April 20, 2012.

7. "Back side of the clock" refers to operating in conditions in which one's circadian clock is reversed. For example, a pilot based in Los Angeles may have flown to Tokyo on the first day of a trip. Just twenty-four hours after arrival in Tokyo, he may be expected to fly from Tokyo to Singapore at night, when his circadian clock makes it feel as though he is just starting the seven-plus-hour flight at 2:00 a.m.

8. If a relief pilot is on duty, the off-duty pilot is allowed to nap in a designated space outside the cockpit.

9. On a two-pilot aircraft. Older, three-pilot planes have different requirements.

10. Atul Gawande, *The Checklist Manifesto* (New York: Metropolitan Books, 2009).

11. Peter Pronovost and Eric Vohr, *Safe Patients, Smart Hospitals: How One Doctor's Checklist Can Help Us Change Health Care from the Inside Out* (New York: Hudson Street Press, 2010).

12. "How the Pilot's Checklist Came About," John Schamel, January 31, 2011, http://www.atchis tory.org/History/checklst.htm, accessed March 21, 2011.

13. "Fatal Accidents and Onboard Fatalities by Phase of Flight Worldwide Commercial Jet Fleet: 2001 through 2010," Boeing, http://www.boeing.com/news/techissues/pdf/statsum.pdf, accessed March 23, 2011.

14. "STRESS . . . At Work," NIOSH, http://www.cdc.gov/niosh/docs/99–101.

15. Robert. M. Sapolsky, *Why Zebras Don't Get Ulcers* (New York: Holt Paperbacks, 2004).

16. Mark Singer, "Task Saturation, Ruthless Ignorance, and the Power of Focus," *No Map. No Guide. No Limits* (blog), March 23, 2010, http://www.nomapnoguidenolimits.com/2010/03/23/task-saturation.

17. V1, also known as decision speed, is arguably the most critical moment during a takeoff. If an engine fails prior to V1 speed, a successful abort on the runway can be made; if an engine fails after V1, the pilot is committed to takeoff, a very technically challenging maneuver. Because of this, V1 cuts (engine failure at V1) are practiced often in the simulator.

18. The simulator is often referred to as "the box."

7. Case Study: Interprofessional Education and Practice at the University of Toronto

1. Ivy Oandasan and Scott Reeves, "Key Elements for Interprofessional Education, Part 1: The Learner, the Educator and the Learning Context," *Journal of Interprofessional Care*, supp. 1 (May 2005): 24.

2. Health Canada, Commission on the Future of Health Care in Canada: The Romanow Commis sion, http://www.hc-sc.gc.ca/hcs-sss/hhr-rhs/strateg/romanow-eng.php.

3. http://www.healthforceontario.ca/WhatIsHFO/AboutInterprofessionalCare/Interprofessional CareEducationFund.aspx.

4. To download tool kit go to http://www.ipe.utoronto.ca/initiatives/ipc/implc/preceptorship. html. For information on DVDs go to http://www.ipe.utoronto.ca/resources/dvd.html.

8. Threat and Error Management

1. Karl W. Weick and Kathleen M. Suttcliffe, *Managing the Unexpected: Assuring High Performance in an Age of Complexity* (San Francisco: Jossey-Bass, 2001), 3.

2. Ibid., 33–34.

3. Ibid., 44.

4. Of course, if an error occurs as the result of an intentional act, such as noncompliance with rules, that is another matter.

5. The takeoff warning will activate when the thrust levers have been advanced to a takeoff setting but the aircraft is not in the appropriate takeoff configuration: e.g., flaps not down, spoilers not armed, gear not centered, or trim not set.

9. Why CRM Worked

1. Peter Pronovost and Eric Vohr, *Safe Patients, Smart Hospitals: How One Doctor's Checklist Can Help Us Change Health Care from the Inside Out* (New York: Hudson Street Press, 2010).

2. Robert L. Helmreich, Ashleigh C. Merritt, and John A. Wilhelm, "The Evolution of Crew Re-source Management Training in Commercial Aviation," *International Journal of Aviation Psychol-ogy* 9 (1) (1999): 19–32.

3. Airline dispatchers must be licensed by the FAA and have extensive knowledge of meteorology and aviation, to a level comparable to that of the holder of an airline transport pilot license. They

are responsible for planning and monitoring the progress of a flight. The pilot in command and the dispatcher are both legally responsible for the safety of a flight. A dispatcher is the "big picture" person on the ground and provides assistance and support to pilots in flight. For example, if an aircraft were forced to divert (change destination) because of weather, mechanical malfunction, or medical emergency, the dispatcher would help the pilot sort through his destination alternatives, taking into account weather, maintenance support, aircraft replacement options, and even political considerations.

4. *Occupational Outlook Handbook, 2010–11 Edition*, Bureau of Labor Statistics, "Flight Attendants," http://www.bls.gov/oco/ocos171.htm; "Aircraft Pilots and Flight Engineers, http://www.bls.gov/oco/ocos107.htm.

5. Although crews are typically compensated at a daily rate that would be less than they would expect to make while flying, if they are in training for an extended period, such as for a new aircraft checkout (four to six weeks), their pay would be the same or similar to their flight pay.

6. Smaller companies may subcontract CRM course development and training to independent training providers such as Patrick's company, CRM LLC.

7. J. Bryan Sexton, Eric J. Thomas, and Robert L. Helmreich, "Error, Stress, and Teamwork in Medicine and Aviation: Cross-Sectional Surveys," *BMJ* 320 (2000): 745–46.

8. H. Heinrich, D. Petersen, and N. Roos, *Industrial Accident Prevention: A Safety Management Approach*, 1st ed. (New York: McGraw-Hill, 1931); European Organisation for the Safety of Air Navigation, *Safety and Quality Relationship Guidelines*, March 7, 2001, 27.

9. James Reason, "Human Error: Models and Management," *BMJ* 320 (March 18, 2000): 768.

10. For a longer discussion of error see James Reason, *Human Error* (Cambridge: Cambridge University Press, 1990).

11. FAA, Advisory Circular No. 120-51C, 10/30/98, http://www.crm-devel.org/resources/ac/ac120_51c.htm, accessed June 4, 2012.

12. J. Richard Hackman, *Leading in Teams: Setting the Stage for Great Performances* (Cambridge, MA: Harvard University Press, 2002), 224.

13. Edgar H. Schein and Warren G. Bennis, *Personal and Organizational Change through Group Methods* (New York: Wiley, 1965), 44–45.

14. Amy C. Edmondson, "Managing the Risk of Learning: Psychological Safety in Work Teams," in *International Handbook of Organizational Teamwork and Cooperative Learning*, ed. M. A. West, D. Tjosvold, and K. G. Smith (New York: Wiley, 2003), 258.

15. Amy C. Edmondson and Josephine P. Mogelof, "Examining Psychological Safety in Innovation Teams: Organizational Culture, Team Dynamics, or Personality?" in *Creativity and Innovation in Organizational Teams*, ed. Leigh L. Thompson and Hoon Seok Choi (Mahwah, New Jersey: Lawrence Erlbaum Associates, 2005).

16. A. Pawlowski, "Why Aren't More Women Airline Pilots?" CNN Travel, http://articles.cnn.com/2011-03-18/travel/female.airline.pilots_1_women-airline-pilots-american-airlines-captain-helen-richey?_s=PM:TRAVEL, accessed April 16, 2012.

17. Rogello Saenz and Louwanda Evans, "The Changing Demography of U.S. Flight Attendants," Population Reference Bureau, June 2009, http://www.prb.org/Articles/2009/usflightattendants.aspx.

18. John Nance, *Why Hospitals Should Fly: The Ultimate Flight Plan to Patient Safety and Quality Care* (Bozeman: Second River Healthcare Press, 2008).

19. For a more detailed discussion of staffing ratios as they apply to nursing see Suzanne Gordon, John Buchanan, and Tanya Bretherton, *Safety in Numbers: Nurse-to-Patient Ratios and the Future of Health Care.* (Ithaca: Cornell University Press, 2008).

10. The Problems in Medicine

1. Geraint H. Lewis, et al. "Counterheroism, Common Knowledge, and Ergonomics: Concepts from Aviation That Could Improve Patient Safety," *The Milbank Quarterly* 89, no. 1 (2011): 4–38.

2. Jerome Groopman, *How Doctors Think* (Boston: Houghton Mifflin, 2007), 27–32 (emphasis added).

3. Atul Gawande, *Better: A Surgeon's Notes on Performance* (New York: Metropolitan Books, 2007), 4.

4. Suzanne Gordon, *Nursing against the Odds: How Healthcare Cost Cutting, Media Stereotypes and Medical Hubris Undermine Nurses and Patient Care* (Ithaca: Cornell University Press, 2006).

5. Atul Gawande. "Personal Best: Should Everyone Have a Coach?," *New Yorker*, October 3, 2011, 44–53.

6. Ibid., 50.

7. Ibid. Emphasis added.

8. Ibid., 53.

9. *Occupational Outlook Handbook, 2010–11 Edition*, Bureau of Labor Statistics, "Physical Therapist Assistants and Aides," http://www.bls.gov/oco/ocos167.htm.

10. Lucien L. Leape, et al., "Perspective: A Culture of Respect, Part 1: The Nature and Causes of Disrespect by Physicians," *Academic Medicine* 87, no. 7 (July 2012): 1, http://journals.lww.com/academicmedicine/Abstract/publishahead/Perspective___A_Culture_of_Respect,_Part_1___The.99620.aspx, accessed June 2, 2012.

11. For an excellent discussion on how bullying or stereotyping impacts workers in health care see Claude Steele, *Whistling Vivaldi and Other Cues about How Stereotypes Affect Us* (New York: Norton, 2010).

12. Daniel Kahneman, *Thinking, Fast and Slow* (New York: Farrar, Strauss and Giroux, 2011), 43–44. This book should be required reading for anyone serious about patient safety.

13. Geoffrey C. Bowker and Susan Leigh Star, *Sorting Things Out: Classification and Its Consequences* (Cambridge, MA: MIT Press, 2000), 5.

14. SOAP (subjective, objective, assessment, plan) notes are a method used by health care providers to document assessment and treatment plans for patients in the medical record.

15. Bonnie O'Connor, "Mandatory Miscommunication: Speech, Status, and Beliefs about Knowledge in American Hospitals," paper presented in panel Lay and Expert Knowledge in the Medical Marketplace, American Folklore Society annual meeting, Nashville, TN, October 2010.

16. Department of Health and Human Services Office of the Inspector General, "Hospital Incident Reporting Systems Do Not Capture Most Patient Harm," January 2012, OEI-0609–00091. http://oig.hhs.gov/oei/reports/oei-06-09-00091.asp, accessed April 16, 2012.

17. "Medication Errors Injure 1.5 Million People and Cost Billions of Dollars Annually," National Academy of Sciences News Release, July 20, 2006, http://www8.nationalacademies.org/onpinews/newsitem.aspx?recordid=11623.

18. For a detailed discussion of the case of this 15-year-old boy who underwent elective surgery for a relatively minor condition and died five days later, see "The Lewis Blackman Case," Quality and Safety Education for Nurses, http://www.qsen.org/video.

19. Lorelei Lingard, "Rethinking Competence in the Context of Teamwork," in *The Question of Competence: Reconsidering Medical Education in the Twenty-First Century*, ed. Brian D. Hodges and Lorelei Lingard (Ithaca: Cornell University Press, 2012).

20. Harvey C. Sax et al., "Can Aviation-Based Team Training Elicit Sustainable Behavior Change?" *Archives of Surgery* 144 (12) (December 2009): 1133–37.

21. Lucien L. Leape, et al. "Perspective: A Culture of Respect, Part 1: The Nature and Causes of Disrespect by Physicians," *Academic Medicine* 87, no. 7 (July 2012), http://journals.lww.com/academicmedicine/Abstract/publishahead/Perspective___A_Culture_of_Respect,_Part_1___The.99620.aspx, accessed June 2, 2012.

22. David R. Gifford, Rhode Island Department of Health, letter to Timothy J. Babineau, MD, CEO of Rhode Island Hospital, October 26, 2010, 1. "Findings," October 26, 2010, pdf document at http://www.health.state.ri.us/hospitals/about/investigations/.

23. Ibid., 1.

24. Rhode Island Department of Health, "Statement of Deficiencies" (appended to letter referenced in #21, above), Item Z105, page 3 of 17.

25. Rhode Island Department of Health, "Statement of Deficiencies," Item Z115, p. 6 of 17.

26. David R. Gifford, Rhode Island Department of Health, letter to Timothy J. Babineau, MD, CEO of Rhode Island Hospital, October 26, 2010, 1. "Findings" October 26, 2010, pdf document at http://www.health.state.ri.us/hospitals/about/investigations/

27. Linda Flynn, *The State of the Nursing Workforce in New Jersey: Findings from a Statewide Survey of Registered Nurses* (Newark, New Jersey: The New Jersey Collaborating Center for Nursing, 2007), 19.
28. Peter Pronovost and Eric Vohr, *Safe Patients, Smart Hospitals: How One Doctor's Checklist Can Help Us Change Health Care from the Inside Out* (New York: Hudson Street Press, 2010), 31–33.
29. Ibid., 35.
30. Sorrel King, *Josey's Story: A Mother's Inspiring Crusade to Make Medical Care Safe* (New York: Atlantic Monthly Press, 2009).
31. Institute of Medicine, *Crossing the Quality Chasm: A New Health System for the 21st Century* (Washington, DC: National Academy Presses, 2001), 419–26.
32. These are family medicine and general internal medicine. See Lars E. Peterson et al., "Training on the Clock: Family Medicine Residency Directors' Responses to Resident Duty Hours Reform," *Academic Medicine* 81 (12) (December 2006): 1032–37; Rebecca Harrison and Elizabeth Allen, "Teaching Internal Medicine Residents in the New Era: Inpatient Attending with Duty-Hour Regulations," *Journal of General Internal Medicine* 21 (5) (2006): 447–52.
33. Ann E. Rogers et al., "The Working Hours of Hospital Staff Nurses and Patient Safety," *Health Affairs* (July–August 2004): 202–11; Alison M. Trinkoff et al., "How Long and How Much Are Nurses Now Working?" *American Journal of Nursing* 106 (4) (2006): 60–71.
34. Alison M. Trinkoff and Jeanne Geiger-Brown, "Sleep-deprived Nurses: Sleep and Schedule Changes in Nursing," in *First, Do Less Harm: Confronting the Inconvenient Problems of Patient Safety*, ed. Ross Koppel and Suzanne Gordon (Ithaca: Cornell University Press, 2012), 168–79.
35. J. Bryan Sexton, Eric J. Thomas, and Robert L. Helmreich, "Error, Stress, and Teamwork in Medicine and Aviation: Cross-Sectional Surveys," *BMJ* 320 (2000): 745, 746.
36. TeamSTEPPS, Instructor Guide, AHRQ Pub. No. 02-0020, June 2006, Specialty Scenarios, 19.
37. Ibid., Specialty Scenarios, 27
38. Ibid., Specialty Scenarios, 33.
39. Ibid., Specialty Scenarios, 61.
40. Lucien L. Leape, et al. "Perspective: A Culture of Respect, Part 1: The Nature and Causes of Disrespect by Physicians," *Academic Medicine* 87, no. 7 (July 2012): 6, http://journals.lww.com/academicmedicine/Abstract/publishahead/Perspective___A_Culture_of_Respect,_Part_1___The.99620.aspx, accessed June 2, 2012.
41. Anita L. Tucker and Amy C. Edmondson, "Why Hospitals Don't Learn from Failures: Organizational and Psychological Dynamics that Inhibit System Change," *California Management Review* 45, no. 2 (Winter 2003): 55–72.

11. Conclusion

1. Pilots—most pilots—routinely brief approach scenarios in great detail. The general consensus is that things are happening very rapidly very close to the ground, and it is crucial that every detail of "the plan" has been discussed and understood by everyone before they actually execute the approach.
2. Earl L. Wiener, Babara G. Kanki, and Robert L. Helmreich, eds., *Cockpit Resource Management* (San Diego: Academic Press, 1993).
3. Captain Chesley "Sully" Sullenberger with Jeffrey Zaslow, *Highest Duty: My Search for What Really Matters* (New York: William Morrow, 2009), 211–15.
4. A "fix" is a geographical point in space. Flight plans are generated with a set of fixes extending from the airport of origin to the airport of destination. Points with navigational significance are circled.
5. Pilots for both airlines eventually started flying together, so they had to be using common procedures.
6. "United Pilots: Rushed New Procedures Hurt Safety," Joshua Freed, Yahoo!Finance, September 26, 2011, http://finance.yahoo.com/news/United-pilots-Rushed-new-apf-1992527133.html?x.
7. Books such as Daniel Gilbert's *Stumbling on Happiness* and Daniel Kahneman's *Thinking Fast and Slow* should be required reading for all those in health care.

8. Charles R. Denham, et al., "An NTSB for Health Care—Learning from Innovation: Debate and Innovate or Capitulate," *Journal of Patient Safety* 8, no. 1 (March 2012): 1–14, www.journalpa tientsafety.com.

9. Geraint H. Lewis et al., "Counterheroism, Common Knowledge, and Ergonomics: Concepts from Aviation That Could Improve Patient Safety," *Milbank Quarterly* 89 (1) (2011): 4–38.

10. Ibid., 4 (emphasis added).

11. Ibid.

12. Lewis et al., "Counterheroism," 21.

13. Mike Rose, *The Mind at Work* (New York: Penguin, 2005).

14. Lorelei Lingard, "Rethinking Competence in the Context of Teamwork," in *The Question of Competence: Reconsidering Medical Education in the Twenty-First Century*, ed. Brian D. Hodges and Lorelei Lingard (Ithaca: Cornell University Press, 2012).

15. American Association of Critical Care Nurses and Vital Smarts, *Silence Kills* (2005).

16. "TeamSTEPPS: Team Strategies to Enhance Performance and Patient Safety," Heidi King et al., AHRQ, accessed September 25, 2011, www.ahrq.gov/downloads/pub/advances2/.../Advances-King_1.pdf,9.

17. Ivy Oandasan and Scott Reeves, "Key Elements for Interprofessional Education, Part 1: The Learner, the Educator and the Learning Context," *Journal of Interprofessional Care* 1 (May 2005): 24. Emphasis added.

18. Daniel Kahneman, *Thinking, Fast and Slow* (New York: Farrar, Strauss and Giroux, 2011), 43–44.

19. Lucien L. Leape, et al., "A Culture of Respect, Part 2: Creating a Culture of Respect," *Academic Medicine* 87, no. 7 (July 2012), http://journals.lww.com/academicmedicine/Abstract/publisha head/Perspective___A_Culture_of_Respect,_Part_2__.99622.aspx.

20. CRICO, http://www.rmf.harvard.edu/patient-safety-strategies/communication-teamwork/index.aspx.

Index

Note: Italic page numbers refer to figures.